NUTRITION SECRETS

Second Edition

Charles W. Van Way III, MD
Ralph Coffey Professor and Chairman
Department of Surgery
University of Missouri-Kansas City
School of Medicine
Chief of Surgery
Truman Medical Center
Kansas City, Missouri

Carol Ireton-Jones, PhD, RD, LD, CNSD, FACN
Nutrition Therapy Specialist
Carrollton, Texas

HANLEY & BELFUS
An Affiliate of Elsevier

HANLEY & BELFUS
An *Affiliate of* Elsevier

The Curtis Center
Independence Square West
Philadelphia, Pennsylvania 19106

Note to the reader: Although the techniques, ideas, and information in this book have been carefully reviewed for correctness, the authors, editor, and publisher cannot accept any legal responsibility for any errors or omissions that may be made. Neither the publisher nor the editor makes any guarantee, expressed or implied, with respect to the material contained herein.

Library of Congress Control Number: 2003110771

NUTRITION SECRETS, 2nd edition ISBN 1-56053-514-8

Printed in the United States

Last digit is the print number: 9 8 7 6 5 4 3 2 1

CONTENTS

I. NUTRITIONAL COMPONENTS

II. BASIC NUTRITION

III. SPECIALIZED NUTRITION

IV. NUTRITION FOR PROMOTING HEALTH AND PREVENTING DISEASE

APPENDICES

CONTRIBUTORS

Kimberly Alexander, RD, LD, CNSD
Clinical Dietitian, Wound and Diabetes Center, Saint Luke's Hospital North, Kansas City, Missouri, and Saint Luke's Hospital South, Overland Park, Kansas

Stanley M. Augustin, MD
Assistant Professor, Department of Surgery, University of Missouri at Kansas City; Truman Medical Center, Kansas City, Missouri

Thomas G. Baumgartner, PharmD, MEd
Gainesville, Florida

Peter L. Beyer, MS, RD
Associate Professor, Department of Dietetics and Nutrition, University of Kansas Medical Center, Kansas City, Kansas

Abby S. Bloch, PhD, RD
Nutrition Consultant, Adjunct Professor, Department of Nutrition and Food Studies, New York University, New York

Charlotte A. Buchanan, RD, LD, CNSD
Clinical Nutrition Specialist, Wesley Medical Center, Wichita, Kansas

Gerard A. Burns, MD, MBA
Chief, Medical Informatics, Department of Medicine and Information Technology, Hackensack University Medical Center, Hackensack, New Jersey

Bill K.W. Chang, MD
Senior Surgery Resident, Department of Surgery, University of Missouri at Kansas City, Kansas City, Missouri

Craig C. Chang, MD
Department of Surgery, Citizens Medical Center, Victoria, Texas

David I. Charney, MD, FACP
Neurology Associates of Dayton, Good Samaritan Hospital, Grandview Hospital, Southview Hospital, and Dayton Heart Hospital, Dayton, Ohio

Pamela Charney, MS, RD, LD, CSND
School of Health-Related Professions, University of Medicine and Dentistry of New Jersey, Newark, New Jersey

Laura Clark, RD, LD, CNSD
Affiliation unknown

Paul G. Cuddy, PharmD
Professor, Department of Medicine, University of Missouri at Kansas City; Truman Medical Center, Kansas City, Missouri

Susan Curtas, RN, MSN
Clinical Nurse Specialist, Department of General Surgery, Cleveland Clinic Foundation, Cleveland, Ohio

Diana S. Dark, MD
Professor of Medicine, Department of Pulmonary Disease and Critical Care Medicine, University of Missouri at Kansas City Medical Center; Saint Luke's Hospital; Truman Medical Center-Hospital Hill, Kansas City, Missouri

Mark H. DeLegge, MD, FACG
Associate Professor of Medicine, Digestive Disease Center, Medical University of South Carolina, Charleston, South Carolina

Animesh Dhar, PhD
Associate Professor, Department of Surgery, School of Medicine, University of Missouri at Kansas City, Kansas City, Missouri

Ellen P. Dooling-McGurk, RPh, BCNSP
Department of Pharmacy, Truman Medical Center-Hospital Hill, Kansas City, Missouri

Theresa A. Fessler, MS, RD, CNSD
Nutrition Support Specialist, Department of Nutrition Services/Digestive Health, University of Virginia Health System, Charlottesville, Virginia

Douglas M. Geehan, MD
Associate Professor, Department of Surgery, University of Missouri at Kansas City; Staff Surgeon, Truman Medical Center, Kansas City, Missouri

Cheryl A. Gibson, PhD
Assistant Professor, Department of Internal Medicine, University of Kansas, Kansas City, Kansas

Ann C. Grandjean, EdD, FACN, CNS
Executive Director, Center for Human Nutrition, Omaha, Nebraska

William S. Harris, PhD
Director, Lipid Research Laboratory, and Professor of Medicine, Saint Luke's Hospital; University of Missouri at Kansas City, Kansas City, Missouri

Thomas S. Helling, MD
Professor and Vice Chairman, Department of Surgery, University of Missouri at Kansas City, Kansas City, Missouri

Thomas S. Helling, Jr., MD
Department of Radiology, Baylor University Medical Center, Dallas, Texas

Benjamin J. Hung, MD
Chairman, Division of General Surgery, Bryan Medical Center; St. Elizabeth's Hospital, Lincoln, Nebraska

Carol S. Ireton-Jones, PhD, RD, LD, CNSD, FACN
Nutrition Therapy Specialist, Carrollton, Texas

Gordon L. Jensen, MD, PhD
Professor of Medicine and Director, Vanderbilt Center for Human Nutrition, Vanderbilt University Medical Center, Nashville, Tennessee

Mary Ann Kaylor, MMSc, RD
Louisiana State University, Shreveport, Louisiana

Howard L. Kremer, MD
Independence Regional Health Center, Independence, Missouri

Scott W. Kujath, MD
North Kansas City Hospital, North Kansas City, Missouri

Marie Ann T. Lansangan, BSN, RN
Metabolic Support Nurse Clinician, Nursing Administration, Truman Medical Center, Kansas City, Missouri

Rifat Latifi, MD
Associate Professor of Clinical Surgery, Director of Surgical Critical Care, and Associate Director of Trauma and Critical Care, Department of Surgery, University of Arizona Health Sciences Center, Tucson, Arizona

George U. Liepa, PhD, FACN
Professor and Head, Department of Human Environmental and Consumer Resources, Eastern Michigan University, Ypsilanti, Michigan

Cynthia L. Lieu, PharmD, BCNSP
Associate Professor of Clinical Pharmacy, School of Pharmacy, University of Southern California, Los Angeles, California

Alan B. Marr, MD
Associate Professor, Department of Surgery, Louisiana State University Health Sciences Center in New Orleans; Medical Center of Louisiana at New Orleans, New Orleans, Louisiana

John M. Miles, MD
Professor of Medicine, Division of Endocrinology, Metabolsim, and Nutrition, Mayo Clinic, Rochester, Minnesota

Kudawashe M. Mushaninga, MS, RD, LD
Clinical Dietitian, Food and Nutrition Services, Truman Medical Center, Kansas City, Missouri

Alyce F. Newton, MS, RD
Area Nutrition Manager, Coram Healthcare, Ellicott City, Maryland

Chau N. Nguyen, MD
Department of Surgery, University of Missouri at Kansas City, Kansas City, Missouri

Pamela A. Orr, MSN, RN, FNP
Truman Medical Center, Kansas City, Missouri

L. Beaty Pemberton, MD
Professor Emeritus, Department of Surgery, University of Missouri at Kansas City School of Medicine; Truman Medical Center, Kansas City, Missouri

Danielle L. Petrocelli, BS, PharmD
Clinical Manager, Pharmacy, Beth Israel Medical Center, New York, New York

Melinda Pine, RD, LD, CNSD
Oncology Nutrition Specialist, University of Kansas Medical Center, Kansas City, Kansas

Angela M. Rialti, RD
Metabolic Support Dietitian, Nutrition Services, Truman Medical Center, Kansas City, Missouri

Joanne Z. Rogers, RN, MSN, CNSN
Clinical Nurse Specialist, Center for Nutrition and Weight Management, Geisinger Medical Center, Danville, Pennsylvania

Vicki M. Ross, MSN, RN
Assistant Research Professor, School of Nursing, University of Kansas, Kansas City, Kansas

Marie-Andree Roy, MSc
Research Assistant, Vanderbilt Center for Human Nutrition, Vanderbilt University, Nashville, Tennessee

Jaime S. Ruud, MS, RD
Nutrition Consultant, Nutrition Link Consulting, Inc., Lincoln, Nebraska

Monique Ryan, MS, RD, CNSD
Private Practice, Evanston, Illinois

David S. Seres, MD
Clinical Instructor, Internal Medicine, Albert Einstein College of Medicine; Beth Israel Medical Center, New York, New York

Ezra Steiger, MD, FACS, CNSP
Clinical Associate Professor of Surgery, Department of General Surgery, Cleveland Clinic Foundation; Case Western Reserve University, Cleveland, Ohio

Charles W. Van Way III, MD
Ralph Coffey Professor and Chairman, Department of Surgery, University of Missouri at Kansas City
School of Medicine; Chief of Surgery, Truman Medical Center, Kansas City, Missouri

Wahid Wassef, MD, FACG
Associate Professor of Medicine, Department of Internal Medicine, University of Massachusetts
Medical School; Director of Endoscopy, University of Massachusetts Memorial Health Care System,
Worcester, Massachusetts

Thomas Whalen, MD
Professor of Surgery and Pediatrics, Robert Wood Johnson Medical School; Robert Wood Johnson
University Hospital, New Brunswick, New Jersey

PREFACE TO THE SECOND EDITION

Although the first edition of *Nutrition Secrets* was edited by one person (CVW), the second edition has two co-editors. One of the main advantages of collaboration is having someone with whom to communicate and to try out new ideas. The two co-editors have worked together for several years on a variety of projects, largely through the American Society of Parenteral and Enteral Nutrition. When Dr. Van Way was Editor of *Nutrition in Clinical Practice*, for example, Dr. Ireton-Jones was one of the Associate Editors. Perhaps the best thing about the collaboration is that the two of us come from fairly different backgrounds. One holds an MD, the other a PhD. One is a surgeon by trade, the other a dietitian. Our backgrounds, areas of expertise, and even our contacts throughout the nutritional community have been both different and complementary. The collaboration, we believe, has added a great deal to this edition.

Preparing a second edition of a successful medical textbook is a bit like the old story of the seventh husband of the much-married movie star. We know what is expected of us, but the challenge is to make it new and interesting. We have added many new authors, modified nearly all of the chapters, and changed the material in the appendices to better reflect current practice. And yes, we have included the Ireton-Jones equations, an omission in the first edition that was pointed out to one of us by the other of us. We sincerely hope that this new edition better fulfills the need of the nutritional community and that it meets with your approval.

Charles W. Van Way III, MD
Carol Ireton-Jones, PhD, RD, LD, CNSD, FACN

PREFACE TO THE FIRST EDITION

Socrates pointed out, 2500 years ago, that the best way to teach is to ask questions. Of course, Socrates was always the one asking the questions. All of us remember being led around on hospital wards or in outpatient clinics, waiting to be asked questions—which we were not sure we could answer. A major purpose of *Nutrition Secrets* is to give the answers to the questions which you are most likely to be asked.

What you have in your hand is a book of questions and answers. It is not the usual kind of nutritional text. Conventional textbooks are good, and all of us use them. But they are not the only way to learn. Nutrition, like other medical sciences, must be learned one fact at a time. A very good way to do that is to concentrate your attention upon a single facet of nutrition as outlined in a key question and its answer.

We, the authors, are dietitians, nutritionists, nurses, pharmacists, and physicians. We are surgeons, internists, and pediatricians. We have written *Nutrition Secrets* for all of our students and colleagues: dietitian students and medical students, medical and surgical residents, nutritionists, pharmacists, physicians, and nurses. We hope it will help satisfy their need for practical knowledge of the many aspects of nutrition. It is sad but true that nutrition is regularly identified as one of the two or three most neglected subjects in medical schools. Pharmacy and nursing schools are little better. And yet there are few things as important to the health of our patients.

In 1986, Charles and Brent Abernathy, surgeons father and son, authored the first edition of *Surgical Secrets*. From their small beginning has grown a series of nearly 40 books. Charles Abernathy died—far too early—in 1994. It is a privilege to those of us who knew Charlie to be able to contribute to this series. To the memory of Charles Abernathy, then, I respectfully dedicate this book.

Charles Van Way III, MD

I. Nutritional Components

1. AMINO ACIDS AND PROTEIN

Stanley M. Augustin, MD, and Charles W. Van Way III, MD

1. What are amino acids?
Amino acids are the building blocks of proteins. Although there are hundreds of amino acids in nature, only twenty occur in proteins in humans. They are organic compounds that contain an amino group ($-NH_2$) and carboxyl group ($-COOH$) on the same alpha-carbon atom.

2. What are the functions of amino acids?
The functions of amino acids include substrates for protein and nucleic acid synthesis, regulation of protein turnover, regulation of enzyme activity, transportation of nitrogen, precursors of signal transduction, regulation of ion fluxes, participation in oxidation-reduction reaction, and precursors for gluconeogenesis, neurotransmitters, protein, and nucleic acids.

3. What is the difference between essential and nonessential amino acids?
Essential amino acids cannot be synthesized by the body and must be a part of the diet to permit growth or to maintain nitrogen balance. Essential amino acids include leucine, isoleucine, lysine, methionine, phenylalanine, threonine, tryptophan, histidine, arginine, and valine. **Nonessential amino acids** can be synthesized by the body either by reductive amination of a keto-acid by NH_4 or by transamination of a carbon chain synthesized in the central pathways of carbon metabolism. Nonessential amino acids include glutamic acid, aspartic acid, asparagine, and alanine. Although many amino acids are nonessential, their dietary intake can be less than optimal. **Conditionally essential amino acids** are derived from metabolism either of other amino acids or of other complex nitrogenous metabolites. Conditionally essential amino acids are cysteine, taurine, tyrosine, proline, serine, glutamine, and glycine.

Essential, Conditionally Essential, and Nonessential Amino Acids

ESSENTIAL AMINO ACIDS	CONDITIONALLY ESSENTIAL	NONESSENTIAL
Leucine	Taurine	Alanine
Isoleucine	Tyrosine	Glutamate
Valine	Cysteine	Asparagine
Lysine	Glycine	Aspartate
Phenylalanine (Tyrosine)	Serine	
Methionine (Cysteine)	Proline	
Threonine	Glutamine	
Tryptophan		
Histidine		
Arginine		

4. What are the branched-chain and aromatic amino acids?
The structure of the different amino acids varies in regard to side chain, size, and charge. Side chains have an important bearing on the stabilization of protein structure and are involved in

other aspects of protein function. The different side chains allow one to group the amino acids into categories. Branched-chain amino acids and aromatic amino acids are hydrophobic and tend to cluster in the center of globular proteins.

The **aromatic amino acids** (phenylalanine, tyrosine, tryptophan, and occasionally histidine) are precursors of neurotransmitters such as dopamine, epinephrine, and serotonin. In liver disease, aromatic amino acids can be precursors to false neurotransmitters that are implicated in hepatic encephalopathy.

The **branched-chain amino acids** (valine, leucine, and isoleucine) are vital in gluconeogenesis. They differ from other amino acids in that they are preferentially taken up by muscle cells rather than the liver. Within the muscle cells they are metabolized to form alanine, which is eventually processed to glucose in the liver.

5. What is protein?

The name *protein* is derived from the Greek word *proteus* and the Latin word *primarius*, literally meaning primary. Proteins are the chemical building blocks that compose our bodies. They are complex molecules made up of one or more chains of amino acids bound by peptide linkages. These amino acids and their interactions among themselves determine the size, shape, and length of each protein molecule.

Proteins do not always exist alone but also are conjugated with other compounds such as nucleic acids, lipids, minerals, and carbohydrates. Proteins form the major constituents of muscle, catalyze all chemical reactions, regulate gene expression, and compose major structural elements of all cells.

6. What is protein's function?

The catalytic functions of proteins are what make life processes possible. Protein functions include movement, acid-base balance, fluid regulation, storage/sequestration, immunity, enzymes, messenger/signals, growth, differentiation, and gene expression. Proteins are classified as fibrous or globular. Fibrous proteins are typically structural in function. Globular proteins are typically enzymes or cell membrane components. Proteins are also important in metabolism. They are the second largest store of energy in the body after fats. Protein provides 4 kcal/gm of energy.

7. What is protein turnover?

All protein in the body exists as either free amino acids or body protein. Protein turnover is the homeostatic mechanism to maintain the balance between protein synthesis and breakdown. The breakdown products of protein are amino acids. Intracellular proteins are broken down via energy-dependent proteasomes. Extracellular and membrane proteins are broken down through endocytosis and a lysosomal pathway. These enter the free amino acid pool of the body.

Only small amounts of free amino acids are found in the body. Sources of free amino acids are dietary protein intake, breakdown products of body protein (particularly skeletal muscle), synthesis of nonessential amino acids, and byproducts of intestinal microbes. The liver via oxidation and deamination metabolizes excess amino acids. The resulting products are the carbon skeletons (which can be used for energy production or converted to adipose) and urea for excretion through the kidney. The net loss or gain of body protein depends on the balance between the degradation and resynthesis of proteins in the body.

8. What is the urea cycle?

The end product of protein catabolism is excretion of nitrogen in the form of urea, which is a small molecule containing two nitrogen groups. Urea is formed from arginine, which splits off its terminal nitrogen groups to form urea and the amino acid ornithine. Ornithine then accepts a nitrogen to become citrulline, which goes on to re-form arginine. The potentially toxic ammonium ion, formed by amino acid metabolism, is thus converted to the inert compound urea. About 80% of the nitrogen excretion in the urine is in the form of urea; the remainder is creatinine, ammonium ion, and other components.

9. What is the daily requirement of protein?

The requirement for protein arises from growth, the need to replace losses, and the need to respond to environmental stimuli. Estimations of protein and amino acid requirements are based on nitrogen balance studies. The current RDA protein requirement is 0.8 gm/kg body weight per day. Essential amino acid intake should be at least 11% for adults and 43% for infants.

10. What are good sources of protein?

The nutritional quality of proteins depends on their essential amino acid composition, digestibility, and absorptive ability. Dietary intake should supply all essential amino acids in proper proportions to help maintain the person as well as repair damage to tissues. Because most food proteins contain many different types of proteins, the protein quality reflects a composite of the amino acids. Animal proteins (meat, milk, eggs, and fish) are regarded as high-quality or complete proteins. Meat and fish can contain 20% protein on a weight basis, whereas eggs contain 14% protein. Milk typically contains 3–5% protein.

Protein can also be derived from plant sources. Legumes (especially soybeans) have the highest percentage of protein per weight (up to 45%), and cereal grains contain 6–20% protein. Unfortunately, plant sources of protein are considered low-quality or incomplete proteins because they lack one or more essential amino acids. Since different plant proteins lack different essential amino acids, a person can obtain complete protein quality and quantity by eating foods that contain complementary proteins such as legumes and grains or legumes and vegetables.

One measure of protein quality is biologic value. It is determined by measuring the amount of nitrogen retained in the body in relation to nitrogen absorbed. The biologic value for an ideal protein is 100. The biologic values of common foods include the following: egg (85), milk (84), fish (76), meat (74), and wheat (66). Another measure of protein quality is its protein efficiency ratio. This ratio compares an animal's weight gain to the amount of protein consumed within a period of time.

11. What are the disease states of protein deficiency?

Protein deficiency (kwashiorkor) rarely occurs as an isolated condition. It is usually accompanied with a deficiency of dietary energy and micronutrients resulting from insufficiency food intake. Protein-energy malnutrition (PEM) is the most widespread form of malnutrition in the world, particularly in underdeveloped countries of Africa, Asia, and Central and South America. In this starved state the body cannibalizes protein for energy. This decrease of lean body mass (metabolically active tissue) reduces the resting energy expenditure.

The signs and symptoms of low and incomplete protein intake (kwashiorkor) in children include stunting, poor musculature, edema, thin and fragile hair, skin lesions, and diarrhea. In adults prominent signs of protein deficiency include expansion of the extracellular fluid compartment causing body edema, hair loss, atrophy of skeletal muscle mass, low serum albumin, immune dysfunction, and hormonal imbalances. Marasmus is the condition of insufficient dietary protein, calories, and nutrients. Symptoms of marasmus include muscle-wasting, absence of fat, reduced growth, hepatomegaly, and dermatosis.

Severe and prolonged deficiency may lead to death, generally by secondary infections. Deficiency of this severity is rare in the United States except as a consequence of pathologic conditions and poor medical management of the acutely ill. More commonly, lesser degrees of protein deficiencies place patients at increased risks from primary diseases and other coincident diseases.

12. Is there protein excess?

Some 30 years ago, a weight-reduction diet was developed which emphasized large amounts of protein, little starch, and no added fat. Following its original form, adherents to the diet were supposed to monitor their urine until they began to show ketone bodies, which was a sign that the body had "switched over" to a protein metabolism. What it actually meant was that the patient was beginning to get into keto-acidosis. This diet was effective, for two reasons. First, limiting one's intake to protein means limiting the calories. Second, a protein diet provides maximum satiety. Patients on relatively modest caloric intake did not get hungry between meals. The acidosis was not especially harmful. This low-carbohydrate diet remains both effective and popular. But in the years since, there have been developed some more sophisticated and more dangerous forms of this diet. A concentrated amino acid preparation is used, with the patient taking very little other food. With careful medical monitoring, this diet has produced spectacular weight reduction. But without monitoring, it has also produced several deaths.

BIBLIOGRAPHY

1. Chiolero RL, Fink MP: Nutritional and metabolic care in the intensive care unit: A feeling of some uncertainty? Curr Opin Clin Nutr Metab Care 5:159–161, 2002.
2. Desai BB: Handbook of Nutrition and Diet. New York, Marcel Dekker, 2000.
3. Food and Nutrition Board, Commission on the Life Sciences, National Research Council: RDA, 10th ed. Washington, DC, National Academy Press, 1989.
4. Gershwin ME, German JB, Keen C: Nutrition and Immunology: Principles and Practice. Humana Press, 1999.
5. Obled C, Papet I, Breuille D: Metabolic bases of amino acids requirements in acute diseases. Curr Opin Clin Nutri Metab Care 5:189–197, 2002.
6. Shils M, Olsen J, Shike M, Ross C: Modern Nutrition in Health and Disease, 9th ed. Philadelphia, Lippincott Williams & Wilkins, 1999.
7. Souba WW: Drug therapy: Nutritional support. N Engl J Med 336:41–48, 1997.
8. Spalholz JE, Boylan LM, Driskell JA: Nutrition: Chemistry and Biology, 2nd ed. Boca Raton, CRC Press, 1999.
9. Young VR, Borgonha S: Adult human amino acid requirements. Curr Opin Clin Nutr Metab Care 2:39–45, 1999.

2. CARBOHYDRATES

Angela M. Rialti, RD, and John M. Miles, MD

1. What are carbohydrates?

Synthesized from carbon dioxide and water, carbohydrates are the most abundant organic molecules on earth. Among the carbohydrates are sugars and starches, which are the major sources of energy in the human diet. Sugars consist of concentrated sweets, fruits, and milk; starches consist of grains and vegetables. Sugars can exist in the form of monosaccharides (glucose, fructose, and honey) or di- and oligosaccharides (sucrose, lactose, galactose, and dextrose). The most abundant sugar in nature is glucose, a monosaccharide, which is a major fuel for most animal species. Most of the carbohydrates found in nature are in the form of polysaccharides, which are high-molecular-weight polymers, and consist of starches and fibers. Starch is a polymeric storage form of glucose found in plants. In animals, glucose is stored as glycogen.

2. What is the difference between pentose and hexose?

Hexose monosaccharides are made up of six carbon atoms. These are the common simple sugars: glucose, fructose, and galactose, as noted above. Pentose monosaccharides have only five carbon atoms. The common pentoses are ribose, xylose, and arabinose. Ribose and deoxyribose are found widely in the body in nucleic acids and nucleotides. Actually, there are sugars containing from three to seven carbon atoms: trioses, tetroses, pentoses, hexoses, and heptoses. However, the most common are the pentoses and hexoses.

3. What are the chief functions of carbohydrates?

Carbohydrates are an important fuel for living organisms. In order to be used as a fuel, the polysaccharide storage form of carbohydrate (starch or glycogen) must be hydrolyzed to monosaccharides (simple sugars). In addition to its role as a fuel, carbohydrate serves as a structural element in bacteria, plants, and animals. Cellulose is the principal structural carbohydrate in plants and is the most abundant polysaccharide in nature. Vertebrate animals lack the enzymes (cellulase) necessary for digestion of cellulose, with the exception of ruminants such as cattle and sheep. In humans, cellulose passes unmolested to the colon, where it is metabolized by colonic bacteria to CO_2, H_2O, methane, and short-chain fatty acids. Short-chain fatty acids are absorbed and used for energy, primarily by the liver. Thus, indigestible carbohydrates can, indirectly, serve as a minor energy source. Carbohydrates, in addition, aid in vitamin and mineral absorption. They have also been shown to be preventative against certain forms of cancer.

There are other kinds of structural polysaccharides. Chitin is the principal component of the exoskeleton of arthropods. In addition, heteropolysaccharides such as hyaluronic acid are the chief component of the extracellular matrix that holds cells together and provides strength and shape in tissues such as bone and cartilage. Heteropolysaccharides can form aggregates with proteins called proteoglycans; these materials are responsible for the viscosity in secretions such as mucus.

4. How important is carbohydrate as a source of energy for humans?

Carbohydrates are the most important source of energy in the diet. In most Western diets, even those considered to be high in fat, carbohydrate comprises 50–60% of the total calories. The remainder is provided by fat (30–40%) and protein (10–20%). In some agrarian cultures, especially in Africa and Asia, carbohydrate provides up to 80% of the total energy in the diet.

5. What is the energy content of carbohydrate?

The energy content of carbohydrate, determined by bomb calorimetry, is approximately 3.8 kcal/gm. An apparent exception is found in the aqueous solutions of glucose that are administered parenterally to hospitalized patients. Because glucose exists in aqueous solutions as a monohydrate (molecular weight = 198) rather than anhydrous glucose (molecular weight = 180), its energy content in this situation is 3.4 kcal/gm. If the 5% dextrose is analyzed, it contains only 4.5% anhydrous glucose. Therefore, the caloric content appears lower because the anhydrous glucose content is actually lower.

6. Why is carbohydrate an essential nutrient?

Carbohydrate is essential primarily because of the high energy requirement of central nervous system tissue (i.e., the brain) in mammals. The brain has limited ability to use noncarbohydrate energy sources. In humans, the brain requires an estimated 100 g of glucose per day—one third to one half of the carbohydrate present in the average diet. Other tissues, such as hematopoietic tissues and white blood cells, are also obligate glucose users.

7. What is the minimum amount of carbohydrate required?

The minimum daily requirement for carbohydrates is 100 gm (380 kcal). This supplies enough energy as glucose to meet the need of the obligate glucose-using tissues and to minimize the breakdown of body protein for gluconeogenesis.

Carbohydrate intake minimizes, but does not eliminate, protein breakdown. Protein breakdown cannot be completely eliminated, even in the unstressed and fasting patient. On the other hand, fat intake has little effect on protein breakdown. Fat does not spare protein. It should be noted, however, that fat emulsions contain about 10% of their caloric content as glycerol, which is a carbohydrate.

8. What is the maximum amount of carbohydrate that can be tolerated?

The maximum rate of glucose utilization is around 4 mg/kg/min, which is approximately 400 g per day (1500 kcal/day) in an average person. If glucose is given in excess, hyperglycemia may result. This can in turn cause osmotic diuresis, excessive free water loss, dehydration, and even death. It is important in patients receiving glucose infusions or total parenteral nutrition (TPN) to keep the infusion rate below the tolerance level. A very good way to accomplish this is to give 30–40% of the calories as fat. This allows the use of TPN formulas containing 10–15 g of glucose per deciliter, rather than the old-fashioned 25 gm/dl. It should be pointed out that giving 2 liters a day of 25% glucose (with added amino acids), as was commonly done in past years, results in a glucose load of 500 gm per day.

Glucose tolerance is decreased by tissue injury, stress, and sepsis. Circulating hormones such as cortisol and the catecholamines can lower the tolerance for glucose. Therefore, the limit of 4 mg/kg/min should be regarded as a ceiling, and the goal of management should be to stay well beneath it.

If glucose is given in amounts exceeding energy needs, excess carbohydrate is converted into fat. This process is called lipogenesis. This process causes carbon dioxide release and may raise the respiratory quotient to an amount over 1.0. This in turn can put excessive stress on a patient with respiratory insufficiency.

9. What are complex carbohydrates?

Complex carbohydrates are digested less quickly than simple carbohydrates. Starch digestion occurs very rapidly in the proximal portion of the small intestine if the starch is presented in a form to which intestinal amylase has easy access. However, certain foods contain starch in a physical form that prevents rapid and complete digestion. There is good evidence, for example, that the starch in a pasta meal is digested rather slowly and that digestion is not complete during small bowel transit. Thus, undigested pasta starch may reach the cecum, where it can serve as a substrate for anaerobic bacterial fermentation. A recent study demonstrated a rapid increase in breath hydrogen shortly after a breakfast consumed 12 hours after a pasta meal. This presumably represents fermentation of undigested starch presented to cecal bacteria due to emptying of the terminal ileum.

10. What are the factors involved in starch absorption?

Amylose and amylopectin are the two types of glucose polymer found in starch. The initial step in starch digestion involves the action of salivary and pancreatic amylase on the α-1,4, linkage in amylose and amylopectin. Amylose is quickly broken down by amylase, but amylopectin is highly branched, and the α-1,6 linkage at the branch points is resistant to amylase. The action of amylase on amylopectin produces dextrins, which are oligosaccharides containing 5–10 glucose molecules. The dextrins are then further hydrolyzed by brush border enzymes in the small intestine.

11. What other functions do carbohydrates serve in foods besides being a source of energy?

A major role of carbohydrates, specifically simple sugars, is to impart sweetness to food. However, starch, structural polysaccharides, and various oligosaccharides serve a variety of other functions. For example, polydextrose is an ingredient that can provide the texture of fat in some foods because of its rheologic properties; it adds texture to such food items as puddings, frostings, and frozen desserts and allows a reduction in fat content without sacrificing "mouth feel" and thus palatability. Carbohydrates can provide hygroscopicity, coating ability, flavor encapsulation, and crystallization inhibition. Polysaccharides can be used as thickeners, stabilizers, emulsifiers, and gelling agents. The food industry has become quite sophisticated in its ability to use carbohydrates in prepared foods for these purposes.

12. What are sorbitol and mannitol?

The alcohol derivatives of certain sugars are called polyhydroxy alcohols. They are used in nutrition for a variety of purposes. The common polyhydroxy alcohols are sorbitol, which is derived from sucrose; mannitol, from mannose; and xylitol, from xylose. They taste sweet but are more slowly absorbed from the gastrointestinal tract than simple sugars. Sorbitol is widely used. Tasting as sweet as glucose, it is absorbed slowly but completely and hence has about the same energy content as the sugars. It is used therapeutically mixed with charcoal to detoxify ingested poisons. The charcoal binds the toxin, and the sorbitol in large dosage induces diarrhea.

13. How are carbohydrates digested?

There are three phases of carbohydrate digestion. In the mouth, salivary amylase begins hydrolysis of starch to dextrins and then to maltose and simple sugars. This process continues in the stomach, although the stomach does not contribute anything new. In the small intestine, pancreatic amylase continues starch hydrolysis. In the intestine, disaccharidases located in the cells of the brush border of the intestinal mucosal cells break down specific disaccharides to simple sugars. Sucrase splits sucrose into glucose and fructose. Lactase splits lactose into glucose and galactose; it is this enzyme that is deficient in the lactose-intolerant individual. As noted elsewhere, this deficiency is found in a majority of the people of the world. Maltase cleaves maltose into two glucose molecules.

The simple sugars are absorbed into the intestinal mucosal cells by an active process closely linked to the sodium-potassium pump. Glucose is transported by a carrier that also carries sodium, driven by the large sodium gradient between the intestinal lumen and the interior of the cell. That gradient in turn is maintained by the Na^+, K^+ ATPase that exchanges intracellular sodium for extracellular potassium, maintaining the low sodium level in the cell.

14. Are there really benefits of the popular low-carbohydrate diet for health and weight loss?

There is not enough research to support or refute this concept completely, although it always comes down to the basic principle, a calorie is a calorie. Weight loss occurs due to a negative energy balance: more calories are expended than consumed. And evidence is showing that weight loss results are likely due to restriction of caloric intake and longer duration of dieting. The American Dietetic Association, the American Heart Association, and other professional organizations have warned the public against the potentially serious medical consequences of low-carbohydrate diets, largely due to the common high-fat, high-protein content.

BIBLIOGRAPHY

1. Asp N-G: Classification and methodology of food carbohydrates as related to nutritional effects. Am J Clin Nutr 61:930S–937S, 1995.
2. Barclay L: Benefits of low-carbohydrate diet still uncertain. Medscape Med News 2003. Available at <http://www.medscape.com>.
3. Binkley RW: Modern Carbohydrate Chemistry. San Diego, Marcel Dekker, 1988.
4. Cashman MD, Wightkin WT: Carbohydrates. In Van Way C (ed): Handbook of Surgical Nutrition. Philadelphia, JB Lippincott, 1992, 30–36.
5. Chinachoti P: Carbohydrates: Functionality in foods. Am J Clin Nutr 61:922S–929S, 1995.
6. Ettinger S: Macronutrients: Carbohydrates, proteins, and lipids. In Mahan LK, Escott-Stump S (eds): Krause's Food, Nutrition, and Diet Therapy, 10th ed. Philadelphia, W.B. Saunders, 2000.
7. Flatt J-P: Use and storage of carbohydrate and fat. Am J Clin Nutr 61:952S–959S, 1995.
8. Gold PE: Role of glucose in regulating the brain and cognition. Am J Clin Nutr 61:987S–995S, 1995.
9. Hirsch J: Role and benefits of carbohydrate in the diet: Key issues for future dietary guidelines. Am J Clin Nutr 61:996S–1000S, 1995.

3. FATS AND LIPIDS

George U. Liepa, PhD, FACN

1. What is the difference between lipids and fats?

Lipids are a large class of compounds, which include fats, oils, waxes, and a variety of other compounds such as cholesterol, phospholipids, and lipoproteins. Their common properties are insolubility in water, solubility in organic solvents, and usability by living organisms.

Fats can be defined in three different ways. Commonly, a fat is anything that is oily to the touch and not soluble in water. Chemically, fats are fatty acids that exist mostly in the form of triglycerides but are also found as monoglycerides, diglycerides and free fatty acids. For nutritional purposes, dietary fats include the previously mentioned fatty acids as well as other lipids. The "other lipid" category includes compound lipids, such as phospholipids and glycolipids; sterols, such as cholesterol; and synthetic lipids, which include medium-chain triglycerides, structured lipids, and fat substitutes.

2. What does a fatty acid look like?

Fatty acids are made up of a chain of carbon atoms with a methyl group (CH_3^-) on one end and a carboxyl group ($COOH^-$) on the other. The individual carbon atoms in the chain have either one or two hydrogen atoms attached. If two hydrogens are attached to each carbon, the chain has the following form:

$$-CH_2-CH_2-$$

If one hydrogen is attached, the carbon is bound to the next carbon in the chain by a double bond and that carbon, in turn, has only one hydrogen atom attached. This is called a double bond, or an unsaturated bond:

$$-CH = CH-$$

Fatty acids are characterized by the length of the carbon chain and by the position of its double bonds. For example, linoleic acid (discussed in questions 4 and 5) has 18 carbons, of which two pairs are linked by double bonds. The first of these double bonds is located six carbons from the methyl end of the chain. Its designation is C18:2 w-6, and it is normally written as C18:2 n-6 or C18:2n6. A less commonly used notation for linoleic acid is 18:2(9, 12).

Unsaturated fatty acids can also exist in one of two stereometric forms. The *cis* form is most commonly found in the diet and is the only form that can be synthesized by animal cells. *Trans* fatty acids are usually found in hydrogenated fats (e.g., margarines, shortenings) and, because they can be synthesized by bacteria, they are found in small amounts in some dairy products.

3. What are the essential fatty acids?

Linoleic and alpha-linolenic acids cannot be synthesized by the human body and are therefore classified as essential fatty acids. If they are omitted from the diet, metabolic malfunctions eventually result with symptoms that include skin rashes and neuropathy. Both of the essential fatty acids can serve as precursors for the synthesis of "hormone-like" compounds called eicosanoids. A wide variety of eicosanoids can be made in the body (discussed in question 5), and these compounds affect a number of parameters, including blood pressure, vascular reactivity, blood clotting, and the immune system.

4. Which of the dietary fats have been shown to have the greatest health benefits?

Dietary fats can be divided into two large families: saturated and unsaturated. The unsaturated fats can be subdivided into monounsaturated fats (MUFA) and polyunsaturated fatty acids (PUFA). The monounsaturated fatty acids contain a single double bond in the ninth position and are classified as omega-9 fatty acids. Oleic acid is the most common omega-9 fatty acid found in the diet. The omega-9 fatty acids are commonly found in both olive and peanut oil and are considered to have a favorable impact in regard to coronary heart disease and possibly cancer.

The PUFA are subdivided into two main groups classified as the omega-3 and omega-6 fatty acid families. The omega-3 fatty acids are built from a linolenic acid base. Initially linolenic acid is synthesized by chloroplasts. When linolenic acid is consumed by cold-water ocean fish and certain other animals (e.g., deer) it can readily be converted into docosahexaenoic acid (DHA; C22:6w3) and eicosapentanoic acid (EPA; C20:5w3). These two fatty acids (EPA and DHA) are commonly marketed as "fish oil." Omega-3 fatty acids, in the form of linolenic acid, are also found in canola and flax oils. The precursor for the omega-6 fatty acid family of compounds is linoleic acid, which is readily converted by animal cells into arachidonic acid. Linoleic acid is primarily manufactured by a wide variety of plant seeds. It is critical that humans consume omega-3 and omega-6 fatty acids in similar amounts because they are used to make hormone like compounds (eicosanoids) that compete for metabolic control in the body. Because seed oils are so prevalent in the American diet, it has been suggested that consumption of omega-3 fatty acids should be increased to prevent the occurrence of coronary artery disease and certain types of cancers.

The United States does not presently have guidelines regarding omega-3 fatty acid intake. The Canadian Guidelines in 1990 were 1.0–1.5 gm/day for omega-3 fatty acids and 7.0–9.0 gm/day of omega-6 fatty acids. In the United States the average daily intake of EPA and of DHA is 0.050 gm/day and 0.080 gm/day, respectively. Both are far lower than the amounts presented in the 1990 Canadian Guidelines. During the past decade a wealth of data has been produced, indicating that 1–2 grams per day of omega-3 fatty acids are good for maintenance of health, whereas up to 10 grams per day may have a significant positive impact on other specific conditions related to mental health. Omega-3 fatty acids also have been shown to be effective in moderating diseases such as rheumatoid arthritis and atopic dermatitis.

5. What are eicosanoids? How are they used in the body?

Eicosanoids are derived from omega-3 and omega-6 fatty acid precursors (linoleic and linolenic fatty acids). The omega-6 eicosanoids include prostaglandin E_1 (PGE$_1$), prostaglandin E_2 (PGE$_2$), and thromboxane A_2. These compounds have a wide number of activities. Thromboxane A_2, for example, causes platelet aggregation, clot formation, and vasoconstriction, all of which promote the hemostatic response to injury. Linoleic acid is found in most vegetable oils, such as corn oil, safflower oil, cottonseed oil, and soybean oil.

Linolenic acid (C18w3) gives rise to the omega-3 (w-3) fatty acids and a wide variety of eicosanoids that include prostaglandin E_3 (PGE$_3$), thromboxane (TXA) A_3, and prostacylin. Prostacylin has nearly the opposite effect from thromboxane A_2. It vasodilates and inhibits platelet aggregation. When linolenic acid and DHA and EPA are consumed, they encourage the formation of the omega-3 family of eicosanoids. This eicosanoid family appears to have cardioprotective effects via decreased blood clotting and decreased blood pressure.

6. What are trans fatty acids? Are they bad for you?

Trans fatty acids are most commonly found in products that include partially hydrogenated vegetable oils (e.g., margarines, shortenings). They are used to make a wide variety of baked foods (e.g., donuts) and fried foods (e.g., potato chips, French fries). French fries contain up to 3.6 grams of trans fats, whereas donuts can contain up to 4.3 grams. In a report released by the Institute of Medicine (a functional arm of the National Academy of Science) during the summer of 2002, scientists recommended that Americans should cut back on trans fatty acid intake. Studies have shown that at autopsy up to 15% of the fatty acids found in human tissues have been in the trans configuration. During the coming year it is anticipated that food labels will have to include trans fatty acid content.

7. What are lipoproteins?

Lipoproteins are a group of compounds that are synthesized in the body and used to transport water-insoluble lipids. Plasma lipoproteins vary greatly in size, depending on the amount of lipid that is contained in a protein "envelope." Their density is dependent on the ratio of lipid to protein; if there is a lot of lipid and a small amount of protein, the density is low. Chylomicrons are large, low-density particles that are formed in the intestine and transport dietary lipid to the liver and other parts of the body after a meal. The chylomicrons that reach the liver are converted into smaller packages called very-low-density lipoproteins (VLDL) and low-density lipoproteins (LDL), which transport fat to the cells. Two primary lipoproteins are clinically important in the transport of cholesterol. Low-density lipoproteins (LDL) carry cholesterol to cells throughout the body, whereas high-density lipoprotein (HDL) carries cholesterol from the cells in the body to the reproductive organs and to the liver for eventual breakdown and elimination. A major objective in the prevention of arteriosclerotic cardiovascular disease is to lower the LDL and raise the HDL Low-density lipoprotein can exist in a variety of modified forms. Two of these forms, low-density lipoprotein of greater density (pattern A) and lipoprotein (a), have gained attention recently. Pattern A LDL is found more frequently in patients with coronary heart disease. Lipoprotein (a) is a modified form of LDL that is produced in the liver and is also found in greater amounts in patients with coronary heart disease. Recent studies have shown that dietary omega-3 fatty acids may help decrease lipoprotein (a) level in the blood stream.

8. What are phospholipids? How are they related to lecithin?

Phospholipids are a class of lipids consisting of long-chain fatty acids, phosphorus, and a nitrogenous base. They are important components of the cell membrane. A commonly consumed phospholipid is lecithin. Phopholipids have both a hydrophobic end, made up of fatty acids, and a hydrophilic end, which contains phosphorus and nitrogen. Lecithin is the fundamental building block of the lipid bilayer that forms cell membranes and can be synthesized in all cells.

Lecithin is found widely in both animal and plant tissues; good dietary sources are liver, egg yolk, soybeans, peanuts, spinach, and wheat germ. Although it is commonly promoted as a dietary supplement, it is not particularly effective in this capacity since it is broken down in the intestine by phospholipase A (lecithinase). Lecithin's nitrogen-containing base, choline, is a lipotrophic factor that is thought to help prevent the accumulation of fat in the body.

9. What is glycolipid?

The glycolipids are compound lipids combining fatty acids with a carbohydrate, such as galactose, and an amino alcohol, such as sphingosine. In general, glycoplipids are found in cell membrane structures. Particular glycolipids (cerebrosides) are found largely in brain tissue.

10. What does acrylamide have to do with dietary fat?

Recently acrylamide was discovered in fried foods that contain primarily carbohydrate. This finding is of interest to clinicians since acrylamide has been shown to be a weak carcinogen when it is fed to rats. Apparently acrylamide is made when asparagine, an amino acid, reacts with carbohydrates at temperatures above 100°C. It is presently not known whether acrylamide, when consumed in foods like French fries and potato chips, exists in quantities that are large enough to cause health problems in humans.

11. What is the function of cholesterol?

While cholesterol is usually classed as a lipid, it is neither a fatty acid nor a triglyceride. It is a member of a class of compounds known as sterols and is composed of carbon, hydrogen, and oxygen bound together in ring structures. Cholesterol is an important component of the body since it forms the molecular starting point for synthesis of the steroid hormones, including cortisol, aldosterone, and sex hormones. Cholesterol is also a precursor for the synthesis of vitamin D and bile acids and is used in the synthesis of cell membranes. Oxidized cholesterol plays a major role in the pathogenesis of cardiovascular disease.

12. What are cholesterol oxidation products? Why are they harmful?

Cholesterol oxidation products (COP) are found in dietary products and can be produced in the body. The most atherogenic variety of COP is oxidized LDL. Oxidized LDL has been shown to be atherogenic in both experimental animals and humans. Treatment for the prevention of COP production includes the use of antioxidants such as vitamin E, vitamin C, and beta carotene.

13. How much fat should be in the diet?
The percentage of fat that one should consume is not firmly established. Fat normally should make up no more than 30% of the calories in the diet, with protein adding no more than 20–25% to the diet and carbohydrates (primarily of the complex variety) making up the rest. The amount of fat in the average American diet has been steadily dropping over the past generation, from 40–45% in 1960s to 34–37% in 1990–1994.

Although this decrease is clearly a good idea, two caveats should be pointed out. First, cutting down the fat percentage is not highly effective at promoting weight loss unless the total caloric intake is appropriate. One can become just as obese on brown rice as on potato chips; one just has to eat more. Second, some of the reduction in fat is simply switching calories from one category to another. An example is the "fat-free" foods that are available. The fat in these foods is usually defined as triglyceride content, which is a narrow definition. But a dish of fat-free ice cream still contains 300–400 calories as carbohydrates, monoglycerides, and diglycerides. This sort of nutritional bookkeeping is both futile and misleading. Fat calories per se do not increase the risk of disease. It is obesity that renders people less healthy, and it is maintenance of normal body weight that should be the objective of nutritional counseling.

BIBLIOGRAPHY

1. Grosvenor MB, Smolin LA: Nutrition from Science to Life. New York, Harcourt College Publishers, 2002.
2. Harris WS, O'Keefe SH: Cardioprotective effects of omega 3 fatty acids. Nutr Clin Pract 16:6–12, 2001.
3. Liepa G, Han-Markey T, Sutton M: Nutritional and health aspects of dietary lipids. In O'Brian RD, Farr WE, Wan PJ (eds): Introduction to Fats and Oils Technology. AOCS Press, 2000.
4. Mahan LK, Escott-Stump S (eds): Krause's Food, Nutrition, and Diet Therapy, 9th ed. Philadelphia, W.B. Saunders, 1996.
5. Murray RK, Granner DK, Mayes PA, Rodwell VW: Harpers Biochemistry. Norwalk, CT, Appleton & Lange, 1990.
6. Palevitz BA: Acrylamide in French fries: How does it get there? Scientist 16(20):23, 2002.
7. Sarubin A: The Health Professionals Guide to Popular Dietary Supplements. American Dietetic Association, 2000.
8. Shils ME, Olson JA, Shike M, Ross AC (eds): Modern Nutrition in Health and Disease. Philadelphia, Lipincott Williams & Wilkins, 1999.
9. Stoll AL: The Omega-3 Connection. New York, Simon & Schuster, 2001.
10. U.S. Department of Health and Human Services, Public Health Services: Healthy People 2000: National Health Promotion and Disease Prevention Objectives, Pub No 91-50212. Washington, DC, U.S. Government Printing Office, 1990.
11. Ziegler EE, Filer LJ (eds): Present Knowledge in Nutrition. ILSI Press, 1996.

4. VITAMINS

Thomas G. Baumgartner, PharmD, MEd, and Charles W. Van Way III, MD

1. What are vitamins?

Vitamins are nutrients that are essential for maintenance of normal metabolic functions and hematopoiesis. Vitamins cannot be synthesized by mammalian cells. They function as cofactors for enzymatic reactions. The water-soluble vitamins play vital roles in the conversion of carbohydrate, protein, and fat into tissue and energy. Thiamin (B_1) acts as a coenzyme in carbohydrate metabolism. Riboflavin (B_2) is a coenzyme in the electron transport system associated with conversion of tissue oxidations into usable energy. Niacin (B_3) serves as a coenzyme in oxidation-reduction reactions in tissue respiration. Pantothenic acid functions as a coenzyme in various metabolic acetylation reactions. Folic acid and cyanocobalamin (B_{12}) are metabolically interrelated. They are essential to nucleic acid synthesis and normal maturation of red blood cells. Ascorbic acid (C) performs a vital function in the process of cellular respiration, is involved in both carbohydrate and amino acid metabolism, and is essential for collagen formation and tissue repair.

Classification of Vitamins

WATER SOLUBLE	LIPID SOLUBLE
Thiamin (B_1)	Vitamin A
Riboflavin (B_2)	Vitamin D
Niacin (B_3)	Vitamin E
Pantothenic acid (B_5)	Vitamin K
Pyridoxal (B_6)	
Biotin	
Cobalamin (B_{12})	
Folic acid	
Ascorbic acid (C)	

The water-soluble vitamins (B-complex and C) are not significantly stored by the body; excess is excreted in the urine. They must be replenished regularly through diet or other means to maintain essential tissue levels. They are rapidly depleted in conditions interfering with their intake or absorption. Lipid-soluble vitamins (A, D, E, K) are better stored in the body. If they are not excreted, as in renal failure, excess may accumulate and cause toxicity. Synthetic and natural vitamins are equivalent in action and exert similar kinetics.

2. What are the biological kinetics of vitamins?

Vitamin Kinetics

Vitamin A	
Absorption:	Duodenum, upper jejunum
Distribution/binding:	Various target organs (not heart or skeletal muscle)
Metabolism:	Enterohepatic = glucuronide, oxidation stored in liver
Excretion:	Urine, feces (metabolite and parent vitamin)
Vitamin D	
Absorption:	Ergocalciferol and cholecalciferol from small intestine; cholecalciferol more completely; bile necessary for absorption
Distribution/binding:	Rapid; chylomicron in lymph; kidneys, adrenals, bones and intestines

(Table continued on next page.)

Vitamin Kinetics (Continued)

Vitamin D (cont.)	
Metabolism:	t 1/2 = 19–25 hrs. for ergocalciferol or cholecalciferol
	t 1/2 = 3–5 days for calcitriol
	Body stores = six months
Excretion:	40% excreted in 10 days in bile; small amount in urine
Vitamin E	
Absorption:	35% absorbed from small intestine
Distribution/binding:	Lymph, all tissues
Metabolism:	Urinary tocopheronic acid and gamma lactone glucuronides
Excretion:	70–80% by liver over seven days; 20–30% urine
Vitamin K	
Absorption:	Small intestine, colon; requires bile (about 50% of total body vitamin K is synthesized in the bowel)
Distribution/binding:	Lymph
Metabolism:	Glucuronide and sulfate conjugates
Excretion:	Bile, urine
Vitamin B_1 (thiamin)	
Absorption:	Small intestine (maximum absorption = 8–15 mg/day)
Distribution/binding:	Heart, brain, liver, kidneys, skeletal muscles
Metabolism:	Degraded by tissues
Excretion:	Excess excreted in the urine unchanged
Vitamin B_2 (riboflavin)	
Absorption:	Small intestine
Distribution/binding:	All tissues; little storage
Metabolism:	Phosphorylation to flavin mononucleotide (FMN)
Excretion:	9% (increased with larger doses) unchanged in urine
Vitamin B_3 (Niacin)	
Absorption:	Throughout the gastrointestinal tract
Distribution/binding:	All tissues, particularly the liver
Metabolism:	N-methyl 2-pyridone 5-carboxamide; N-methyl 4-pyridone 3-carboxamide
Excretion:	Unchanged in urine
Vitamin B_6 (pyridoxine)	
Absorption:	Throughout the gastrointestinal tract (passive transport)
Distribution/binding:	Brain, liver, kidneys
Metabolism:	4-pyridoxic acid in liver
Excretion:	Feces, urine
Vitamin B_{12} (cyanocobalamin)	
Absorption:	Ileum (distal)
Distribution/binding:	Liver, heart, kidney, spleen, brain
Metabolism:	Cobalt complex
Excretion:	Bile (principally), feces, urine
Pantothenic acid	
Absorption:	Throughout the gastrointestinal tract
Distribution/binding:	All tissues
Metabolism:	Not metabolized
Excretion:	70% unchanged in urine
Inositol	
Absorption:	Throughout the gastrointestinal tract
Distribution/binding:	All tissues; brain, heart, and skeletal muscle
Metabolism:	To glucose
Excretion:	Small amount in urine
Choline	
Absorption:	As lecithin (not fully absorbed)

(Table continued on next page.)

Vitamin Kinetics (Continued)

Choline (cont.)	
Distribution/binding:	Liver, peripheral tissues liberate into lymphatics
Metabolism:	Trimethylamine (metabolized by intestinal bacteria)
Excretion:	Feces
Biotin	
Absorption:	Throughout the gastrointestinal tract
Distribution/binding:	Liver and brain
Metabolism:	Metabolizes in urine
Excretion:	Parent compound in feces and urine
Folic acid	
Absorption:	Ileum
Distribution/binding:	Liver, tissue
Metabolism:	Metabolites
Excretion:	Urine
Vitamin C (ascorbic acid)	
Absorption:	Intestine
Distribution/binding:	Plasma, body cells
Metabolism:	Metabolites
Excretion:	Urine after 2 mg/dl plasma concentrations

3. What considerations affect bioavailability of vitamins?

Bioavailability of orally administered vitamins depends on many factors. The most common way of measuring bioavailability is to determine the fraction of an oral dose that reaches the systemic circulation. For micronutrients, however, one must consider the physiological plasma concentration as well as the mechanisms that regulate intestinal absorption and distribution of micronutrients between functional and storage compartments in response to the demand. The rate of exchange between these compartments affects both delivery into the plasma compartment and clearance from it. Monitoring the area under the plasma concentration time curve after oral administration is inadequate to measure bioavailability if the plasma concentration is actively regulated. Bioavailability can be quantified by the rate at which deficiency symptoms are cured or by weight gain during growth. But both of these endpoints are influenced by homeostatic mechanisms, and neither is a very useful way of measuring bioavailability.

Bioavailability varies by age. Pediatric requirements are well worked out and the recommended dietary allowances have been recently revised to include both a 51–70-year and a > 70-year category.

4. What are the requirements for oral intake of vitamins?

Dietary Reference Intake (DRI) (Adults ≤ 50 Years Old)

Biotin	300 μg
Folate	400 μg
Niacin (B_3)	20 mg
Pantothenic acid (B_5)	10 mg
Riboflavin (B_2)	1.7 mg
Thiamin (B_1)	1.5 mg
Vitamin B_6	2 mg
Vitamin A	5,000 iu
Vitamin B_12	6 μg
Vitamin C	60 mg
Vitamin D	400 iu
Vitamin E	30 iu
Vitamin K	80 μg

iu = international units; mg = milligrams; μg = micrograms.

5. What is in a typical multivitamin dose?

This is typical of the dose given to a patient on enteral feeding or used as a routine supplement.

Typical Oral Liquid Multivitamin Dose

A (iu)	D (iu)	B_1 (mg)	B_2 (mg)	B_3 (mg)	B_6 (mg)	B_{12} (µg)	C (mg)	Pantothenic Acid (mg)
3,000	400	10	10	100	4.1	5	200	21.4

6. What vitamins should be given to a patient on parenteral nutrition?

Several preparations meet the new, revised guidelines from the FDA. The major change in these new guidelines is the increase in vitamin K in both adults and children. For both adults and children, vitamin supplements should be given daily when patients are on parenteral nutrition.

7. What vitamins are found in intravenous lipid or propofol?

Lipid emulsions used in parenteral nutrition are lipoprotein-like suspensions that are rich in polyunsaturated fatty acids and vitamin E. It has been hypothesized that vitamin E may act as a pro-oxidant in lipid emulsions, as it is in lipoprotein suspensions. Intralipid is highly susceptible to oxidation. Elevated levels of oxidized lipids can be formed during its clinical use, especially when Intralipid infusion is combined with phototherapy. Because lipid hydroperoxides are cytotoxic and can cause adverse effects, inadvertent infusion of rancid intralipid may add to the numerous problems encountered by premature neonates.

Commercially available intravenous lipid emulsions are largely derived from vegetable oils, which are a natural source of phylloquinone (vitamin K_1). The vitamin K_1 concentrations of 10% emulsions of Intralipid and Liposyn II are 31 and 13 µg/dl, respectively. The concentrations of vitamin K_1 in the 20% emulsions of these products are 62 and 26, respectively, twice that in the 10% emulsions. The amount of vitamin K_1 contained in these intravenous lipid emulsions is substantial. Besides usually meeting the daily requirements, lipid emulsions may have other effects on the vitamin K status of the patient. For example, they may greatly increase the dose of warfarin (Coumadin) required to maintain the prothrombin time within the therapeutic range.

The cell membrane is protected against lipid peroxidation through endogenous antioxidants such as the lipid soluble alpha-tocopherol. The anesthetic agent propofol (2,6-diisopropylphenol) has a chemical structure that is similar to alpha-tocopherol since it also contains a phenolic OH-group. The transient protection of glutathione (GSH) against lipid peroxidation in control liver microsomes is not observed in microsomes deficient in alpha-tocopherol. Introducing propofol (2 and 5 µM) restored the protective effect of GSH. Similar to the control microsomes, the GSH-protective effect did not occur in previously heated microsomes. These results suggest that propofol acts similarly to alpha-tocopherol as a chain-breaking antioxidant in liver microsomal membranes.

8. What vitamins are stable when given with medicinals in parenteral nutrition solutions?

Few studies exist that define the stability of vitamins in total parenteral nutrition (TPN) solutions containing medicinals. Parenteral nutrition (PN) formulas that have been used in medication stability studies frequently were a standardized mix. But the results have been and are extrapolated to any composition solution. In spite of this shortcoming, investigators have sought to identify the stability of medications being used with PN and rarely appreciated the stability of macronutrients and micronutrients in the PN solutions. The vitamins in particular are relatively labile. Detrimental effects can result from the instability of the fragile vitamin ingredients. A PN solution containing 60 g of amino acid, 250 g of dextrose with standard concentrations of electrolytes, trace elements, and vitamins, with or without ranitidine, has recently been shown to contain less than 90% of the initial thiamine concentration. This falls below the USP stability requirement for intravenously administered medications. In the absence of adequate data, the clinician should be wary of giving parenteral medications in the PN solution.

9. What vitamins are associated with which macronutrients?

Different vitamins are associated with particular substrate utilization. The vitamins that play a role in the utilization of each of the macronutrients are presented in the following table.

Vitamin Involvement in Macronutrient Utilization

	A	D	E	B_1	B_2	B_3	B_6	B_{12}	Biotin	FA	PA	C
AA	X	X	X	X	X		X	X	X	X		X
CHO	X			X	X	X		X				
Fat		X				X		X	X		X	

AA, amino acid; CHO, carbohydrate.

10. Why should vitamin megadosing be avoided?

Many of the vitamins can produce significant side effects if they are taken in excess. The fat-soluble vitamins are especially dangerous, as they can accumulate in the body.

VITAMIN	SIDE EFFECTS
Vitamin A	Headache, vomiting, diplopia, alopecia, dryness of mucous membranes, dermatitis, anemia, insomnia, bone abnormalities, bone and joint pain, hepatomegaly, liver damage, hypercalcemia, hyperlipemia, menstrual irregularities, spontaneous abortions, and birth defects.
Vitamin D	Nausea, vomiting, excessive thirst and urination, muscular weakness, joint pain, hypercalcemia, disorientation, and irreversible calcification of heart, lungs, kidneys, and other soft tissues.
Vitamin E	Exacerbation of the coagulation defect produced by vitamin K deficiency caused by either malabsorption or anticoagulant therapy.
Vitamin K	Hemolytic anemia, liver damage, and, in newborns, kernicterus.
Vitamin C	Nausea, diarrhea, kidney stones, mobilization of bone minerals, systematic conditioning to high intakes, and abortion; prooxidant in higher doses.
Vitamin B_1	Gastric upset.
Vitamin B_2	None reported in humans.
Niacin	Vascular dilation, gastrointestinal irritation, increased muscle glycogen utilization, decreased serum lipids, decreased mobilization of fatty acids from adipose tissues, and hepatomegaly.
Nicotinamide	Nausea, heartburn, fatigue, dry hair, sore throat, and inability to focus eyes.
Vitamin B_6	Dizziness, nausea, ataxia, peripheral neuropathy, and systemic conditioning to high intakes.
Folic Acid	Can obscure the diagnosis of pernicious anemia by preventing anemia and permitting nerve damage; may reduce zinc absorption.
Vitamin B_{12}	None reported.
Biotin	None reported.
Pantothenic acid	Occasional diarrhea and edema.
Choline	Nausea, dizziness, diarrhea, depression, excessive cholinergic stimulation, and EKG abnormalities.
Carnitine	Occasional diarrhea.
Inositol	None reported except problems may arise when inositol breakdown is impaired (diabetes mellitus, chronic renal failure, galactosemia, and multiple sclerosis).

11. Who is at high risk for vitamin deficiencies?

Chronic deficiency of various vitamins has been associated with cancer, cardiovascular pathology, cataract, arthritis, disorders of the nervous system, and photosensitivity. The very young, the very old, the stressed, and the chronically ill are most at risk for vitamin deficiencies. It is supposed that each vitamin plays a different role in the pathogenesis of various diseases, depending on the type of damage relevant to a specific disease. Beta-carotene, vitamin E and vitamin C have received much attention, particularly in the prevention of oxidative damage from free radicals. Clinically, thiamin deficiency is the most common; it is seen in chronic alcoholics and chronically undernourished patients. In addition, medications may be associated with vitamin deficiencies.

12. What are dosing considerations in the setting of organ compromise?
Liver disease is associated with deficiencies of the fat-soluble vitamins. In patients with primary sclerosing cholangitis (PSC) being evaluated for liver transplantation, vitamin A deficiency was seen in 82% and deficiencies of vitamin D in 50%. Other hepatic diseases may also be associated with deficiencies of vitamin A since 90% of vitamin is stored in the liver. Significant stores of folate, cobalamin, and vitamin K are also found in the liver.

Vitamin D is activated through both the liver and the kidney. Hypervitaminosis D is an especial hazard in renal failure. Vitamin D is not removed by dialysis. Oxalosis, or calcium oxalate deposition in the tissues, may develop in patients with accumulation of vitamin D and sometimes with parenteral vitamin C. Vitamins A and K can also be elevated and can be osteolytic in renal patients under the right conditions. Folate and cyanocobalamin supplements are needed to preserve the integrity of the erythrocyte. Folate is particularly important to supplement since renal patients have higher homocysteine serum concentrations. Although B_{12} is not removed during dialysis since it is so highly protein-bound, it is still wise to supplement B_{12} since folate supplementation may mask pernicious anemia.

13. What is the effect of vitamins on the immune system?
Tissue damage, enhanced inflammatory mediator production, and suppressed lymphocyte function may occur from inflammation or infection. Antioxidative vitamins, particularly ascorbic acid, and the tocopherols are important for limiting tissue damage and for preventing increased cytokine production. Glutathione is a major endogenous antioxidant and is important for lymphocyte replication. Pyridoxine and riboflavin participate in the maintenance of glutathione status. Pyridoxine is a cofactor in the synthesis of cysteine (the rate-limiting precursor for glutathione biosynthesis) and riboflavin is a cofactor for glutathione reductase. Deficiencies in tocopherol, vitamin pyridoxine, and riboflavin reduce cell numbers in lymphoid tissues of experimental animals and produce functional abnormalities in the cell-mediated immune response. Ascorbic acid and tocopherols exert anti-inflammatory effects in studies in man and animals. In humans, dietary supplementation with ascorbic acid, tocopherols, and pyridoxine enhances a number of aspects of lymphocyte function.

Oxidative stress is implicated in septic shock. The effect of intravenous antioxidant therapy on antioxidant status, lipid peroxidation, hemodynamics, and nitrite in patients with septic shock has been investigated by Galley et al. Thirty patients received either antioxidants or glucose infusion. The antioxidants were N-acetylcysteine plus bolus doses of ascorbic acid and alpha-tocopherol. In the 16 patients receiving antioxidants both heart rate and cardiac index increased, while systemic vascular resistance decreased. This beneficial effect of antioxidants on hemodynamic variables is highly encouraging for the future. Antioxidant administration may be a useful adjunct to conventional approaches in the management of septic shock.

14. How are vitamins involved in wound healing?
Ascorbic acid, iron, zinc, and energy (1 kcal/g collagen synthesized) are principally needed to heal wounds. Many of the biochemical events of wound healing are directly related to the patient's nutritional state. Although the initial local events of inflammation occur normally in any viable tissue, the subsequent reparative capacities of macrophages, fibroblasts, and endothelial cells are seriously impaired by any compromise of local perfusion and oxygenation. In particular, the bacteriocidal capacities of granulocytes are heavily dependent on local perfusion, nutrition, and endocrine status. Wound healing requires appropriate physiologic, nutritional, and endocrine support.

15. What vitamins provide antioxidant action?

Antioxidants are a complex and diverse group of molecules that protect key biologic sites from oxidative damage. They act by removing or inactivating free radicals and other reactive oxygen intermediaries. Both cancer and heart disease may be linked to our dietary intake antioxidants. Beta-carotene has been advocated for both cancer and heart disease. A randomized trial of 22,000 physicians in the U.S. Physicians Health Study, however, showed no differences in the overall incidence of malignant neoplasms or cardiovascular disease, or in overall mortality. In the Beta-Carotene and Retinol Efficacy Trial, with 18,000 subjects, beta-carotene and vitamin A produced a slight *increase* in the risk for lung cancer. Beta-carotene is not currently recommended.

Vitamin E (alpha-tocopherol) is thought to have a role in prevention of atherosclerosis through inhibition of oxidation of low-density lipoprotein. Some epidemiological studies have shown an association between high dietary intake or serum concentrations of alpha-tocopherol and lower rates of ischemic heart disease. In patients with symptomatic coronary atherosclerosis, alpha-tocopherol treatment substantially reduced the rate of non-fatal myocardial infarction after one year.

Selected Antioxidant Enzymes and Coenzymes

Enzyme Antioxidants

Superoxide dismutase
(Mn-containing superoxide dismutase, Cu-Zn-containing superoxide dismutase)
Glutathione peroxidase (selenium-dependent)
Glutathione-S-transferase
Glutathione reductase
Catalase

Coenzyme Antioxidants

Vitamin A
Vitamin C
Vitamin E
Ubiquinol (reduced form of coenzyme Q)

16. Who is at risk for elevated homocysteinemia?

Homocysteine is a sulphur-containing amino acid which, at high plasma concentrations, predisposes to thrombosis and induces focal arteriosclerosis. Mild increases in plasma homocysteine may predispose to atherosclerosis. Causes of mild increases in plasma homocysteine are usually dietetic deficiencies in protein, folic acid, vitamin B_6 or B_{12}, probably combined with a genetic alteration in the enzyme methylene-tetrahydrofolate reductase. Plasma homocysteine is an independent risk factor for myocardial infarction (see chapter 15, Nutrition and the Heart). Patients receiving large doses of niacin for hyperlipidemia may also have elevated serum homocysteine.

BIBLIOGRAPHY

1. Aarts L, van der Hee R, Dekker I, et al: The widely used anesthetic agent propofol can replace alpha-tocopherol as an antioxidant. FEBS Lett 357(1):83–85, 1995.
2. Baumgartner TG: Clinical Guide to Parenteral Micronutrition. Melrose Park, IL, Fujisawa, Inc., 1997.
3. Baumgartner TG, Henderson GN, Fox J, et al: Stability of ranitidine and thiamine in parenteral nutrition solutions. Nutrition 13(6):547–553, 1997.
4. Dietary Reference Intakes for Calcium, Phosphorus, Magnesium, Vitamin D, and Fluoride. Washington, DC, National Academy Press, 1997.
5. Dietary Reference Intakes for Thiamin, Riboflavin, Niacin, Vitamin B_6, Folate, Vitamin B_{12}, Pantothenic Acid, Biotin, and Choline. Washington, DC, National Academy Press, 1999.
6. Dietary Reference Intakes for Vitamin C, Vitamin E, Selenium, and Carotenoids. Washington, DC, National Academy Press, 2000.
7. Filiberti R, Giacosa A, Brignoli O: High-risk subjects for vitamin deficiency. Eur J Cancer Prev 6(Suppl 1): S37–S42, 1997.

8. Galley HF, Howdle PD, Walker BE, et al: The effects of intravenous antioxidants in patients with septic shock. Radic Biol Med 23(5):768–774, 1997.
9. Grimble RF: Effect of antioxidative vitamins on immune function with clinical applications. Int J Vitam Nutr Res 67(5):312–320, 1997.
10. Gutteridge JM: Antioxidants, nutritional supplements and life-threatening diseases. Br J Biomed Sci 51(3):288–295, 1994.
11. Helphingstine CJ, Bistrian BR: New Food and Drug Administration requirements for the inclusion of vitamin K in adult parenteral multivitamins. J Parenter Enteral Nutr 27:220–224, 2003.
12. Hennekens CH, Buring JE, Manson JE, et al: Lack of effect of long-term supplementation with beta carotene on the incidence of malignant neoplasms and cardiovascular disease. NEJM 334(18): 1145–1149, 1996.
13. Hunt TK: The physiology of wound healing. Ann Emerg Med 17(12):1265–1273, 1988.
14. Lennon C; Davidson KW; Sodowski JA et al. The vitamin K content of intravenous lipid emulsions. J Parenter Enteral Nutr 17(2):142–144, 1993.
15. Neuzil J, Darlow BA, Inder TE, et al: Oxidation of parenteral lipid emulsion by ambient and phototherapy lights: potential toxicity of routine parenteral feeding. J Pediatr 126(5 Pt 1):785–790, 1995.
16. Omenn GS, Goodman GE, Thornquist MD, et al: Effects of a combination of beta carotene and vitamin A on lung cancer and cardiovascular disease. NEJM 334 (18):1150–1155, 1996.
17. Stephens NG, Parsons A, Schofield PM, et al: Randomised controlled trial of vitamin E in patients with coronary disease: Cambridge Heart Antioxidant Study (CHAOS). Lancet. 347(9004):781–786, 1996.
18. Verhoef P, Stampfer MJ, Buring JE, et al: Homocysteine metabolism and risk of myocardial infarction: Relation with vitamins B-6, B-12, and folate. Am J Epidemiol 143(9):845–859, 1996.

5. TRACE ELEMENTS

Charles W. Van Way III, MD

1. What are trace elements?

A number of elements are present in the body in small amounts but are essential for the body's functioning. Unlike the macrominerals such as sodium and potassium, the requirements for trace elements are less than 100 mg/day. Most, but not all, of the trace elements are metals. They are frequently components of enzymes. Many are essential components of the diet but are required in such small amounts that deficiency states are rarely seen. Others, such as iron and iodine, can be sufficiently rare in the diet that their intake may be inadequate.

2. Which trace elements are essential?

Currently, the essential trace elements are iron, zinc, copper, manganese, chromium, cobalt, molybdenum, selenium, fluoride, and iodine. Recommended daily allowances (RDA) have not been established for all of them. Continuing research indicates that trace elements previously not known to be essential have been determined to be important. The table summarizes the trace elements which are known to be essential, and those known to be present, but not necessarily essential.

ESSENTIAL	POSSIBLY ESSENTIAL
Iron (Fe)	Silicon (Si)
Iodine (I)	Vanadium (V)
Zinc (Zn)	Nickel (Ni)
Copper (Cu)	Tin (Sn)
Manganese (Mn)	Cadmium (Cd)
Chromium (Cr)	Arsenic (As)
Cobalt (Co)	Aluminum (Al)
Selenium (Se)	Boron (B)
Molybdenum (Mo)	
Fluoride (F)	

A major impetus to progress in this area has been the widespread use of total parenteral nutrition (TPN) over the past 25 years. When all nutrients are given in a chemically defined intravenous formula, deficiencies become apparent relatively quickly. And with children and adults both being supported by TPN over periods of years, the demonstration of previously undetermined requirements has been frequent.

3. Which trace elements should be added to intravenous nutrition solutions?

Current recommendations are zinc, copper, chromium, manganese, and selenium. Iron must also be given, but by the intramuscular route. The exact amounts given daily at one hospital are as follows:

Zinc	5 mg
Copper	2 mg
Chromium	20 µg
Manganese	0.5 mg
Selenium	100 µg

This regimen is representative of good practice throughout the country, but the exact amount of each element varies.

21

4. What are the requirements for iron?

The adult human contains 3–5 grams of iron. About 70% of this is in hemoglobin, 5% in myoglobin, and the rest in enzymes or in the plasma pool bound to transferrin, the iron transport protein. Recycling of iron from old red cells is quite efficient, with 90% of the iron being re-used in the synthesis of new hemoglobin, so requirements are relatively small. Men require about 10 mg/day. Women require about 15 mg/day, with requirements going up during pregnancy to 30 mg/day. Iron deficiency is the most common deficiency syndrome and the normal diet is only marginally adequate. Good sources of iron include liver, oysters, shellfish, meat, poultry, and fish. Whole grain products and dried beans are good plant sources.

5. Is it possible to take in too much iron?

The iron content of the body is regulated by absorption, transport, and storage. Absorption in particular is controlled by how much apoferritin—iron binding protein—is present in the intestinal mucosa. Much of the iron ingested in the diet is not absorbed, although if the body's reserves are low, a much higher proportion is absorbed. But under certain conditions, the body can accumulate excess iron. This produces *hemosiderosis*, a condition in which iron is deposited in the tissues. The cause may be excessive intake or absorption, or excessive turnover of red blood cells. *Hemochromatosis*, a rare genetic disease, is characterized by iron overload. Finally, repeated transfusions for such diseases as renal failure or sickle cell anemia may bypass the normal regulation of iron absorption and result in excess iron.

6. What are the roles of zinc in the body?

There are only two or three grams of zinc in the human body, but it is a cofactor in enzymes that are involved in both synthesis and degradation of carbohydrates, fats, proteins, and nucleic acids. It is found in cellular nuclei, where it is involved with both RNA and DNA. It is present in bone. Zinc deficiency causes poor healing and, in children, growth retardation. The requirements for zinc are 12 mg/day for women, 15 mg/day for men. The best sources of zinc are meat, fish, poultry, and milk products, as well as beans, whole grain products, and nuts.

7. Why is iodine essential?

Iodine is used in the synthesis of thyroxin, the thyroid hormone. The main dietary source is seafood. It is also found in meats but this depends upon the amount of iodine available to the animal; similarly, the amount in vegetables depends on the amount in the soil. Iodine deficiency produces goiters in adults and mental retardation (cretinism) in children. These diseases used to be quite common in people living inland, far from the sea, where there was little iodine in the food chain. This was especially true for some of the landlocked countries in Europe, such as Switzerland. This problem has been solved in many places by such expedients as iodization of salt and by the use of iodine-containing disinfectants, coloring agents, and conditioners of bread dough. In many countries, such as Canada, it is mandatory to put iodine in the salt. Nonetheless, it is estimated that over one billion people in the world are at risk for iodine deficiency.

The RDA for iodine is 150 µg/day for adults and adolescents, with an increase to 175 µg/day during pregnancy and 200 µg/day during lactation.

8. What is the function of copper in the body?

Copper in the body is found in the liver, brain, kidneys, and heart. It is found in the plasma incorporated into a globulin, *ceruloplasmin*, which is active in iron absorption. There is no RDA; rather, there is an "estimated safe and adequate daily dietary intake" (ESADDI). This is a designation used where there is too little data available to allow an RDA to be assigned. The ESADDI is 1.5–3 mg/day for adolescents and adults. Copper is found in shellfish and organ meats, dried beans, cereals, fruits, and poultry. There is copper in the drinking water from the copper piping used in most residences.

9. What place does chromium have in glucose metabolism?

Chromium was discovered to be essential about 20 years ago by detecting abnormalities of glucose metabolism in patients on long-term TPN. Since then, it has become apparent that chromium is important to glucose regulation. It is a cofactor of insulin and appears to facilitate insulin binding to the cell membrane. Further, it is thought to be a component of the so-called *glucose tolerance factor*, which has a role in maintaining normal blood glucose. Chromium is also involved in the regulation of triglyceride levels. The ESADDI for chromium is 50–200 µg/day. Good sources are brewer's yeast, oysters, liver, and potatoes, as well as seafood, whole grain products, bran, meat, and poultry. Deficiency of chromium causes insulin resistance and may be a contributing factor in some cases of maturity-onset diabetes.

10. What is the function of manganese?

Manganese is located in liver, bone, pancreas, and pituitary; within the cells, it is found in the nucleus and mitochondria. It is a component of enzymes, including *glutamine synthetase, superoxide dismutase*, and *pyruvate carboxylase*. There is about 20 mg of manganese in the adult body. Deficiency produces weight loss, dermatitis, and nausea. In animals, interference with sexual and reproductive functions has been reported. ESADDI is 2–5 mg/day for adults.

11. Why is cobalt important?

The only known function for cobalt is as a component of vitamin B_{12} (*cobalamin*). As such, it is involved in the maturation of red blood cells. Vitamin B_{12} deficiency produces a characteristic macrocytic anemia. The more serious *pernicious anemia* is produced by an inability to absorb vitamin B_{12}. There is no RDA for cobalt *per se*, since it is contained in vitamin B_{12}. Sources are meats; for this reason strict vegetarians may become vitamin B_{12} deficient. However, the deficiency takes 3–6 years to develop and can be easily treated with vitamin B_{12} injections.

12. What is selenium deficiency?

Selenium is a component of *glutathione peroxidase*. This enzyme, present both in intracellular and extracellular forms, is found in almost all cells, and widely in body fluids. Glutathione peroxidase is both an antioxidant and a free radical scavenger, acting to detoxify tissue peroxides. Selenium deficiency has been observed largely in children receiving TPN for a long time. Deficiency takes years to develop. Symptoms include muscle weakness, pain, and tenderness. Selenium deficiency has been found in patients with cystic fibrosis. It may be related to cancer mortality and perhaps to cardiac disease. The RDA for selenium is 55–70 µg/day in adults, or about 1 mg/kg/day.

13. What enzymes contain molybdenum?

Molybdenum, like many trace elements, is an essential component or cofactor of a number of enzymes, in particular *xanthine oxidase*, which converts the end product of purine metabolism (adenosine, guanosine, etc.) to uric acid. *Sulfite oxidase* metabolizes cysteine and methionine. A congenital deficiency of sulfite oxidase has been reported, producing severe brain damage. These are enzymes which catalyze oxygen-reduction reactions. Molybdenum is a cofactor in a number of enzymes which act upon amino acids. It activates the fat-clearing factor *lipoprotein lipase*. The ESADDI is 75–250 µg/day for adults.

14. Why is fluoride added to drinking water?

Fluoride has been found to prevent dental caries. For that reason, it has been added to the drinking water widely throughout the United States and elsewhere. The incidence of dental caries has indeed dropped, for several reasons. Areas without fluoride are decreasing and fluoride is also widely used in toothpaste and in topical fluoride products. The fluoride content of foods has risen, especially when fluoridated water has been used in food processing or has appeared in the food chain. Interestingly, cooking food in Teflon-coated pans increases fluoride content because Teflon is a fluoride-containing polymer. The ESADDI for fluoride is 1.5–4 mg/day for adults.

Reportedly, the average intake in areas of the United States with fluoridated water is 1.7 mg/day and, without, 0.9 mg/day.

BIBLIOGRAPHY

1. Baumgartner T: Trace elements in clinical nutrition. Nutr Clin Pract 8:251, 1993.
2. Deitel M (ed): Nutrition in Clinical Surgery. 2nd ed. Baltimore, Williams & Wilkins, 1985.
3. Fischer JE (ed): Total Parenteral Nutrition. 2nd ed. Boston, Little, Brown, 1991.
4. Heimburger DC, Weinsier RL: Handbook of Clinical Nutrition. 3rd ed. St. Louis, Mosby-Year Book, 1997.
5. Lang CE (ed): Nutritional Support in Critical Care. Rockville, MD, Aspen, 1987.
6. Latifi R, Dudrick SJ (eds): Current Surgical Nutrition. Austin, R.G. Landes, 1996.
7. Mahan LK, Escott-Stump S (eds): Krause's Food, Nutrition, and Diet Therapy. 9th ed. Philadelphia, W.B. Saunders, 1996.
8. Van Way CW (ed): Handbook of Surgical Nutrition. Philadelphia, J.B. Lippincott, 1992.
9. Williams SR: Nutrition and Diet Therapy. 7th ed. St. Louis, Mosby-Year Book, 1993.

6. MINERALS AND ELECTROLYTES

Stanley M. Augustin, MD, Benjamin J. Hung, MD, and
Charles W. Van Way III, MD

1. What are minerals?

Minerals are inorganic chemicals that are required by the body in small amounts for the maintenance of life. There are approximately 20 minerals recognized as essential for humans. Macrominerals exist in the body at levels greater than 0.005% of body weight and are required at levels of 100 mg or more per day. The essential macrominerals include calcium, magnesium, phosphorus, and major electrolytes. Microminerals are less than 0.005% of body weight and only a few milligrams or less per day are required. The microminerals include iron, zinc, copper, selenium, iodine, cobalt, manganese, fluoride and chromium.

Most minerals function as cofactors in enzymatic reactions and as osmotic factors maintaining fluid balance. Other functions of minerals are acid-base balance, nerve transmission, structural components, and maintaining resting membrane potentials.

2. What do sodium, potassium, and chloride have in common?

They are monovalent electrolytes involved primarily in the osmolarity of body fluids. These elements determine the volumes of the intracellular and extracellular fluids.

3. What is the function of sodium?

Sodium is the main extracellular cation. Total body sodium is 70 grams. The concentration of sodium (135–145 mEq/L) is the main factor that determines the extracellular osmolarity. Sodium is actively pumped out of cells via the sodium-potassium pump. Sodium is found as well in bone lattice.

4. What are the characteristics of sodium absorption and excretion?

Sodium is absorbed from dietary sources completely within the small bowel. The body tries to actively conserve sodium. Its excretion via the kidney is related to total serum osmolarity and volume status through the influence of antidiuretic hormone, aldosterone, and atrial natreutic peptide.

5. What are the daily RDA requirements of sodium?

Between 500 and 2000 mg of sodium are required per day. This amount should be lower in people with diseases associated with fluid retention, such as congestive heart failure, renal failure, and peripheral edema.

6. What are the consequences of sodium excess?

Sodium excess is caused by increased intake and renal retention. Sodium excess increases the extracellular fluid resulting in edema in the interstitial space.

7. What is the consequence of sodium deficiency?

Sodium deficiency causes a reduction in the extracellular fluid. This reduction is usually accompanied by decreased tissue perfusion, muscle weakness, fatigue, and CNS symptoms.

8. What is the function of potassium?

Potassium is the main intracellular cation with a concentration of 140–150 mEq/L; the extracellular concentration is only 3.5–5.0 mEq/L. Total body potassium is 3000–4000 mEq or 150 grams. It is actively pumped into the cell via the sodium-potassium pump. Along with sodium, it is critical for resting membrane potential and acid-base balance. Additionally it helps regulate muscle activity, neuromuscular activity, and cardiac contraction.

9. What are the characteristics of potassium absorption and excretion?
Potassium is absorbed from dietary sources throughout the small bowel. Its excretion is via the kidney with a smaller amount through sweat and stool.

10. What are the daily RDA requirements of potassium?
The minimal daily requirement is 2000 mg or 50–80 mEq/L via intravenous fluids. This amount is approximately 1 mEq/L per kilogram. It is found in high concentrations in fruits, vegetables, fresh meats, legumes, nuts, and beans.

11. What are the consequences of potassium excess?
Hyperkalemia causes muscle weakness secondarily to loss of cellular depolarization, paralysis, and cardiac arrhythmias. Because the total amount of potassium in the extracellular fluid is so small, a relatively minor change in absorption or excretion can result in a dangerous increase in its level. Potassium absorption is proportional to the amount in the gut. The most common cause of potassium excess is impaired excretion as seen in renal failure.

12. What are the consequences of potassium deficiency?
Hypokalemia causes muscle weakness and cardiac arrhythmias. It alters the resting membranes potential by making the cell hyperpolarized. Potassium depletion is found in numerous conditions, such as malnutrition, diarrhea, and vomiting. Prolonged gastric suction causes hypokalemia indirectly. All of these conditions are associated with high losses of sodium. As the kidney tries to conserve sodium, potassium is excreted via the sodium-potassium pumps. This tendency toward potassium loss as a consequence of sodium loss has two beneficial characteristics. The potassium in the intracellular space remains in balance with the sodium in the extracellular space. Additionally, it preserves sodium, which is the substance being lost. Treatment of sodium loss and dehydration must include replenishment of the potassium stores. The potassium deficit is usually as large or larger than the sodium deficit.

13. What is the function of chloride?
Chloride is the main extracellular anion. Extracellular concentration is 95–105 mEq/L. Along with sodium it helps maintain osmotic pressure in the serum. It functions in acid-base balance via chloride-bicarbonate buffer within red blood cells and neural cells. It is found in highest concentration in gastric acid as hydrochloric acid (HCl) and spinal fluid.

14. What are the characteristics of chloride absorption and excretion?
Because its intake is usually associated with sodium, chloride absorption is similar to sodium absorption. It is absorbed within the small intestine and excreted via the kidneys, although it is not as tightly regulated as sodium.

15. What is the daily RDA requirement of chloride?
Chloride is commonly ingested with sodium as sodium chloride (NaCl). The requirement is 750 mg per day.

16. What do calcium, phosphorus, and magnesium have in common?
These elements are involved primarily in the normal physiology of the bony skeleton as the primary mineral elements. Because these minerals are involved in numerous physiologic and biochemical processes such as neuromuscular excitation, enzyme activation, coagulation, and membrane permeability, close monitoring of levels of these minerals is essential in critical illness.

17. What is the function of calcium?
Calcium is the main mineral of bone and teeth in the form of hydroxyapatite. Total body calcium is 1000–1200 grams of 1.5–2% of body weight. The amount of calcium within the skeleton changes with age, body size, and body composition. Additional functions of calcium include muscle contraction, intracellular transmission, and coagulation cascade.

18. What are the characteristics of calcium absorption and excretion?

Normal daily intake of calcium is 1–3 grams. It is absorbed in the duodenum and colon under the influence of vitamin D. Only 10% of ingested calcium is absorbed; the rest passes out in the stool. Calcium excretion occurs via the kidneys, although most calcium is conserved by renal absorption.

19. What are the characteristics of calcium regulation?

In the bloodstream the normal plasma concentration is 9–11 mEq/L. One-half of calcium is nonionized and inactive bound to plasma proteins. The other half is ionized (Ca^{2+}) and active in neuromuscular activity.

Regulation appears directed at maintaining the plasma-ionized calcium within a normal range. Parathyroid hormone causes increased calcium absorption. It mobilizes bone stores and decreases renal excretion by promoting absorption in the distal tubule. Calcitonin is produced by the C-cells of the thyroid gland. It decreases the releases of calcium from the bone, thus lowering the plasma calcium level. Vitamin D promotes calcium absorption from the gastrointestinal tract.

20. What is the relationship of albumin and calcium?

Only ionized calcium is active in bodily functions, and the body regulates ionized calcium. Laboratory analyzers obtain total calcium that includes ionized calcium and calcium bound to plasma proteins. If the albumin is low, the total calcium will be low even though the ionized levels may be normal. This can be corrected by adding 0.8 mEq/dl to the measured calcium result for every 1-mg/dl drop of albumin below 4 mg/dl.

21. What is the daily RDA requirement of calcium?

The recommended calcium intake is 400–1200 mEq per day. Calcium is found in dairy products, green leafy vegetables, legumes, nuts, and whole grains. The daily requirement is higher in women than in men. Lactating women require a higher amount, and osteoporosis, which is common in elderly women, may be prevented by calcium supplementation.

22. What is the consequence of calcium excess?

The most common causes of hypercalemia are cancer, immobilization, hyperthyroidism, and hyperparathyroidism. The mean effects are decreased activity of nerve and muscle cells, causing weakness and fatigue. Other manifestations include anoxeia, nausea, vomiting, hypertension, and urinary stones. These effects are more pronounced if the levels rise in a rapid manner vs. a slow manner. Many patients can tolerate high levels if they occur over many months.

23. What is the consequence of calcium deficiency?

Common causes include hypoparathyroidism, hypomagnesemia, malabsorption, vitamin D deficiency, and alcoholism. Calcium deficiency causes excessive contraction of muscles, leading to tetany, paraesthesias, seizures, and cardiac arrhythmias. Long-term systemic calcium deficits lead to osteoporosis.

24. What is the function of magnesium?

Magnesium is an important intracellular cation. It is involved in numerous enzyme processes as well as muscle contraction and nerve conduction. Along with calcium, magnesium is found within the skeleton.

25. How is magnesium found in the body?

Total body magnesium is 20–30 grams. Normal plasma concentration is 2.0 mEq/L. Approximately 60% is ionized, 25% is protein-bound, and the other 15% is complexed.

26. What are the characteristics of magnesium absorption and excretion?

Normal daily intake is 250 mg. Magnesium is absorbed within small bowel even with low dietary intake but is load-dependent. At higher levels of intake absorption is decreased, while at lower levels absorption is increased. Its absorption by the bowel is related to vitamin D and parathyroid hormone. The kidney conserves magnesium extensively.

27. What is the daily RDA requirement for magnesium?
Magnesium is found in vegetables, nuts, legumes, dairy products, and fruit. Daily intake is 250–350 mg but only 40% is absorbed.

28. What is the consequence of magnesium deficits?
Hypomagnesaemia occurs in poor dietary intake, hyperthyroidism, hyperparathyroidism, potassium deficiency, hyperaldosteronism, protein malnutrition, and short-bowel syndrome. Similar to potassium, low levels of magnesium can cause cardiac arrhythmias, paresthesias, weakness, seizures, and confusion.

29. What is the consequence of magnesium excess?
Hypermagnesaemia occurs commonly in renal failure. It causes hyperflexia and results in abnormal bone collagen matrix formation by delaying its crystallization.

30. What is the function of phosphorus?
Total body content is 500–800 grams. Phosphate is the most common intracellular anion. Extracellular concentration is 2.4 mEq/L. The majority of phosphorus is nonionized as phosphate and located in bone. In addition to bone physiology, phosphorus is involved in generation of adenosine triphosphate (ATP) and is complexed to lipids, proteins, and sugar.

31. What are the characteristics of phosphorus absorption and excretion?
Phosphorus is absorbed in the jejunum. Its absorption is increased in the presence of vitamin D. Its excretion is related to levels of calcium and parathyroid hormone via the renal tubules.

32. What is the daily RDA requirement for phosphorus?
The RDA requirement is 800 mg. Only 1% of the phosphorus turns over each day. High concentrations are found in milk, meat, poultry, fish, and cereals.

33. What is the consequence of phosphorus deficiency?
Phosphorus deficiency contributes to respiratory failure, secondary to inability to generate ATP, osteomalacia, myopathy, leukocyte dysfunction, and growth failure.

BIBLIOGRAPHY

1. Desai BB: Handbook of Nutrition and Diet. New York, Marcel Dekker, 2000.
2. Food and Nutrition Board, Commission on the Life Sciences, National Research Council: RDA, 10th ed. Washington, DC, National Academy Press, 1989.
3. Pemberton LB: Treatment of Water, Electrolyte, Acid-Base Disorders in the Surgical Patient. New York, McGraw-Hill, 1994.
4. Prelack K, Sheridan R: Micronutrient supplementation in the critically ill patient: Strategies for clinical practice. J Trauma 51:601–620, 2001.
5. Shils M, Olsen J, Shike M, Ross C: Modern Nutrition in Health and Disease, 9th ed. Philadelphia, Lippincott Williams & Wilkins, 1999.
6. Souba WW: Drug therapy: Nutritional support. N Engl J Med 336:41–48, 1997.
7. Spallholz JE, Boylan LM, Driskell JA: Chemistry and Biology, 2nd ed. Boca Raton, FL, CRC Press, 1999.
8. Weinsier RL, Heimburger DC: Handbook of Clinical Nutrition, 3rd ed. St. Louis, Mosby, 1996.

7. FIBER

Charlotte A. Buchanan, RD, LD, CNSD

1. What is fiber?
Fiber is material from plant cell walls that is resistant to digestion by enzymes of the human small intestine. Fiber is often classified according to its solubility in water. Water-soluble fibers (pectin, gums, mucilages, and some hemicelluloses) tend to be efficiently broken down by bacteria in the colon. Water-insoluble fibers (lignin, cellulose, and the remaining hemicelluloses) pass through the body mostly unchanged. Dietary fiber is a complex mixture of both.

2. How does the colon digest fiber?
Soluble fiber is still undigested when it reaches the colon. It is attacked by bacteria that ferment the polysaccharides to produce gases (carbon dioxide, hydrogen, methane, and volatile fatty acids). Unfortunately, gas production is a byproduct of a high fiber diet. The good news is it can be minimized if fiber intake is increased gradually, allowing intestinal microflora to adapt.

3. What is the recommended daily fiber intake?
Infants: The amount recommended is controversial. On one hand, fiber is not recommended in large amounts (foods containing 31 grams per serving), because of the need for a high-calorie, nutrient-dense diet for adequate intake and growth. However, a recent study by Ross Laboratories suggested that caloric intake was not compromised in infants 6–20 weeks of age by the addition of 9.1 grams of fiber/L of formula.
Children: Age plus 5 grams per day (beginning at age 2–age 18).
Adults: 20–35 grams per day.

4. How much fiber is consumed by adults in the United States?
Men: 16.6–20.0 grams per day
Women: 12.5–14.7 grams per day
Fiber intake was reported from Third National Health and Nutrition Examination (NHANE) Survey, 1988–91. This is improved from a mean of 11.1 grams per day for men and women on the Second NHANE Survey eight years earlier (1980–84).

5. What are the usual food sources of dietary fiber?

FOOD	PORTION	FIBER CONTENT (GRAMS)
Fruits		
Banana	1 medium	2.7
Pear w/skin	1 medium	4.0
Prunes	5 dried prunes	3.0
Raisins	1 cup	2.0
Vegetables		
Broccoli	1 cup, cooked	2.3
Corn	1 cup, cooked	2.0
Green beans	1 cup, cooked	2.2
Lettuce	1 cup	1.0
Peas	1 cup, cooked	2.2
Potato	1 medium	4.8

(Table continued on next page.)

29

FOOD	PORTION	FIBER CONTENT (GRAMS)
Legumes		
Kidney beans	1 cup, cooked	3.2
Navy beans	1 cup, cooked	3.3
Breads and cereals		
White bread	1 slice	0.4
Whole wheat bread	1 slice	1.5
Brown rice	1 cup	2.0
Popcorn	2 cups	1.4
Bran flakes	1 cup	5.0
Shredded wheat	1 cup	3.9
Nuts and seeds		
Almonds	10 nuts	1.9
Peanuts	10 nuts	2.2

Pennington, Bowes & Church, 16th ed., 1994.

6. How do you tell patients to increase fiber in their diet?
• Eat at least 5 fruits and vegetables per day.
• Use whole grain breads and cereals rather than white bread and sugary cereals.
• Eat bran cereal daily.
• Add beans 1–2 times per week.
• Finally, tell them that when they increase fiber, they should also increase fluid intake by a minimum of 2 glasses of water per day.

7. Does a high-fiber diet affect nutrient absorption?
Not generally. There has been concern that (1) some dietary fiber contains phytate (inositol hexaphosphate) that may form insoluble compounds with vital minerals, and (2) oxalates may interfere with the absorption of iron. But it is unlikely that a nutrient deficiency would occur from a high-fiber diet if an adequate, balanced diet is consumed. The human body adapts to the continued intake of relatively high amounts of dietary fiber. There is a period of compensation lasting 8–10 weeks after starting a high-fiber diet. The body also compensates for the decreased availability of phytate-bound minerals by increasing absorption.

8. What are the mechanical and metabolic effects of soluble and insoluble fiber?

EFFECT	SOLUBLE	INSOLUBLE
Delays gastric emptying	Yes	No
Increases fecal bulk and frequency of bowel movements	Yes	Yes
Regulates colonic transit time	Yes	Yes
Slows glucose absorption from small intestine	Yes	No
Reduces postprandial blood glucose levels	Yes	No
Lowers serum total cholesterol and LDL cholesterol	Yes	No

9. What are the specific effects upon the gastrointestinal tract?
Dietary fiber promotes normal bowel function by interacting with various substrates and effectors of transit time and nutrient absorption. Insoluble fibers produce a laxative effect, increase transit time and fecal bulk. Addition of fiber to treat constipation is an effective, inexpensive treatment, especially for the elderly population. However, a select group of constipated patients classified as "slow transit constipation" do not respond at all to a fiber regimen. It may also be necessary to prescribe a bowel stimulant for individuals with a long history of chronic constipation

because of the possibility of decreased contractile function. It is important to note that a failure to increase water consumption with fiber intake can actually result in constipation.

10. What conditions can be improved by increasing fiber intake?

Diseases of the colon	Diabetes mellitus
Constipation	Hyperlipidemia
Hemorrhoids	Obesity
Diverticulosis	

Diabetes mellitus: An increase in fiber has been proven to improve glycemic control and increase sensitivity to insulin. May allow a reduction in medication due to improved control.

Obesity: Fiber provides a feeling of fullness and may aid in long-term weight management.

Hyperlipidemia: The addition of soluble fiber, especially oat bran, has produced reductions in serum lipid levels. The addition of $\frac{2}{3}$–1 cup of oat bran per day can reduce serum low-density-lipoproteins (LDL) by 10–20%.

11. Can a high-fiber diet aid in prevention of disease?

Probably. An increase in dietary fiber may help prevent heart disease and cancer (particularly colon cancer). Of course, a low-fat diet, weight control, exercise, stress management, and the avoidance of smoking helps, too. Fiber is very good, but it won't do everything.

12. Does fiber help reduce diarrhea in enteral feedings?

Yes. Fiber-free formulas can contribute to gut mucosal atrophy, especially in the distal portion of the small bowel, and in the colon. Atrophy can lead to diarrhea, dehydration, electrolyte imbalance, and lack of nutrient absorption. There are many other causes of diarrhea, including antibiotics or other medications, Clostridium difficile, food intolerance, or simple interference with the normal gut flora. But fiber is important. Most fiber-containing formulas on the market use soy polysaccharides because they help to prevent clogging and they are not affected by heat processing. Fiber-enriched infant and enteral formulas (soy-polysaccharides) have also been effective in the treatment of diarrhea and can assist in achieving normal laxation in children on long-term enteral nutrition.

BIBLIOGRAPHY

1. Anderson JW, Smith BM, Gustafson NJ: Health benefits and practical aspects of high-fiber diets. Am J Clin Nutr 59(5 Suppl):1242S–1247S, 1994.
2. Bass DJ, Forman LP, Abrams SE, Hsueh AM: The effect of dietary fiber in tube-fed elderly patients. J Gerontological Nrsg 22(10):37–44, 1996.
3. Glinsmann WH, Bartholmey SJ, Coletta F: Dietary guidelines for infants: a timely reminder (Review). Nutr Rev 54(2 Pt 1):50–7, 1996.
4. Gorman MA, Bowman C: Position of the American Dietetic Association: health implications of dietary fiber. JADA 93(12):1446–1447, 1993.
5. Gray DS: The clinical uses of dietary fiber. Am Family Physician 51(2):419–426, 1995.
6. Homann HH, Kermen M, Fuessenich C, Senkal M, Zumtobel V: Reduction in diarrhea incidence by soluble fiber in patients receiving total or supplemental enteral nutrition. JPEN 18(6):486–490, 1994.
7. Labarthe DR: Dietary fiber. Further epidemiological support for a high-intake dietary pattern (editorial; comment). Circulation 94(11):2696–2698, 1996.
8. Minaker KL, Harari D: Constipation in the elderly. Hosp Practice 30(5):67–70, 73–76, 1995.
9. Reese JL, Means ME, Hanrahan K, Clearman B, Colwell M, Dawson C: Diarrhea associated with nasogastric feedings. Oncl Nrsg Forum 23(1):59–66, 1996.
10. Sinkler S, Reitmeier CA, Mills L: Addition of pectin and temperature influence the viscosity of some tube-feeding formulas. JADA 94(1):85–86, 1994.
11. Voderholzer WA, Schatke W, Muhldorfer BE, Klauser AG, Birkner B, Muller-Lissner SA: Clinical response to dietary fiber treatment of chronic constipation. Am J Gast 92(1):95–98, 1997.
12. Williams CL, Bollella M: Is a high-fiber diet safe for children? Peds 96(5 Pt 2):1012–1019, 1995.

II. Basic Nutrition

8. DIETARY PRINCIPLES AND THE FOOD GUIDE PYRAMID

Abby S. Bloch, PhD, RD

1. What are the Dietary Guidelines for Americans?

These guidelines serve as the government's recommendations for maintaining the health of the general population. The dietary guidelines are used as the basis of nutrition standards for the federal government's food and nutrition programs as well as the basis for nutrition education messages for the general public.

The Dietary Guidelines for Americans is mandated to be reviewed every 5 years by the U.S. Department of Agriculture (USDA) and U.S. Department of Health and Human Services (HSS). The last review was completed and published in May, 2000. An advisory committee selected by the secretaries of USDA and HHS reviewed peer-reviewed scientific literature and found that substantial knowledge available since the 1995 guidelines were issued warranted a revision.

The 2000 guidelines were developed around three basic messages: **A**im for fitness, **B**uild a healthy base, and **C**hoose sensibly for good health (**ABC**). Then guidelines were developed from these three messages.

Dietary Guidelines for Americans, 2000

1. Aim for fitness
   - Aim for a healthy weight.
   - Be physically active each day.
2. Build a healthy base
   - Let the pyramid guide your food choices.
   - Choose a variety of grains daily, especially whole grains.
   - Choose a variety of fruits and vegetables daily.
   - Keep food safe to eat.
3. Choose sensibly
   - Choose a diet that is low in saturated fat and cholesterol and moderate in total fat.
   - Choose beverages and foods to moderate your intake of sugars.
   - Choose and prepare foods with less salt.
   - If you drink alcoholic beverages, do so in moderation.

2. What is the food guide pyramid?

In 1992, the food guide pyramid was created by the USDA as a graphic with a 29-page accompanying text to accompany the original 1990 dietary guidelines. Its original intent was as a teaching tool to be used by the general healthy population as a guide for food choices and portion sizes. It provides the number of recommended servings for five major food groups.

Although the dietary guidelines have been revised twice since the pyramid was developed, it has not undergone revision since its creation in 1992. Although it is currently being reassessed, no date for a revision has been determined.

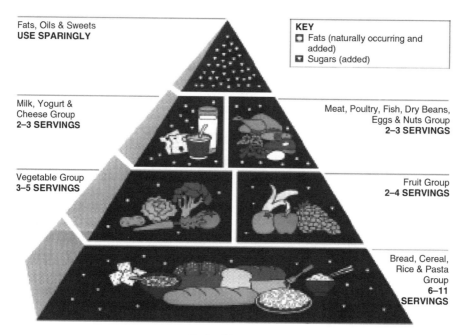

Food guide pyramid.

3. Is the food guide pyramid still valid?

Recently nutrition and health professionals have begun to question the usefulness of the pyramid. It is no longer consistent with the current guidelines.

A concern of many nutrition experts is the basic premise of the pyramid. The emphasis on carbohydrates at the base of the pyramid provides too many carbohydrates without distinguishing between healthy carbohydrates vs. sugars and refined carbohydrates. Many agree with Dr. Walter Willett, chair of the Nutrition Department, and Dr. Meir Stampfer, chair of the department of Epidemiology at Harvard's School of Public Health, that the pyramid does not reflect the basic science currently known and that it conveys the wrong message. With emerging science questioning the need to restrict fat, many also believe that the pyramid's message to avoid fat is incorrect.

4. What are the limitations of the pyramid?

Whereas the new dietary guidelines emphasize eating whole grains and moderate amounts of healthy fats, the pyramid does not convey this message. The pyramid gives the message that all fats are bad and all complex carbohydrates are good, all proteins are nutritionally equivalent, and dairy products should be encouraged. These messages are not consistent with current research.

One limitation of the pyramid is the way in which it is frequently used as a stand-alone educational piece. When it is used this way, the information can be distorted and an incorrect message conveyed in terms of portions, amounts, and sizes as well as individual food choices. People may look at the base and think that they can consume anywhere from 6 to 11 servings per day from the bread, cereal, rice, and pasta group. A person consuming about 1,600 calories per day should have about 6 servings from the grain group; a person consuming 2,200 calories per day should have about 9 servings; and a person consuming 2,800 calories per day should have about 11 servings. However, most people do not make these distinctions.

The message that resonates with individuals using the pyramid is that eating lots of starch is good and eating any fat is bad. Nutrition experts such as Dr. Willett believe that none of those perceptions are accurate. By emphasizing the intake of carbohydrates, the pyramid may be contributing to the current rise in obesity and diabetes.

5. Are other pyramids available?

Yes. There are over two dozen different pyramids from the California Cuisine Food Pyramid, Mediterranean Diet Pyramid, and Soul Food Pyramid to various ethnic pyramids and the vegetarian pyramid. Both Dr. Walter Willett, Fredrick John Stare Professor of Epidemiology and Nutrition at the Harvard School of Public Health, and Dr. David Heber, Director, UCLA Clinical Nutrition Research Unit, and Chief, Division of Clinical Nutrition for the Center for Human Nutrition at UCLA, have developed pyramids that they believe better reflect healthy eating. Willett's Healthy Eating Pyramid puts daily exercise and weight control at the base, recommends eating whole-grain foods at most meals, and suggests eating vegetables "in abundance." He places emphasis on plant oils, such as olive, canola, and soy, and gives fish and poultry a higher profile than red meat, which he recommends eating sparingly. All pyramids encourage the consumption of lots of vegetables and fruits, although some distinguish between high- and low-glycemic fruits to limit the amount of sugar consumed. Most health professionals recognize the need for Americans to limit their intake of sugar, sugar products, and refined carbohydrates, such as breads/flour and starches (e.g., white rice, white potatoes, pasta).

Despite this acceptance, the National Academy of Sciences recently released a significant revision of the macronutrient recommendations for carbohydrates, proteins, fats, fiber, and physical activity. The 2002 dietary recommendations are in ranges rather than specific amounts of each macronutrient.

1. Healthy Americans should eat:
   - 45–65% of the total caloric intake from carbohydrates
   - 20–35% from fat
   - 10–35% from protein
   - No safe level of consumption was given for either trans fats or saturated fats. The advise was to limit both.
2. Fiber intakes for adults up to the age of 50:
   - 38 grams for men
   - 25 grams for women
3. For adults > 50 the recommendation was to consume:
   - 30 grams of fiber for men
   - 21 grams form women
4. Physical activity was increased to 1 hour of exercise daily.
5. Added sugars found in soft drinks, candy, baked goods, and desserts were permitted for up to 25% of total calories.

It seems that these recommendations do not encourage people to select healthy choices of any of the macronutrients and to limit less desirable choices within each category. In addition, the suggestion that up to 25% of total calories as added sugar is acceptable seems excessive in light of the rampant obesity and diabetes epidemic currently seen in the U.S.

6. What should be recommended to my patients?

The 2000 Dietary Guidelines may be reasonable to follow without using the current food guide pyramid. Health professional should encourage people to eat healthy choices of all macronutrients, including moderate amounts of both fats and healthy carbohydrates, that provide maximum nutrient and phytochemical benefits. Maintaining a healthy weight and incorporating exercise or physical activity into daily activities is also important.

BIBLIOGRAPHY

1. Food and Nutrition Board, Institute of Medicine, National Academy of Sciences: Dietary Reference Intakes for Energy, Carbohydrates, Fiber, Fat, Protein and Amino Acids (Macronutrients). Washington, DC, National Academy Press, 2002.
2. Food and Nutrition Information Center: Pyramids for Ethnic/Cultural, Special Audiences. Available at <http://www.nal.usda.gov/fnic/etext/000023.html>.

3. McCullough ML, Feskanich D, Stampfer MJ, et al: Diet quality and major chronic disease risk in men and women: Moving toward improved dietary guidance. Am J Clin Nutr 76:1261–1271, 2002.
4. Willett WC, Skerrett PJ, Giovannucci EL: Eat, Drink, and Be Healthy: The Harvard Medical School Guide to Healthy Eating. New York, Simon & Schuster, 2001.
5. Willett WC, Stampfer MJ: Rebuilding the Food Pyramid. New York, Scientific American, 2003.
6. USDA Food Guide Pyramid: Information and guidelines about the food pyramid, including basics about the food groups and servings. Available at <http://www.nal.usda.gov:8001/py/pmap.htm>.
7. U.S. Dietary Guidelines for Americans: Nutrition and Your Health: Dietary Guidelines for Americans, 5th ed. 2003. Available at <http://www.nal.usda.gov/fnic/dga/>.

9. THE NUTRITIONAL CARE PROCESS

Charles W. Van Way III, MD

1. What is the nutritional care process?

The nutritional care process is a systematic approach to meeting the nutritional needs of a particular patient. While the process can be broken down into discrete and identifiable steps (see question 2), it must incorporate the following actions:

1. Considering a patient's history, present state of nutrition, and disease status
2. Identifying individual nutritional needs
3. Planning a nutritional strategy that will meet both the general and particular needs of the patient
4. Providing food or more exotic nutritional components
5. Evaluating the results in order to provide corrective feedback
6. Facilitating discharge or transfer to another level of care

This process has been the foundation for the practice of clinical nutrition for a generation. Several years ago, the Joint Commission for Accreditation of Health Care Organizations (JCAHO) formally outlined standards for the nutritional care process in hospitals and other health care organizations. As part of that process, the discrete steps involved in the process were defined.

The process is parallel to and has many features in common with the medical therapeutic process. Both start with a history, both include physical and laboratory examinations, both focus on a therapeutic prescription designed to meet the needs of the patient, and both incorporate evaluation and corrective feedback. There are, of course, significant differences between the two. Medicine is concerned with disease and its treatment, while nutrition is concerned with foods in all of their forms and with their effects on the body. Everyone must eat, while only a relative few must be treated for any particular disease. Nonetheless, the processes are similar.

2. What are the steps in the nutritional care process?

Viewing the process as a system, it is useful to divide it into five discrete steps or tasks. Each of these has subtasks.

1. Assessment
   - Perform nutrition screening
   - Assess patient by means of diet history and multidisciplinary assessment
   - Formulate nutrition care plan
2. Order support
   - Determine route of delivery
   - Order nutrition therapy
   - Determine patient's preferences within constraints of order
   - Transmit order
3. Preparation and distribution
   - Receive order in dietary services or pharmacy
   - Prepare order
   - Distribute to patient care unit (or home site)
   - Review preparation process for quality control
4. Administration
   - Administer nutrition to patient
   - Observe patient for compliance with orders and for complications
5. Monitoring and feedback
   - Monitor each patient daily
   - Reassess patient and nutritional plan

- Change orders as necessary
- Review entire nutritional care process for performance improvement
- Plan for transition to next site of care (or discharge to home)
- Educate patient and family as appropriate

3. What is the nutritional screening process?

It is a requirement of the JCAHO that all patients admitted to a health care facility—hospital, skilled nursing facility, or home health care agency—be evaluated for nutritional needs. This can be done in a variety of ways. Most facilities use nursing service personnel for the initial screening. The nursing database includes information such as body weight, recent weight loss, and the presence of diseases such as diabetes and renal failure. There may be other basic elements of the diet history. If this preliminary screen reveals that the patient may have specialized nutritional needs or may be malnourished, then further action is taken. Sometimes an intermediate screening is done by nutritional technicians. Eventually, the patient has a formal nutritional consultation by a registered dietitian. This consultation includes a detailed diet history, laboratory studies for nutritional assessment, and the formulation of a nutritional care plan for the patient. Further nutritional care may involve the preparation of specialized diets or physician-ordered aggressive enteral nutritional support or total parenteral nutrition.

4. What are the elements of a diet history?

The diet history is a specialized and focused medical history. It must include the following elements:

- Weight history, emphasizing recent changes
- Eating habits and food intake, again emphasizing recent changes
- Food intolerances, allergies, and specific religious or personal exclusions
- Physical activity and exercise
- Systemic and endocrine diseases related to nutrition, such as diabetes
- Gastrointestinal diseases
- Evidence of poor nutrition, such as pressure sores and poor wound healing
- Concurrent drug therapy, including nonprescription drugs and nutrition supplements

While not always necessary, a 3-day or 1-week food record can be helpful in dealing with particularly difficult problems.

The diet history is a part of the overall process of nutritional assessment (see Chapter 29). A complete nutritional assessment includes laboratory studies relevant to nutrition, such as albumin and prealbumin levels, as well as such physical measurements as skinfold thickness.

5. What is a nutrition care plan?

A nutrition care plan is a specific formulation of nutrients to meet the special requirements of a particular patient. It should specify energy requirements, protein requirements, percentage of calories as fat, and any special or unusual micronutrient requirements. The nutritional care plan is usually outlined by the dietitian, but components such as total parenteral nutrition may require the patient's physician to order the nutrition or another physician to consult on the patient's management. The nutrition care plan is dynamic, and changes are expected as the patient responds to nutrition and medical therapy.

6. What is an order support system?

The order support system covers the process of specifying and ordering food or other nutrients for patients. It encompasses all the steps between formulation of the nutrition care plan and arrival of the order for food at the kitchen. It includes writing the diet order, interviewing the patient about food preferences, and transmitting both the order and the food preferences (menu card) to the kitchen.

Despite the reputation of hospital food services, hospital dietitians generally do a good job in assessing patient needs, and hospital food services usually prepare food that is at least as palatable as other institutional fare. The order support system is truly a weak link. For example, consider the food ordering process from the patient's standpoint. He or she will pick items off a menu in the evening or early in the morning and then receive the food many hours later. How many restaurants would stay in business if they required customers to place their food order when they called in for reservations? The order support system is, as the current jargon would have it, an opportunity for improvement. Of course, other steps in the process, such as transportation and delivery of food, can and often are equally weak links.

7. Who prepares nutritional orders?

The obvious answer would be the kitchen. However, a lot of diets are prepared outside the kitchen, and just who prepares them varies from hospital to hospital. The institution's pharmacy usually prepares total parenteral nutrition orders. Enteral formulas, used for tube feedings and nutritional supplements, may be prepared by pharmacies, regular kitchens, or specialized formulation kitchens. They also may be prepared on the floor by nursing personnel. Sterility of the process, training of the personnel, and quality control of the mixing process are management issues. Many hospitals used canned, premade preparations to avoid these preparation issues. Enteral preparations are like the proverbial stepchild. Often, neither dietary services nor the pharmacy wants to prepare them.

8. How is quality assurance carried out?

Quality assurance in nutrition services involves two very different programs: first, maintaining quality food preparation and second, performance improvement for the entire nutritional care process. Maintaining quality food preparation involves monitoring the entire process of food preparation, distribution, and administration to the patient to make sure that no errors are being made and that the food service is as good as possible. Total parenteral nutrition preparation is subject to the same sort of program, which is usually managed as part of the quality assurance program of the pharmacy. TPN preparation is held to the same standards as any other intravenous fluids or drugs.

Performance improvement for the entire nutritional care process is far more complicated. Indicators covering the whole process have been published, but monitoring the system is time-consuming and difficult. Indicators tend to ask questions, such as, "Are patients getting screened properly," which can be both helpful and valid. However, larger issues may be so difficult to measure that they become lost. Is nutritional therapy meeting its goal? Has the patient been enabled to change bad eating habits? Has nutritional therapy reinforced medical therapy in an appropriate manner? Integrated management of the entire nutritional care process is rarely achieved in acute care hospitals.

9. What is the transition process?

The transition process is the last step in the nutritional care of a patient. It is the process by which the patient is sent home or to another facility. Discharge planning is another term for the transition process, but discharge planning carries the implication of ending at the time of discharge, while the transition process carries over into the next phase of the patient's care. After all, nobody just goes home and never comes back to see the doctor. Well, almost nobody. The transition process includes education of the patient and family, medical counseling on such issues as drug-nutrient interactions and insulin dosage, and follow-up care. Often, home health care is helpful to ensure that the patient continues to eat an appropriate diet. If the patient is transferred to another facility, nutritional assessment and diet prescription information can be sent with the patient, so the next facility does not have to start with a blank slate.

The transition process is often neglected. It is common to see patients sent home or referred to a home health care agency with only sketchy verbal instructions. Even for such complex therapies as home TPN, the coordination between hospital and home health care agency may be poor or nonexistent. The transition process is where the patient can achieve lasting benefit from his or her nutritional care in the hospital. It should be recognized as an important part of the nutritional care process.

BIBLIOGRAPHY

1. Kushner RF, Ayello EA, Beyer PL, et al: National Coordinating Committee clinical indicators of nutrition care. J Am Dietetic Assn 94:1168–1177, 1994.
2. Williams SR (ed): Nutritional assessment and therapy in clinical care. In Nutrition and Diet Therapy, 7th ed. St. Louis, Mosby, 1993.
3. Mahan LK, Escott-Stump S (eds): The nutrition care process. In Krause's Food, Nutrition, and Diet Therapy, 9th ed. Philadelphia, WB Saunders, 1996.

III. Specialized Nutrition

10. PEDIATRIC NUTRITION
Angela M. Rialti, RD, and Thomas Whalen, MD

1. What differences must one consider in nutritional assessment of the infant and child?
The predominant difference in assessment of nutritional status and provision of nutrients in both health and disease is the need to consider growth. Growth is fastest in the neonate and infant. The cost of such normal development is a considerable increase in caloric needs with a lesser increase in requirements for certain substrates and minerals. Growth charts developed by the National Center for Health Statistics (NCHS) are widely used to assess and track a child from birth to 18 years of age. These charts give percentiles for weight/height, height/age, and age/head circumference—and lately for BMI.

Certainly psychological differences will make some difference in the provision of nutritional support. Poor tasting enteral formulae will almost never be voluntarily taken in amounts needed, yet nasoenteric tubes may be pulled out all too frequently, or at least lead to the necessity of troublesome restraints.

2. What are the calorie requirements for infants up to age 18?
Various approaches lead to an estimate of the calories needed for any age patient. Judgment of adequacy of such estimates is covered below. However, as a first and simplest impression one may use 100 kilocalories per kilogram for the first 10 kilograms, 50 kcal for the next 10 kg, and 20 kcal/kg after that. As in any other age patient, mitigating circumstances should be considered. A septic post-operative neonate breathing room air will require more, while the pharmacologically paralyzed one-year-old on extracorporeal membrane oxygenation (ECMO) without infection may need less.

A guide to calorie needs may be seen in the following table.

Suggested Kcal Goals

AGE (YEARS)	KCAL REQUIREMENTS (KCAL/KG)
Premature	120
0–0.5	108
0.5–1	98
1–3	102
4–6	90
7–10	70
11–14	(F) 47, (M) 55
15–18	(F) 40, (M) 45

3. What are the fluid needs of the neonate?
There are at least four bases for determination of fluid needs of the neonate. These are by body surface area, by body weight alone, by caloric expenditure with requisite fluid needs, and by multiple physiologic parameters. Each has intrinsic problems and none is completely accurate

when used alone. As in any age patient, such formulas lead to an initial approximation that must then be continuously adjusted based on feedback from physiologic systems. In its simplest form, caloric expenditure is perhaps the soundest approach that is readily and easily utilized. Set against the known conversion of one milliliter of water being necessary for one calorie of the body's metabolism, it is then easiest for the neonate or any child up to 10 kg in weight to use 100 ml/kg of weight as the first approximation of fluid needs.

4. What are the protein needs of the infant and child?
In all of nutrition support there remains controversy about whether protein is directed as an anabolic building block or as a fuel source. Obviously both descriptions can and do apply, and may vary in any given physiologic circumstance. Yet clearly the younger the child, the more one will see provided protein as a substrate for body protein construction during the all important growth phase. The need for protein thus will decrease as the child ages, and a guide to protein requirements may be seen in the following table.

Suggested Protein Goals

AGE (YEARS)	PROTEIN REQUIREMENTS (GM/KG)
Premature	2.5–3.5
0–0.5	2.2
0.5–1	1.6
1–3	1.2
4–6	1.1
7–10	1.0
11–14	(F) 46, (M) 45 (gm/day)
15–18	(F) 44, (M) 59 (gm/day)

5. Do the usual considerations of time without enteral intake change for the infant and child?
Definitely. The consideration of growth in the child and continuing organogenesis in the neonate mandate that the usual time lines considered in the adult be shaved in half. Thus if the normal practice in the adult is to estimate that a period without nutritional intake will be at least five days before consideration of specialized nutritional support, in the neonate and child that time frame should be diminished to two to three days.

6. How is intravenous access gained in the neonate?
Concurrent with the development of parenteral nutritional support, access to the circulatory system for provision of nutrients became a key challenge. A surgical approach was generally accepted for many years, with cutdowns performed upon any of a number of relatively easily accessed veins (external jugular, common facial, saphenous at the groin, etc.). As the length of time necessary for parenteral support became longer and longer, the need for multiple sites for catheters increased. Catheters have been placed in a multitude of veins including the inferior epigastric, intercostals, and even directly into the atrium.

Over the past several years the most common approach has become percutaneously inserted central venous catheters in even the smallest of micropremies. Both operatively implanted and percutaneously inserted long-term catheters are made of Silastic, impregnated with barium so as to become radiopaque.

7. What are the complications of these intravenous lines?
The two most common complications of long-term intravenous catheters are infection and mechanical failure. Catheter infection is almost universal for a hospitalized infant with an indwelling catheter and a serious illness. The most common organism for such an infection has

become *Staphylococcus epidermidis*. Despite the relatively inert characteristics of Silastic, the catheter always remains a foreign body. A small clot of fibrin invariably forms on the tip of these catheters and the interstices of the fibrin provide a safe harbor for bacteria and fungi from leukocytes. Thus colonization is extremely frequent and, given a sufficient generation of microorganisms, infection will frequently result. A course of antibiotics will frequently diminish the colony count to a sufficiently low level so as to ameliorate the outward signs of infection and even produce negative peripheral (and sometimes through-the-catheter) blood cultures, but the nidus of the infection will persist in the fibrin clot. Experimental support for diminution of recurrent infection with urokinase lysis of the fibrin clot has been shown.

Mechanical problems with catheters include catheter blockage as well as catheter breakage or leakage. Blockage is most commonly seen with blood clots at the tip, which may sometimes be reopened with a thrombolytic agent. Other sources of obstruction include mineral precipitants, predominantly from parenteral nutrition solutions, which may be cleared with the use of dilute hydrochloric acid. Any obstruction may lead to catheter disruption if forceful irrigation against that distal obstruction is attempted. Finally, catheters may frequently be either broken or dislodged.

8. Is the use of a special formulation of amino acid proteins necessary in the neonate?

The definition of an essential amino acid is one that cannot be manufactured by the body and therefore one that must be exogenously supplied. Of the twenty identified amino acids there are eight accepted as essential, yet, in addition, the infant is unable to synthesize histidine and therefore it too is considered essential in infancy. Furthermore the *premature* neonate is unable to generate tyrosine and cystine so they, too, are to be considered essential in that age group.

Many if not all of the same arguments used for inclusion or exclusion of glutamine and arginine that are seen in discussions of nutritional support for adults also apply in pediatrics. Probably the use of glutamine is even more important in the neonate due to the rapid growth of the gastrointestinal tract.

A parenteral formula that has an amino acid profile akin to that of breast milk is a logical choice in the neonate, especially the premature neonate. It should be noted however that, while many scientific variables have been shown to be positively influenced by the use of such formulas and while these are the variables one would most like to change in order to influence the outcome of the neonate, significant changes in what is in the modern era viewed as outcomes has not been overwhelmingly demonstrated.

9. How much fat should there be in the diet of an infant or child?

While the trend is widespread to limit the amount of fat to avert both weight gain and disease, there are compelling reasons in the young to ensure that there is an adequate source of fat in the diet. This goes well beyond the simple provision of essential fatty acids and is predicated upon the need for fat in normal neural development. What balance may be struck between this need and that of early seeds of atherogenesis remains to be elucidated. As a guide, the composition of breast milk is probably the best benchmark, and that is 45 grams of fat per liter. Another guideline to follow is to provide 30–55% of daily calories from fat.

10. What differences in minerals are to be taken into account in the infant and child?

Following from the rapid growth of the neonate and infant is the need for "growth minerals" in a significantly higher amount than the adult daily recommended requirement. Foremost among these are calcium and phosphorus, and this is especially so in the premature neonate. The neonate should receive up to 3 mEq/Kg per day of calcium while the child requires up to 20 mEq/day and the adolescent 15 mEq (total dose, *not* per kg). Similarly, for magnesium the neonate requires up to 1.0 mMol/kg per day, the child and adolescent up to 24 mEq/day total.

11. Does prematurity affect these recommendations?

To a considerable degree, prematurity alters nutritional recommendations. Several important distinctions must be made in the approach to enteral nutrition of the premature infant. Foremost is immaturity of the neonatal suck response that may obviate normal oral feeding. Gavage feeding is therefore very common in prematurity. Neonates less than one kilogram in weight will generally begin with oral feedings of from one to six ccs of sterile water. Increases are administered slowly with increments of just one to two ccs with each feeding to a goal of at least 100 cc/kg/24 hours and a caloric goal that will then increase that amount further.

12. Does the premature gut absorb normally?
The maturity of the intestinal tract is a major factor in the overall care of the premature neonate. In addition, the stressed premature neonate remains at risk for necrotizing enterocolitis, and one of the important factors in this still enigmatic insult is nutrient substrate in the lumen of the intestine. Sufficient length may not have been achieved to allow enough absorption for growth and, within whatever length there is, there may be physiologically insufficient mucosa. Constant drip feeding may overcome a significant amount of this disadvantage, but not all, and parenteral nutritional supplementation is often necessary.

13. What anatomic considerations in the infant affect nutritional support?
The single greatest anatomic immaturity that must be considered is the imcompetence or at least immaturity of the lower esophageal sphincter. In addition, neurologically-coordinated suck, swallow, and preventive gag may not be fully operational before 33 weeks post-conceptional age.
Therefore oral feedings must be delayed and even intragastric or gavage feeds may be dangerous if significant gastroesophageal reflux is present. Many will then use a tube placed past the ligament of Treitz for nasojejunal feeding.

14. What are the different formulas used in premature infants, term infants, and children?
The predominant "formula" used in the neonate is breast milk. Although the approximate composition is well known, there may, of course, be situational variations. Breast milk is highly recommended for the first year of life due to its high nutritional value and immunologic characteristics. It has a caloric density of 20 kcal/oz or 0.67 kcal/ml. When fed to a premature infant, who has greater needs, a human milk fortifier must be used. These fortifiers provide the additional calories, protein, vitamins, and minerals necessary for the proper growth and development of the child. In addition, due to the low iron content of breast milk, iron should always be supplemented for both preterm and term infants.
Formula companies go to great lengths to develop products that are as close to breast milk as possible. Common commercial formulas are based on whey and casein as protein. Most formulas also have a caloric density of 20 kcal/oz. Intolerance of such exogenous protein is not uncommon or, at least, is commonly diagnosed. Soy formulas are thus quite common at the same caloric density. When soy intolerance is expected, casein hydrolysate formulas are also available. A recent development provides formulas enriched with the components DHA and ARA (docosahexaenoic acid and arachidonic acid respectively), natural in breast milk. Research suggests they support mental and visual development. These are also available as standard, soy, and premature formulations.
Premature and transition formulas are also available. Preterm formulas are appropriate for infants < 1800 gm and provide 24 kcal/oz. Transition formulas are ideal for preterm infants > 1800 grams throughout the first year of life. These contain 22 kcal/oz. Higher caloric concentrations can be achieved as needed up to 30 kcal/oz by the addition of a carbohydrate source, such as Polycose, and/or a fat source, such as MCT oil.

15. How does one assess efficacy of nutritional support in children?
The essential elements of nutritional assessment in pediatrics are the same as those in adults. Specifically, the history of the patient's disease with particular attention to the nutritional history should be obtained, combined with physical examination and certain biochemical markers. Emphasis is made on the measurement of height and ratios of weight for height. The well-known percentiles produced from the data collected by the National Center for Health Statistics

are invaluable over time with a chronic illness. In the acute setting, even neonates have been shown to be amenable to measurement of indirect calorimetry when specialized metabolic carts are employed. Measures must be taken to obviate the effect of ventilatory leak around the uncuffed endotracheal tubes that are always used in infants and small children.

16. What are the most common indications for specialized nutritional support in children?
The overwhelming indication for specialized nutritional support and especially the provision of parenteral nutrition across the pediatric age spectrum is prematurity. Many pediatric nutrition support teams will find from 50–75% of their patients present with this primary indication. Other indications that are particular to a pediatric population include short bowel syndrome with its accompanying deleterious effects on growth, pediatric inflammatory bowel disease, and pediatric oncology (with a decreasing distribution of leukemia, lymphoma, neurologic malignancy, and intra-abdominal solid tumors). Pediatric trauma is a polysystem process, with head trauma the most important component. Specialized enteral nutritional support should be undertaken as quickly as possible in these patients.

17. Is short bowel syndrome approached differently in the pediatric population?
The first successful report of total parenteral nutrition in the modern era by Dudrick, Wilmore, and colleagues was that of a surgical neonate treated at the Children's Hospital of Philadelphia. Short bowel syndrome presents several challenges in children beyond the already formidable ones seen in adults. Primary among these is the additional consideration of growth failure. In the neonate and infant, however, there is a phenomenon not seen in the older patient of actual compensatory lengthening of the gastrointestinal tract rather than just villous hypertrophy. Dramatic examples have been reported of near normal length of the GI tract at one year of life with less than ten centimeters of small bowel as a neonate. Even allowing for the confounding factors that one would see of inflammatory shortening of the residual bowel at the initial operation, these reports clearly demonstrate dramatic lengthening.

18. Are there any different ethical considerations in withdrawal of nutrition and hydration in the pediatric population?
Third-party consent always draws more attention than consent by the affected individual, and rightly so. Until the pediatric patient attains the age of legally recognized majority, there is a statutory requirement that mandates someone to speak for that child. In such a circumstance, motivation ideally will be pure but in reality must be thoroughly examined. Confounding such a problem is the recognized widely held emotional belief that the dying child is somehow "cheated" in comparison with the adult who has led a "full life." Finally, the adolescent as an emerging adult presents significant issues when the individual cannot legally be involved in the consent process, or may present explicit objection to the parent's decision. As much as possible, that adolescent should be drawn into a process of assent even when legal consent is not an issue.

BIBLIOGRAPHY

1. Baer MT, Harris AB: Pediatric nutrition assessment: identifying children at risk. J Am Diet Assoc 97(10 Suppl 2):S107–S115, 1997.
2. Canete A, Duggan C: Nutritional support of the pediatric intensive care unit patient. Curr Opin Pediatr 8(3):248–255, 1996.
3. Chathas MK, Paton JB: Sepsis outcomes in infants and children with central venous catheters: percutaneous versus surgical insertion. J Obstet Gynecol Neonatal Nurs 25(6):500–506, 1996.
4. Ford EG: Nutrition support of pediatric patients. Nutr Clin Pract 11(5):183–191, 1996.
5. Goldsmith B: Nutritional assessment in pediatric patients: how can the laboratory help? Pediatr Pathol Lab Med 16(1):1–7, 1996.
6. Heird WC: Amino acid and energy needs of pediatric patients receiving parenteral nutrition. Pediatr Clin North Am 42(4):765–789, 1995.
7. Miller TL: Malnutrition: metabolic changes in children, comparisons with adults. J Nutr 126(10 Suppl): 2623S–2631S, 1996.

 8. Pirenne J: Short-bowel syndrome. Medical aspects and prospects of intestinal transplantation. Acta Chir Belg 96(4):150–154, 1996.
 9. Schears GJ, Deutschman CS: Common nutritional issues in pediatric and adult critical care medicine. Crit Care Clin 13:669–690, 1997.
10. Trahms CM: Nutrition in infancy. In Mahan LK, Escott-Stump S (eds): Krause's Food, Nutrition, and Diet Therapy, 10th ed. Philadelphia, W.B. Saunders, 2000, pp 204–207.
11. Zemel BS, Stallings VA, Riley EM: Evaluation of methodology for nutritional assessment in children: anthropometry, body composition, and energy expenditure. Annu Rev Nutr 17:211–235, 1997.

Website
www.meadjohnson.com

11. ADOLESCENT NUTRITION

Charles W. Van Way III, MD, and Carol Ireton-Jones, PhD, RD, LD, CNSD, FACN

1. How much does the adolescent grow from 12 to 18 years of age?

Typically, there is a 5 to 7 year period of rapid growth, during which the adolescent will gain about half of their final adult weight. During the peak two years of the growth spurt, growth is as rapid as in early childhood. This peak occurs at around 12 in girls and around 15 in boys. It is associated with the onset of sexual maturity. After this is reached, growth tapers off until the late teens in girls and the early twenties in boys.

2. How much should adolescents be fed?

Energy needs in girls reach a level of 2200 kcal/day at age 11 to 12 and stay at that level through adolescence. Boys, with their later growth peak, start out at 2500 kcal/day and go up to 3000 kcal/day during the period of maximum growth, dropping back to adult levels during the late teens and early twenties. Protein needs are increased, with girls requiring 44–46 gm/day, and boys rising from 45 gm/day early in adolescence to 59 gm/day from 15 to 18. Protein remains around 15% of the total energy needs.

Anyone who has raised an adolescent will testify to the large amounts of food which they consume. This can be deceptive. The above requirements are large by comparison to their intake during late childhood but are not so large as to justify excessive intake. In fact, a major problem in adolescence is the avoidance of excessive weight gain. Food habits and physical activity participation developed during adolescence continue into adulthood. Adolescents should be encouraged to participate in physical activities at school and after. Healthy food habits should be based on eating a variety of foods in moderation. Portion size, food labels, and healthy snacks should be discussed rather than focusing on food restriction to encourage a healthy body weight. Resources are available at www.eatright.com, the website of the American Dietetic Association.

3. What minerals are important to bone growth in adolescence?

Some 45% of the overall skeletal growth occurs during adolescence. Calcium requirement in adolescents is therefore elevated to 1200 mg/day, with boys requiring somewhat more than girls. Zinc and magnesium are also required, both of which are incorporated into the growing skeleton.

Girls, under the influence of estrogen, show an increase in bone density as well as bone size during adolescence. This increase is 11% in white girls, and 34% in black girls. It has been suggested that the lowered incidence of osteoporosis in adult black women may be due to this greater increase in bone density during adolescence.

4. Is iron required in both boys and girls?

Yes, but the requirements in girls as they go through menarche are somewhat greater. While boys have a peak of iron utilization during their growth spurt, they drop to the adult male levels in late adolescence. Girls, on the other hand, require adult female levels of iron from age 12 onward (see Chapter 5, Trace Elements).

5. Which vitamins are likely to be needed in supplemental amounts?

A number of the B complex vitamins, specifically thiamin, riboflavin, and niacin, are required in large amounts to meet high energy requirements and to support muscle synthesis. Vitamin D is crucial to support the rapid skeletal growth. Deficiency of vitamin D is harmful anytime during childhood but requirements are at or above adult levels during adolescence. Vitamins A, C, E, B_6, and folate, are required in adult amounts (see Chapter 4, Vitamins).

None of these should require supplementation in individuals consuming a healthy and balanced diet. Since most parents have little control over the dietary practices of their adolescents, however, it is probably wise to give a multivitamin capsule with iron daily.

6. What vitamins and minerals are most often deficient in the adolescent diet?

Deficiencies can be seen in adolescents for a variety of reasons. Calcium and zinc may be inadequate. Magnesium, copper, and manganese may be low in females. Intake of vitamin A, B_6, C, folate, and riboflavin are often decreased below the RDA. There is a relatively higher incidence in adolescent girls of macrocytic anemia from folic acid deficiency.

7. What is the adverse effect of pursuit of thinness in boys and girls?

This has been of some interest to a number of investigators. In one survey, about 75% of girls were actively trying to either control or lose weight and about 10% exhibited behavior consistent with eating disorders, from occasional bulimia to clinical anorexia. Among boys, about 40% were trying to manage their weight, with 15% trying to lose weight and 25% trying to gain weight. A number of nutritional ills have been attributed to this search for thinness among adolescent girls. These include vitamin and mineral deficiencies, inadequate caloric intake, insufficient protein intake, and exercise-induced amenorrhea.

8. What is the adverse effect of alcohol?

Alcohol consumption among adolescents has always been a problem. From the nutritional standpoint, alcohol represents carbohydrate calories which are not accompanied by an adequate amount of vitamins and minerals. Chronic alcohol use often inhibits the absorption of other nutrients. In particular, folic acid deficiency is often found in association with chronic alcohol use.

9. Honestly, now—just how bad are the eating habits of teenagers?

Teenagers have eating habits that are similar to adults, unfortunately. They like to eat too many high-fat, high-calorie meals at fast food restaurants. While many adolescents continue to participate in athletics and exercise regularly, it is during the teenage years that the athletically inclined are separated out from the rest, and many of the rest simply stop exercising.

Adolescents generally get enough protein and calories but they are often deficient in vitamins and minerals. Girls, because they often try to maintain thinness, seem to do somewhat less well than boys. Boys simply eat more and usually get enough nutrients as a result. The popular perception of adolescents as terrible eaters is probably an example of projection—in truth, most adolescents mirror the eating behaviors of their parents and other adults around them.

10. How prevalent are overweight and obesity in adolescents?

Over the last 10 years, the percentage of overweight children ages 6–17 has increased from 5 to 11 percent. This has occurred due to a decrease in physical activity more so than an increase in intake of calories. However, there are many reasons for the increased body weight including family history, inactivity, and poor food habits. A registered dietitian working with the physician and family can provide a beneficial approach to adolescent weight management. Resources for dietitians can be found by calling the local hospital or at www.eatright.com—find a nutrition professional in your area.

BIBLIOGRAPHY

1. Casper RC, Offer D: Weight and dieting concerns in adolescents: Fashion or symptom? Pediatrics 86:384, 1990.
2. Gilsanz V, et al: Changes in vertebral bone density in black girls and white girls during childhood and puberty. N Engl J Med 325:1597, 1991.
3. Heimburger DC, Weinsier RL: Handbook of Clinical Nutrition. 3rd ed. St. Louis, Mosby, 1997.
4. Mahan LK, Escott-Stump S, (eds): Krause's Food, Nutrition, and Diet Therapy. 9th ed. Philadelphia, W.B. Saunders, 1996.
5. Mahan LK, Rees JM: Adolescent Nutrition. St. Louis, Times/Mirror Mosby, 1984.
6. Tsui JC, Nordstrom JW: Folate status of adolescents: Effects of folic acid supplementation. J Am Diet Assoc 90:1551, 1990.
7. Williams SR: Nutrition and Diet Therapy, 7th ed. St. Louis, Mosby, 1993.

12. OLDER PERSONS

Marie-Andrée Roy, MSc, Joanne Z. Rogers, RN, MSN, CNSN,
and Gordon L. Jensen, MD, PhD

1. What are the greatest nutritional problems in the older population?
Paradoxically, both malnutrition and obesity. Studies suggest that one third or more of hospitalized older adults meet criteria for protein-calorie malnutrition. The same is true for those in nursing homes and other long-term care facilities. Estimates for malnutrition in community-dwelling persons are less than 10%. The prevalence of obesity is alarming with more than 68% overweight (BMI ≥ 25) and 31% obese (BMI ≥ 30) older Americans by the NHANES 1999–2000 survey. Although the prevalence of obesity has increased in all age groups since the NHANES III survey, the most dramatic change (more than 12%) was observed for people between 60 and 69 years of age. Either malnutrition or obesity may adversely affect quality of life and independent functioning for older persons. Health may also be affected by specific nutrient deficiencies.

2. What nutrients are of particular importance?
The water-soluble vitamins of particular interest for older adults include C, B_6, B_{12} and folate. Although there is no evidence to suggest vitamin C absorption or utilization is impaired in older persons, this vitamin may be effective in protecting against stress-related and degenerative diseases. Inadequate intake is the principal cause of vitamin C deficiency, though high doses of salicylates may also cause depletion. Supplementation with large doses of vitamin C may have serious side effects and is not recommended.

Vitamin B_6 deficiencies have been observed in those taking antagonistic medications or abusing alcohol. This vitamin has a significant role in immune function, so replacement therapy is warranted.

Vitamin B_{12} deficiency is a concern in older persons because it may be associated with megaloblastic anemia, impaired cognitive function, dementia, neuropsychiatric disorders or nonspecific complaints of lethargy and malaise. Older persons often eliminate red and organ meats from their diet, fearing the fat and cholesterol content, but these foods are a major dietary source of B_{12}. Physiologic changes may decrease the absorption or bioavailability of B_{12}, and deficiency may be observed in those with pernicious anemia, achlorhydria, gastric resection, or ileal surgery or disease.

Folate deficiency is common among older adults and megaloblastic anemia may result. Typical causes include inadequate intake, alcoholism, medications, or malabsorption syndromes.

Elevated homocysteine concentrations have been found to be associated with low levels of folate, vitamin B_6 or vitamin B_{12}. Hyperhomocysteinemia may be related to increased risk of coronary and vascular diseases, stroke, and dementia, so there may be opportunity to decrease disease burden by supplementation of these vitamins.

Vitamin D is the most common fat-soluble vitamin deficiency for older persons. Home-bound or institutionalized persons are particularly at risk. Low dietary intake, especially of milk products, and decreased sun exposure contribute to low levels. The roles of vitamin D in maintaining bone health and facilitating calcium absorption make it a very important dietary component.

Iron deficiency in older persons is usually due to inadequate iron intake and blood loss associated with hemorrhage and chronic disease. The absorption of nonheme iron is reduced secondary to the hypochlorhydria of atrophic gastritis. Vitamin C deficiency may also impair iron absorption.

3. What methods are available to screen older persons for nutritional risk?
Nutrition screening of the older person is an important part of each individual's overall care. Recognition of malnutrition by physicians is notoriously poor, especially in the older population.

It is important to identify and treat nutritional disorders, thereby preventing or ameliorating many chronic diseases or disabilities.

There has been limited investigation in nutritional screening of community-dwelling population of older adults. A variety of screening tools were developed by consensus and widely disseminated. Many have not been well studied and validated. The Nutrition Screening Initiative (NSI) was begun in 1990 as a national effort to improve identification and treatment of nutritional concerns of older persons. The DETERMINE Your Nutritional Health Checklist is a 10-item, single-page, self-reported checklist addressing risk factors such as weight change, dietary habits, chronic diseases, dentition, polypharmacy, living environment, resources, and functional status. Although initially developed as a self-screening and awareness tool, the Checklist is now being used in a variety of settings for which it was never intended.

The NSI has also produced higher level screens intended for further evaluation of older persons at risk for poor nutritional status. The Level I screen was designed for use by allied health professionals and includes a recorded height, weight and detailed questions regarding weight change, dietary habits, living environment, and functional status. The Level II screen, developed for clinical settings, collects additional diagnostic information including anthropometrics, laboratory data (serum albumin and cholesterol), medication use, relevant clinical features, and mental/cognitive status.

The Mini Nutritional Assessment (MNA) is an 18-item nutrition screening and assessment tool designed for older people. It includes body mass index, anthropometric indices, weight loss, living environment, medication use, dietary habits, and self-assessment of health and nutrition. Cross-validation studies completed on the MNA have shown that scores were significantly correlated with dietary, anthropometric and biological nutritional parameters. A shorter version of the original MNA, called MNA Short-Form, has recently been released. The MNA Short-Form is a quick 6-item questionnaire used as a screening instrument and prompt for more extensive nutritional assessment.

4. What are valid indicators of nutritional risk status in older persons?

Nutrition screening items that have been associated with functional compromise and health care resource use include weight loss or underweight status, eating difficulties (poor dentition or difficulty swallowing), polypharmacy, low albumin, and older age.

5. What physiologic changes associated with aging affect nutritional status?

As part of the normal aging process, many changes occur in the human body that may negatively influence the intake, absorption, or utilization of nutrients. Consideration of these factors may result in more positive treatment outcomes.

Taste, smell, and thirst play crucial roles impacting the oral intake of older persons. Decreases in taste buds and papilla on the tongue, decrease in taste and olfactory nerve endings, and changes in taste and smell thresholds will lessen interest in food and affect its palatability in the older person. Oral health is a key factor in the ability to ingest nutrients. Poor-fitting dentures, an edentulous state, gingival lesions or mucous membrane erosions will hamper intake. The risk of mortality has been found to correlate with the number of oral health problems. Thirst responses tend to be impaired with increasing age. This may lead to inadequate intakes of water and subsequent dehydration.

Gastric emptying and other gastrointestinal functions have been found to decline with aging. Atrophic gastritis is frequently reported among older persons and is associated with decreased secretion of hydrochloric acid and intrinsic factor, which impairs the bioavailability of vitamin B_{12}, calcium, iron, folic acid, and possibly zinc.

Although the liver tends to decrease in mass and blood flow with aging, its functions appear to be relatively well preserved. Recent research suggests that there is no age-related change in albumin synthesis and concentration in healthy subjects. Low albumin concentrations observed among older people should be attributed to other precipitating factors, such as underlying inflammatory conditions or disease.

Age-related changes in the skin can lead to decreased efficiency of vitamin D synthesis. If this is combined with decreased sun exposure and inadequate intake, deficiency is likely.

Some older persons may experience a decline in physical functioning or cognition. These factors may affect their ability to plan balanced meals, shop for groceries, or prepare or consume meals.

6. Is a change in lean body mass a normal part of the aging process?

Advancing age is associated with well-documented changes in body composition, including reduction in lean body mass (sarcopenia) and increase in body fat.

It remains unclear whether sarcopenia is a normal part of the aging process or the result of possible causal elements, such as suboptimal protein intake or sedentary lifestyle. Suggested age-related factors include altered cytokine regulation, decrease in endogenous growth hormone production, decreased androgen and estrogen secretion, and loss of alpha motor neurons from the spinal column. Administration of trophic factors (growth hormone and testosterone) and resistance strength training have been successful in increasing skeletal muscle mass. Supplementation of protein or other nutrients is of uncertain benefit and warrants further evaluation.

Preconceived societal expectations regarding reduced activity levels in older persons promote a sedentary life-style. Inactivity may lead to an increase in intraabdominal (visceral fat) obesity, a risk factor for insulin resistance, hypertension, dyslipidemia and coronary artery disease. These diseases, and associated functional impairments, may lead to further muscle disuse. A decline in muscle strength has been found to contribute to falls and frailty among older persons.

7. Are there Recommended Daily Allowances (RDAs) of nutrients for older persons?

The Food and Nutrition Board of the Institute of Medicine has recently released the Dietary Reference Intakes (DRIs), a set of updated and new reference values including Recommended Dietary Allowance (RDA), Adequate Intake (AI), Tolerable Upper Intake Level (UL), and Estimated Average Requirement (EAR). Dietary Reference Intakes are presented for 16 life stage groups including stages for ages 51 through 70 and over 70 years. This is a more appropriate set of reference values for older persons than the former 1989 RDA, which did not include breakdowns after age 51 and were based on extrapolations of requirements for healthy young adults. Among DRI categories, the RDA should be used as a goal for an individual's daily intakes. Adequate Intakes (AI) are used when there is no associated RDA value for a specific nutrient. Table 1 summarizes RDAs and AIs for people over 50 years.

Table 1.   Dietary Reference Intakes (DRIs) for Micronutrients for Older Persons

NUTRIENT	MALE 51–70 YR	MALE > 70 YR	FEMALE 51–70 YR	FEMALE > 70 YR
Calcium (mg)	1200*	1200*	1200*	1200*
Phosphorus (mg)	700	700	700	700
Magnesium (mg)	420	420	320	320
Vitamin D (µg)	10*	15*	10*	15*
Fluoride (mg)	4*	4*	3*	3*
Thiamin (mg)	1.2	1.2	1.1	1.1
Riboflavin (mg)	1.3	1.3	1.1	1.1
Niacin (mg)	16	16	14	14
Vitamin B_6 (mg)	1.7	1.7	1.5	1.5
Folate (µg)	400	400	400	400

(Table continued on next page.)

Table 1.   Dietary Reference Intakes (DRIs) for Micronutrients for Older Persons (Continued)

NUTRIENT	MALE 51–70 YR	MALE > 70 YR	FEMALE 51–70 YR	FEMALE > 70 YR
Vitamin B$_{12}$ (µg)	2.4	2.4	2.4	2.4
Pantothenic acid (mg)	5*	5*	5*	5*
Biotin (µg)	30*	30*	30*	30*
Choline (mg)	550*	550*	425*	425*
Vitamin C (mg)	90	90	75	75
α-Tocopherol (mg)	15	15	15	15
Selenium (µg)	55	55	55	55

Recommended Dietary Allowances (RDA) are presented in ordinary type and Adequate Intakes (AI) are followed by an asterisk (*).
Adapted from Dietary Reference Intakes for Calcium, Phosphorus, Magnesium, Vitamin D, and Fluoride. National Academy Press, Washington, DC, 1997. Dietary Reference Intakes for Thiamin, Riboflavin, Niacin, Vitamin B$_6$, Folate, Vitamin B$_{12}$, Pantothenic Acid, Biotin, and Choline. National Academy Press, Washington, DC, 1999. Dietary Reference Intakes for Vitamin C, Vitamin E, Selenium, and Carotenoids, National Academy Press, Washington, DC, 2000.

8. What are the macronutrient requirements for older persons?

Energy requirements in older persons have been found to decrease by 70 (women) to 100 (men) kilocalories per decade. This decline results from decreased lean body mass as well as decreased physical activity. In the DRIs, the daily energy requirement goal set for individuals is called Estimated Energy Requirement (EER), a new term that is equivalent to EAR. The EER is defined as "the dietary energy intake that is predicted to maintain energy balance in healthy, normal weight individuals of a defined age, gender, weight, height and level of physical activity consistent with good health." As a result, EER should be determined individually according to levels of activity and no RDA is given for a specific age group. For example, a sedentary woman of 70 years old measuring 5'3" with a weight of 141 pounds would have an EER of 1627 kcal, whereas the requirement would be 2103 kcal for an active woman of the same age and size.

Equations for Estimated Energy Requirements (EER)

Male: EER = 662 – 9.53 × Age [y] + PA × (15.91 × Weight [kg] + 539.6 × Height [m])
Female: EER = 354 – 6.91 × Age [y] + PA x (9.36 × Weight [kg] + 726 × Height [m])
Where PA is the physical activity coefficient:
PA = 1.00   Sedentary
PA = 1.11   Low active
PA = 1.25   Active
PA = 1.48   Very active

The current RDA for protein for elderly is 0.8 gm/kg/day, which is the same as for younger adults. Protein requirements may be higher in case of injuries, stress, inflammation or infection. DRIs for protein, carbohydrate, total fiber, and fatty acids are summarized in Table 2. To reduce the occurrence of chronic disease and provide adequate intakes of essential nutrients, Acceptable Macronutrient Distribution Ranges (AMDR) have been proposed and are presented in Table 3. There are no specific AMDRs for older adults and they are the same as for younger adults.

Table 2.   Dietary Reference Intakes for Macronutrients in Older Persons

NUTRIENT	MEN 51–70 YR	MEN > 70 YR	WOMEN 51–70 YR	WOMEN > 70 YR
Energy (kcal/d)[†]	Individually	Individually	Individually	Individually
Carbohydrates (g/d)	130	130	130	130
Fiber (g/d)	30*	30*	21*	21*

(Table continued on next page.)

Table 2.   Dietary Reference Intakes for Macronutrients in Older Persons (Continued)

NUTRIENT	MEN		WOMEN	
	51–70 YR	> 70 YR	51–70 YR	> 70 YR
Protein (g/d)[‡]	56	56	46	46
Fat	ND[//]	ND[//]	ND[//]	ND[//]
n-6 PUFA (g/d)	14[*]	14[*]	11[*]	11[*]
n-3 PUFA (g/d)	1.6[*]	1.6[*]	1.1[*]	1.1[*]
Saturated fat, trans fatty acids and cholesterol	As low as possible for all age groups			

Recommended Dietary Allowances (RDA) are presented in ordinary type and Adequate Intakes (AI) are followed by an asterisk (*).
[†] Estimated Energy Requirement (EER)
[‡] Based on 0.8 gm protein/kg body weight for reference body weight.
[//] ND = not determinable since insufficient data to determine a defined level of fat intake at which risk of inadequacy or prevention of chronic disease occurs.
Adapted from Institute of Medicine, Food and Nutrition Board: Dietary Reference Intakes for Energy, Carbohydrate, Fiber, Fat, Fatty Acids, Cholesterol, Protein, and Amino Acids (Macronutrients). Washington, DC, National Academy Press, 2002. This report can be accessed at www.nap.edu.

Table 3.   Acceptable Macronutrient Distribution Ranges (AMDR) for Adults

MACRONUTRIENT	PERCENT OF ENERGY
Fat	20–35
n-6 polyunsaturated fatty acids* (linoleic acid)	5–10
n-3 polyunsaturated fatty acids* (α-linoleic acid)	0.6–1.2
Carbohydrate	45–65
Protein	10–35

* Approximately 10% of the total can come from longer-chain n-3 or n-6 fatty acids.
Adapted from Institute of Medicine, Food and Nutrition Board. Dietary Reference Intakes for Energy, Carbohydrate, Fiber, Fat, Fatty Acids, Cholesterol, Protein, and Amino Acids (Macronutrients). Washington, DC, National Academy Press, 2002. This report can be accessed at www.nap.edu.

9. Will nutrition supplements decrease the risk of hip fractures in older adults?
   Hip fracture is a devastating injury, causing crippling and even death in older persons. The contribution of calcium and vitamin D to bone health has been the focus of considerable research. Several studies have shown that intakes of these nutrients fall below the DRI in both community and institutional settings. A combined supplement of calcium and vitamin D may help to prevent hip and nonvertebral fractures. To raise their intakes to the recommended amount (1200 mg), older persons should be encouraged not only to increase their consumption of dietary calcium and vitamin D (see Table 1) but also to consider daily supplementation. The use of estrogen replacement and other pharmacologic therapies (e.g., biphosphonates) has gained increasing attention in the prevention and treatment of osteoporosis and hip fractures. Physical activity is also important in reducing the risk of hip fractures through improvement in muscle strength, balance and mechanical load on bone.

10. Should older persons take vitamin and mineral supplements?
   It has been estimated that between 50% and 75% of older Americans, particularly women, take some form of vitamin or mineral supplement on a regular basis. While this can be overdone, supplementation in modest doses does no harm and probably does some good. A daily standard multivitamin with minerals is definitely recommended for those who have inadequate intake, disturbed absorption, or increased tissue requirements. Supplementation for nursing home residents may also be considered. Megavitamin consumption should be avoided because of associated toxicity.

11. What is the meaning of a low cholesterol in an older person?

Hypocholesterolemia (< 160 mg/dl) is a nonspecific indicator of poor health status. Chronic diseases, malignancies, undernutrition, respiratory diseases, increased complications and mortality have all been associated with low cholesterol levels. This condition appears to be independent from dietary intakes in many clinical settings and should rather be attributed to ongoing cytokine-mediated inflammatory response, particularly interleukin-6 (IL-6).

12. How does polypharmacy affect nutritional status?

Older persons often have multiple medical conditions and may be taking several prescription and over-the-counter medications concurrently. Medications may affect food intake and alter nutrient metabolism and excretion. A complete review of medications, including supplements, herbal and other natural products, is required to clarify possible drug-nutrient interactions.

Common Drugs and Drug Classes
That May Cause Nutritional Depletion and Deficiency

DRUG CLASS	DRUG	DEFICIENCY
Antacids	Sodium bicarbonate, aluminum hydroxide	Folate, phosphate, calcium, copper
Anticonvulsants	Phenytoin, phenobarbital, primidone Valproic acid	Vitamins D and K Carnitine
Antibiotics	Tetracycline Gentamicin Neomycin	Calcium Potassium, magnesium Fat, nitrogen
Antibacterial agents	Boric acid Trimethoprim Isoniazid	Riboflavin Folate Vitamin B_6, niacin, Vitamin D
Antimalarials	Pyrimethamine	Folate
Anti-inflammatory agents	Sulfasalazine Colchicine	Folate Fat, Vitamin B_{12}
Anticancer drugs	Methotrexate Cisplatin	Folate, calcium Magnesium
Anticoagulants	Warfarin	Vitamin K
Antihypertensive agents	Hydralazine	Vitamin B_6
Diuretics	Thiazides Furosemide Triamterene	Potassium, magnesium Potassium, calcium, magnesium Folate
H_2-receptor antagonists	Cimetidine Ranitidine	Vitamin B_{12}
Cholesterol-lowering agents	Cholestyramine Colestipol	Fat Vitamin K, vitamin A, folate, vitamin B_{12}
Laxatives	Mineral oil	Carotene, retinol, vitamins D and K
	Phenolphthalein Senna	Potassium, fat, calcium
Oral contraceptives	Estrogens, progestogens	Vitamin B_6, folate, vitamin C
Tranquilizers	Chlorpromazine	Riboflavin

Reprinted with permission from Rosenberg I: Nutrition and aging. In Hazzard W, et al (eds): Principles of Geriatric Medicine. New York, McGraw-Hill, 1994.

13. What role does nutrition play in immune function in older persons?

Protein malnutrition and deficiencies of vitamin B_6, zinc, or antioxidants can impair immune function. Older persons exhibit increased susceptibility to infection and to certain cancers, which may be related to the age-related decline in the function of the immune system. Studies among institutionalized and community dwelling older persons suggest that micronutrient supplementation, most notably of vitamin B_6, zinc and low doses of vitamin E can improve immune response.

14. Can nutrition influence vision in older persons?

Visual impairment is common among older persons. There is an increasing body of evidence from epidemiological studies about the protective effect of long-term use of vitamin supplementation, particularly antioxidants, on the development of cataracts. However, clinical studies of antioxidant supplementation, such as vitamin C, E and β-carotene have yielded inconsistent results, and it is not yet possible to associate a specific nutrient with protection, if any, against cataracts. For this reason, recommendations for taking high doses of antioxidants as a protection against cataracts are not certain at this time.

Among people over 65 years, age-related macular degeneration (ARMD) is the leading cause for visual impairment and blindness in the United States. Recent evidence suggests that the risk of progression for certain categories of ARMD can be reduced with supplementation of antioxidants (vitamins C and E and β-carotene) and zinc.

15. Describe "failure to thrive" in a geriatric population.

Failure to thrive is an age-related syndrome that is among the most prevalent of all late-life diseases. The National Institute on Aging describes failure to thrive as "a syndrome of weight loss, decreased appetite and poor nutrition, and inactivity, often accompanied by dehydration, depressive symptoms, impaired immune function, and low cholesterol." It has also been linked to deterioration in other social and environmental conditions. Causes for this syndrome are believed to be related to underlying physical and/or cognitive conditions and a decline in social functioning. Although it has received increasing attention in the past decade, categorization of failure to thrive into a well-defined syndrome has not yet been possible. Some have suggested replacing this construct by a set of four potentially treatable contributing domains: (1) impaired physical functioning, (2) undernutrition, (3) depression, and (4) cognitive impairment.

16. How helpful are supplements in meeting the nutritional requirements of older persons?

Supplements are widely advertised and often used, but they are not always helpful. Those that are nutritionally sound may actually promote intake of additional calories and nutrients. But when using supplements, some people will decrease the intake of other foods, resulting in little or modest increase in calories ingested. Cost and palatability may preclude consistent use. If the objective of supplementation is to increase lean body mass, then the intervention should also include prescribed exercise.

17. What programs are available to help meet the nutritional needs of community-dwelling older persons?

A variety of community resources are available to the older person with nutritional concerns. Referring the person to the Area Agency on Aging (AAA) will allow access to programs such as Meals on Wheels, the Salvation Army, food kitchens, and food banks. The location of the AAA nearest the person can be found through the Eldercare Locator website at www.eldercare.gov or by calling 1-800-677-1116.

Depending on income, the person may be eligible for food stamps, but many older persons are reluctant to accept this assistance. A growing number of senior centers and adult daycares are available in communities and provide balanced meals to those who attend.

Nutritional supplements may be made available to older persons free of charge or at reduced cost. If the person has cancer, the American Cancer Society may provide free nutritional supplements.

Veterans may also be eligible for assistance through the VA healthcare system. Manufacturers of supplements often provide toll-free numbers to call for ordering of their product with home delivery. Encouraging the utilization of these resources may enhance nutritional intake for those with reduced access to good nutrition.

BIBLIOGRAPHY

1. Age-Related Eye Disease Study Research Group (AREDS): A randomized, placebo-controlled, clinical trial of high-dose supplementation with vitamins C and E and beta carotene for age-related cataract and vision loss: AREDS Report no. 9. Arch Ophthalmol 119:1439–1452, 2001.
2. Age-Related Eye Disease Study Research Group (AREDS): A randomized, placebo-controlled, clinical trial of high-dose supplementation with vitamins C and E, beta carotene, and zinc for age-related macular degeneration and vision loss: AREDS Report no. 8. Arch Ophthalmol 119:1417–1436, 2001.
3. Beattie BL, Louie V, Dwyer J: Nutrition and health in the elderly. In Reichel W (ed): Care of the Elderly: Clinical Aspects of Aging. Baltimore, Williams and Wilkins, 1995.
4. Bergland A, Kirkevold M: Thriving—a useful theoretical perspective to capture the experience of well-being among frail elderly in nursing homes? J Adv Nurs 36:426–432, 2001.
5. Burns J, Jensen G: Malnutrition among geriatric patients admitted to medical and surgical services in a tertiary care hospital: Frequency, recognition and associated disposition and reimbursement outcomes. Nutrition 11:245–249, 1995.
6. Chandra RK: Influence of multinutrient supplementation on immune responses and infection-related illness in 50–65y old individuals. Nutr Res 22:5–10, 2002.
7. Chandra RK: Nutrition and the immune system from birth to old age. Eur J Clin Nutr 56 (Suppl 3):S73–S76, 2002.
8. Chernoff R: Effects of age in nutrient requirements. Clin Geriatr Med 11:641–651, 1995.
9. Chapuy MC, Pamphile R, Paris E, et al: Combined calcium and vitamin D3 supplementation in elderly women: Confirmation of reversal of secondary hyperparathyroidism and hip fracture risk: The Decalyos II Study. Osteoporos Int 13:257–264, 2002.
10. Evans W, Cyr-Campbell D: Nutrition, exercise and healthy aging. J Am Diet Assoc 97(6):632–638, 1997.
11. Feskanich D, Willett W, Colditz G: Walking and leisure-time activity and risk of hip fracture in postmenopausal women. JAMA 288:2300–2306, 2002.
12. Fiatarone MA, O'Neill EF, Ryan ND, et al: Exercise training and nutritional supplementation for physical frailty in very elderly people. N Engl J Med 330:1769–1775, 1994.
13. Flegal KM, Carroll MD, Ogden CL, Johnson CL: Prevalence and trends in obesity among US adults, 1999–2000. JAMA 288:1727–1761, 2002.
14. Fu A, Sreekumaran Nair K: Age effect on fibrinogen and albumin synthesis in humans. Am J Physiol 275 (Endocrinol Metab 38):E1023–E1030, 1998.
15. Gloth FM, Gundberg CM, Hollis BW, et al: Vitamin D deficiency in homebound elderly persons. JAMA 274(21):1683–1686, 1995.
16. Goichot B, Schienger JL, Grunenberger F, et al: Low cholesterol concentrations in free-living elderly subjects: Relations with dietary intake and nutritional status. Am J Clin Nutr 62:547–553, 1995.
17. Guigoz Y, Vellas B, Gary PJ: Assessing the nutritional status of the elderly: The mini nutritional assessment as part of the geriatric evaluation. Nutr Rev 54(Suppl):S59–S65, 1996.
18. Institute of Medicine, Division of Health Promotion and Disease Prevention: Extending Life, Enhancing Life: A National Research Agenda on Aging. Washington, DC, National Academy Press, 1991.
19. Institute of Medicine, Food and Nutrition Board: Dietary Reference Intakes for Thiamin, Riboflavin, Niacin, Vitamin B6, Folate, Vitamin B12, Panothenic acid, Biotin, and Choline. Washington, DC, National Academy Press, 1998.
20. Institute of Medicine, Food and Nutrition Board: Dietary Reference Intakes for Calcium, Phosphorus, Magnesium, Vitamin D, and Fluoride. Washington, DC, National Academy Press, 1997.
21. Institute of Medicine, Food and Nutrition Board: Dietary Reference Intakes for Vitamin C, Vitamin E, Selenium and Carotenoids. Washington, DC, National Academy Press, 2000.
22. Institute of Medicine, Food and Nutrition Board: Dietary Reference Intakes for Energy, Carbohydrate, Fiber, Fat, Fatty Acids, Cholesterol, Protein, and Amino Acids (Macronutrients). Washington, DC, National Academy Press, 2002.
23. Meydani S, Meydani M, Blumberg JB, et al. Vitamin E supplementation and in vivo immune response in healthy elderly subjects. JAMA 277:1380–1386, 1997.
24. Noel MA, Smith TK, Ettinger WH: Characteristics and outcomes of hospitalized older patients who develop hypocholesterolemia. J Am Geriatr Soc 39:455–461, 1991.
25. The Nutrition Screening Initiative: Incorporating nutrition screening and interventions into medical practice. Washington DC: The Nutrition Screening Initiative, 1994.

26. Rubenstein LZ, Harker JO, Salva A, et al: Screening for undernutrition in geriatric practice: Developing the short-form mini-nutritional assessment (MNA-SF). J Gerontol A Biol Sci Med Sci 56:M366–372, 2001.
27. Reuben D, Greendale G, Harrison G: Nutrition screening in older persons. J Am Geriatr Soc 43:415–425, 1995.
28. Rudman D, Feller AG, Nagraj HS, et al: Effects of human growth hormone in men over 60 years old. N Engl J Med 323:1–6, 1990.
29. Russell R: New views on the RDAs for older adults. J Am Diet Assoc 97:515–518, 1997.
30. Sarkisian CA, Lachs MS: "Failure to thrive" in older adults. Ann Intern Med 124:1072–1078, 1996.
31. Satia-Abouta J, Kristal AR, Patterson RE, et al: Dietary supplement use and medical conditions: The VITAL Study. Am J Prev Med 24:43–51, 2003.
32. Singh N, Clements K, Fiatarone M: A randomized controlled trial of progressive resistance training in depressed elders. J Gerontol Biol Sci Med Sci 52(1):M27–M35, 1997.
33. Snyder PJ, Peachey H, Hannoush P, et al: Effect of testosterone treatment on body composition and muscle strength in men over 65 years of age. J Clin Endocrinol Metab 84:2647–2653, 1999.
34. Vellas B, Guigoz Y, BAumgartner M, et al: Relationships between nutritional markers and the mini-nutritional assessment in 155 older persons. J Am Geriatr Soc 48:1300–1309, 2000.
35. Wood R, Suter P, Russell: Mineral requirements of elderly people. Am J Clin Nutr 62:493–505, 1995.

13. NUTRITION IN PREGNANCY

Alyce F. Newton, MS, RD

GENERAL CONSIDERATIONS

1. What is the role of preconception nutrition evaluation and counseling in pregnancy?
Maternal nutrition plays a role in certain types of fetal malformations or spontaneous abortion. Because these abnormalities occur so early in pregnancy (during organogenesis), modifications must be made before pregnancy begins. In diabetes, incidence of congenital defects can be reduced by bringing the blood glucose under good control prior to pregnancy. As evidenced by the 1991 Medical Research Council Vitamin Study in Great Britain,[1] administration of folic acid before conception and during early gestation reduced the incidence of neural tube defects by 71%. Women of childbearing age with phenylketonuria (PKU) can prevent mental retardation and microcephaly in their infants by following a low-protein, amino acid modified diet before and throughout pregnancy.[2]

In addition, women with low body weight and poor nutritional status prior to pregnancy often have problems such as low birth-weight infants, premature spontaneous rupture of membranes, infection, and anemia. Overweight women are more likely to have fetal death, diabetes, hypertensive disorders, labor abnormalities, and fetal macrosomatia. Overweight women are also at increased risk for cesarean section. Prepregnancy counseling is necessary to prevent these problems. Ideally a woman should achieve a body weight within 90–120% of ideal prior to conception. Physical activity should be encouraged for all women of childbearing age, preferably for at least 30 minutes daily. Health benefits include weight management, improved psychological well-being and physical fitness, and reduced risk of adult-onset diabetes, cardiovascular disease, and other chronic diseases linked with obesity.[3,4]

During prepregnancy counseling, identification of other risk factors which may directly affect the outcome of the pregnancy is possible, such as hypertension, heart disease, autoimmune diseases, smoking, excessive use of alcohol, use of street drugs and use or exposure to toxins.[3] A review of alternative medicines used, including herbal and botanical supplements, should be included; few randomized clinical trials have examined the efficacy and safety of herbal and botanical products during pregnancy.[5]

2. What are the general nutrition guidelines for pregnancy?
The developing fetus is influenced most by diet between 17 and 56 days after conception, but many women do not know that they are pregnant until they are beyond this period. Therefore, the diet should be optimal before pregnancy, emphasizing the importance of preconception counseling for weight loss, smoking cessation, reduced alcohol consumption and elimination of social or street drugs. All women who wish to become pregnant should consume 400 µg per day of synthetic folic acid from fortified foods (cereals and other grains), oral supplements, or both. Folate is found naturally in a variety of foods. Both synthetic and naturally occurring folate should be consumed for at least 1 month prior to conception to prevent neural tube defects such as spina bifida. Once pregnant, 1 mg folic acid is the tolerable upper limit from the combination of food and supplement. Pregnant women aged 14–18 should not consume greater than 800 µg/day from foods and supplements combined. If a woman has a personal or family history of neural tube defect, 4 mg folic acid daily for 1 month prior to pregnancy and during the first three months of pregnancy is recommended. Excessive vitamin A as a supplement or medication (i.e., Retin-A and Accutane) should be discontinued prior to conception due to risk of birth defects.[6,7]

During the second and third trimesters, adults and older adolescents usually require an additional 300 kcal/day and adolescents < 14 years require an additional ~500 kcal/day. However, these recommendations vary, depending on prepregnancy weight, maternal age, rate of weight gain, and individual metabolism. In developed countries, normal and overweight women may require less than the recommended additional 300 kcal/day, particularly those with a sedentary lifestyle. Therefore, appropriate weight gain and appetite often indicate sufficient energy intake. Eating disorders may appear as low weight gain in the second trimester, or persistent Hyperemesis Gravidarum. Low weight gain in the second or third trimesters is associated with a higher risk of intrauterine growth retardation and in the third trimester, preterm delivery.[4]

3. What is appropriate weight gain during pregnancy?
The Institute of Medicine (IOM) has published weight gain recommendations based on the body mass index (BMI = weight/height squared or kg/m^2).[4] Weight gain should begin after 12 weeks.

Weight Goals based on Prepregnancy BMI (kg/m^2)[4,11]

BMI	Normal BMI = 19.8–26 (90–120% of ideal weight)	Underweight BMI = < 19.8 (< 90% ideal)	Overweight BMI = 26–29 (120–130% ideal)	Obese BMI > 29 (> 135% ideal)	Twin Pregnancy	Triplet Pregnancy
Goal	25–35 lb	28–40 lb	15–25 lb	15 lb	24–45 lb	50 lb

4. Describe general food guidelines for pregnancy.
Based on the Dietary Guidelines and the Food Guide Pyramid during Pregnancy,[8] generally 9 servings of bread, cereal, rice, or pasta; 4 servings of vegetables; 2 servings of fruit; 2–3 servings of mild, cheese, calcium-fortified beverage, or yogurt; and 2 servings of meat, fish, poultry, legumes, eggs, and nuts are recommended. The whole grains, leafy green and yellow vegetables, and fruit supply necessary vitamins, minerals, and fiber. Protein, zinc, iron, and magnesium are found in the high-protein foods, including meat and legumes, and calcium can be found in the dairy products, along with protein, vitamin D, other vitamins, and minerals. Vegetarians should be sure to consume adequate protein such as peas, beans, and rice; grains and legumes or grains and seeds in addition to soy protein. Iron, calcium, and vitamin B_{12} intake may be low depending on the types of foods consumed. Vegetarians who consume eggs and dairy products (lacto-ova vegetarians) are less likely to have nutrient deficiencies. Multivitamin-mineral supplements are recommended.[11]

5. Do pregnant adolescents have special nutritional requirements?
An older (> 14 yr) adolescent who consumes a well-balanced diet; does not smoke or use alcohol or street drugs; and has achieved most of her growth prior to pregnancy has nutrient requirements similar to an adult. However, a nutritional assessment is crucial as soon into the pregnancy as possible. In addition to the nutritional status, this assessment identifies other early modifiable risk factors, such as lack of access to health care and social and psychological situations detrimental to pregnancy.[9,10] Pregnant teenagers should be advised early on about what constitutes a good diet, due to their tendency to make poor food choices, eat a lot of fast food, skip meals, and use alcohol, tobacco, and street drugs. A specific program should be clearly outlined, and they should be allowed to gain weight at the upper limits of the recommended ranges, unless they are obese. Vitamin and mineral supplementation including folic acid, iron and calcium should be initiated.[11]

In an effort to provide optimal nutrition to this group of patients, all pregnant adolescents should be encouraged to enroll in the federal Special Supplemental Food Program for Women,

Infants and Children (WIC). The Expanded Food and Nutrition Education Program (EFNEP) and the National School Lunch and Breakfast Programs are especially important for pregnant teenagers. Pregnant teens should be seen regularly by nutrition counselors and specialists who can intervene to help prevent detrimental behaviors, which may influence the outcome of the pregnancy.[11]

6. What are potential nutrition-related effects of tobacco, alcohol and street drugs?[4,11]
   1. Impaired fetal growth and development (e.g., fetal alcohol syndrome).
   2. Decreased maternal food intake, which may be due to decreased appetite (cocaine and amphetamines are appetite suppressants), substitution of the substance for food (alcohol), lack of money to spend for food, or any combination of the above .
   3. Increased nutrient requirements. Tobacco increases metabolism and the need for vitamin C and folate; alcohol impairs the absorption or utilization of several nutrients and may impair the placental transport of certain nutrients.
   4. Drug use may be related to concern about body size and anxiety about gaining too much weight. Eating disorders may also occur.
   5. IV drug use is associated with incidence of HIV/AIDS, which may be transmitted to the fetus during pregnancy and postpartum breastfeeding.[11]

7. What are common questions asked by women about gastrointestinal issues during pregnancy?
   Nausea and vomiting. "Morning sickness" is one of the most common complaints during the first trimester, generally without detrimental effect on mother and fetus. However, hyperemesis gravidarum (HG) occurs in 1.3% of all pregnancies and is a serious problem.[12] The Table below offers suggestions to mildly ill patients. In addition, identification and removal of certain triggering events, such as strong odors, heat, noise, exhaustion, and anxiety-producing events, may help control the vomiting events. Certain FDA Pregnancy Category B antiemetic drugs, such as Antivert, Reglan, Zantac, and Zofran, may be helpful, along with Category C drugs Phenergan and Compazine and Category A drugs, pyridoxine and vitamin B_6.

Managing Nausea and Vomiting Associated with Pregnancy[12]

EATING ACTION	FOOD CHOICES	OTHER ACTIONS
Small frequent meals every 2–3 hr	According to preference[21]: bland, sweet, crunchy, sour, salty	Minimize noxious odors from food, perfume, detergents, and others around you
Avoid sudden movements; stay seated after eating to avoid reflux	Easily digested foods include rice, pasta, noodles, potatoes, cereals, fruit, bread	Use relaxation techniques to manage stress and anxiety
Liquids separate from solids	Clear liquids—jello, tea, ginger ale, broth	Take frequent periods of recumbent rest
Slowly sip a carbonated beverage while nauseated	Low-fat proteins include lean meat and poultry, broiled fish, eggs, beans	Prepare cold foods to avoid cooking odors; microwave and open a window or turn on a fan

Heartburn.[11] The following guidelines are often helpful:
• Consume small, low-fat meals and snacks, and eat slowly.
• Consume low-fat snacks, such as toast, crackers, and fruit, as needed for extra energy and nutrients.
• Drink fluids mainly between meals.
• Decrease or avoid spices, chocolate, peppermint or spearmint, and greasy, fried foods.
• Avoid tobacco, alcohol, caffeine, and carbonated beverages.
• Avoid lying down for 1–2 hours after eating or drinking.
• Wear loose-fitting clothing.

Constipation[11] The following guidelines may be helpful:
• Drink 2–3 quarts of fluids daily, including water, milk, juice, and soup.
• Warm or hot fluids are often helpful right after waking up.
• Eat high-fiber cereals and other whole grains, legumes, fruits, and vegetables.
• Prunes, prune juice, and figs may also be helpful.
• Engage in physical activity such as walking and swimming.

8. Describe common food aversions and cravings.

Common food aversions include coffee, tea, fried or fatty foods, highly spiced foods, meat, and eggs. Energy intake/weight gain may be reduced. Food cravings include chocolate, citrus fruits, pickles, chips, and ice cream. Energy intake/weight gain may be increased.[11]

9. What is pica?

Pica is the practice of eating nonfood substances, such as clay, dirt (geophagia); laundry starch, soap, ashes, chalk, paint, burnt matches, baking soda; and freezer scrapings (pagophagia). This practice often has cultural or ethnic roots and may be present during pregnancy. Exposure to lead or other dangerous toxins may occur.[11] Suggestions to avoid pica include:
• Referral to qualified counselor or therapist.
• Suggest safe foods commonly craved, such as sour pickles, chocolate, citrus fruits, chips, or ice cream.
• Chew on frozen fruit juices instead of ice.

VITAMIN AND MINERAL SUPPLEMENTATION

10. Should vitamin and mineral supplements be recommended during pregnancy?

Yes.[11] However, it has not been proved that routine vitamin and mineral supplementation in pregnancy makes any difference in neonatal and maternal outcomes in patients who have ideal body weight and flawless dietary habits and do not smoke, use street drugs, or consume excessive alcohol. Since few patients can claim these characteristics, prenatal vitamins with a variety of B vitamins, vitamin A, 30 mg iron, and 1 mg folic acid should be taken daily. Vitamin and mineral supplements should be chosen with care, and the tolerable upper limits should not be exceeded for vitamins and minerals due to unknown effects.[4]

11. What are the best food sources of iron?

Iron is absorbed in greater amounts during pregnancy than in the nonpregnant state, and non-heme iron absorption is enhanced by an increased intake of fruits rich in ascorbic acid. Foods such as lean red meat, fish, and poultry are good sources of heme iron, and dried fruits and iron-fortified cereals are good sources of nonheme iron. However, tea, coffee, whole-grain cereals, and legumes should be consumed separately from iron-fortified foods and iron supplements, since they inhibit iron absorption.[11,13]

12. How is iron deficiency anemia assessed in pregnancy?

The hemoglobin levels of all patients should be checked at the first prenatal visit and then periodically throughout the pregnancy. Results may vary slightly by labs, but generally a patient is considered anemic if her hemoglobin is < 11 gm% or she has a hematocrit of 33% or less during the first and third trimesters. During the second trimester, the level is slightly lower, at 10.5 gm of hemoglobin and 31.5% hematocrit. For patients who smoke or live at high altitudes, the acceptable lower levels are about 0.5% gm higher. At these cut-offs, a serum ferritin should be drawn to determine if iron deficiency anemia is truly present. Ferritin levels below 20 µg/L indicate iron deficiency. In patients who have demonstrated iron deficiency, 60–120 mg of supplemental iron is recommended daily until the anemia is corrected.[11,13]

13. List good dietary sources of folic acid for prevention of neural tube defects.

Green leafy vegetables, oranges and orange juice, cauliflower, bananas, broccoli, fortified breakfast cereals, whole wheat bread, legumes, and liver.[11]

14. Why is vitamin A supplementation a concern during pregnancy?

Vitamin A is essential to normal reproduction, and its deficiency is a worldwide problem (primarily outside the U.S.). Because of this knowledge, many more women are using various dietary supplements of vitamin A. However, there is an association between high doses of vitamin A and its derivatives (such as Retin-A and Accutane) and congenital defects. The minimum teratogenic dose is probably at least 25,000–50,000 IU daily. The National Research Council's Committee on Dietary Allowances recommends the equivalent of 2700 IU per day. Dietary intake of vitamin A in the United States appears to be adequate in most situations. In patients whose intake may be low, no more than 5000 IU per day should be given, and this amount is supplied in prenatal vitamins.[7]

15. How can women with lactose intolerance increase calcium intake to achieve the recommended intake of 1000–1300 mg/day?

Adequate amounts of vitamin D are important in enhancing absorption of calcium in any form. A calcium-vitamin D supplement may be needed for women who are not able to consume calcium-containing foods and/or have inadequate exposure to sunlight. Calcium-containing or fortified foods include various beverages with supplemental calcium (juices, soy, and rice drinks); yogurt with active, live cultures; aged hard cheese; lactase-treated milk (ready-bought or use of tablets or drops); and cultured buttermilk. Nonmilk products for calcium sources include sardines, canned salmon, tofu, collards, bok choy, turnip greens, waffles, pancakes, corn tortillas processed with calcium salts, and dried beans.[11]

NUTRITIONAL CONSIDERATIONS IN DIABETIC PREGANCY

16. When should pregnant women be screened for diabetes?

All pregnant patients with no identifiable risk factors should be screened for diabetes at about 28 weeks' gestation. Gestational diabetes mellitus (GDM) appears after 24 weeks in 7% of all pregnancies. GDM increases the risk of macrosomia, which may lead to difficult labor, shoulder distocia, and cesarean delivery. In patients with a family history or other risk factors, screening should be done as early as possible, even during prepregnancy counseling.[11,14]

17. How is diabetes screening performed?

A random (nonfasting) loading dose of 50 gm glucose is given to the patient, and a blood sugar sample is drawn 1 hour later. Values to 140 mg/dl are considered normal, and no further testing is needed unless the patient has other risk factors. For values over 140 mg/dl, the patient is referred for a 3-hour glucose tolerance test. A fasting blood sugar is drawn, the patient is asked to ingest 75 gm of glucose, and blood samples are drawn at 1, 2, and 3 hours. Normal values, depending on the lab, are considered to be < 190 mg/dl at 1 hour, < 165 mg/dl at 2 hours, and < 145 mg/dl at 3 hours. The fasting level should be < 105 mg/dl. Different values are used at different institutions for triggering the diagnosis of gestational diabetes. Often two abnormal values or a fasting blood sugar over 105 mg/dl (goal) is consistent with the diagnosis of gestational diabetes, and the postprandial blood sugar should be 120 mg or below.[14,15]

18. What risk factors should trigger a glucose screen prior to 28 weeks?

• Any history of diabetes
• Previous birth of a macrosomatic, malformed, or stillborn baby
• Hypertension
• Persistant glycosuria
• Maternal age 30 years or older
• Previous gestational diabetes
• Marked obesity

19. What are the General Guidelines for the Management of Pregnant Diabetics?
The American Diabetes Association has published guidelines for managing diabetes during pregnancy.[15] Good blood glucose control is important for women with preexisting diabetes prior to conception. Hemoglobin A1c levels less than 1% above normal range is desirable. In obese women (BMI > 30), 25 kcal/kg/day is the recommended energy intake, with restriction of carbohydrate to 35–40% of total calories. Moderate exercise and medical nutrition therapy can often maintain desired glucose levels in gestational diabetics, but insulin is recommended if glycemic control is not maintained. Oral hypoglycemic agents are generally not recommended during pregnancy due to observed malformations. All diabetic patients should meet with a qualified dietetics professional to develop an individualized diet plan.[11]

SPECIAL NUTRITIONAL PROBLEMS IN PREGNANCY

20. How common are nausea, vomiting, and hyperemesis gravidarum?
Nausea and vomiting occur frequently during the early weeks of pregnancy and may affect 50–90% of all pregnant women. However, among some women they may persist until 17 weeks' gestation, and in about 5% of all patients they persist until term. Approximately 1.3% of all pregnant patients develop severe symptoms, known as hyperemesis gravidarum (HG) and require intravenous fluids, electrolytes, antiemetics, and parenteral or enteral nutrition support. The symptoms diminish after the birth of the baby or if the pregnancy is terminated.[12]

21. What are the symptoms of HG before 20 weeks' gestation?
• Weight loss > 5% of prepregnancy weight
• Fluid/electrolyte abnormalities
• Acid/base imbalance
• Ketonuria
• Severe cases may display neurologic disturbances, and liver, renal, esophageal, and retinal damage.

22. Which conditions should be eliminated before HG is diagnosed?
• Pancreatitis, appendicitis, cholelithiasis, hepatitis, Crohn's disease
• Ulcers, gastroenteritis, intestinal obstruction, hepatobiliary disease
• Hyperthyroidism, hyperparathyroidism
• Molar/ectopic pregnancy

23. What causes HG?
HG has an unclear etiology; it may be related to elevated hormone levels, gastrointestinal abnormalities, thyroid dysfunction, and/or psychological/social factors. Risk factors include nulliparity, prior HG, increased body weight, and multiple gestation. HG has a high social and financial cost, with millions of productive hours lost due to illness.[16]

24. List the goals of treatment to achieve birth of a healthy baby.[12]
• Alleviate HG symptoms to resume usual activity.
• Resume adequate oral intake.
• Maintain adequate rate of weight gain.
• Ensure stable electrolyte and fluid balance.
• Promote normal fetal growth and development.
• Avoid ketosis.
• Maintain blood sugar < 120 mg/dl.
• Provide adequate protein, calories, vitamins, minerals, and trace elements.
• Maintain positive nitrogen balance.
• Avoid complications related to use of enteral and parenteral therapy.

25. How is HG treated?

Restoration of fluid and electrolyte balance, along with decreased emesis, is the initial plan of treatment. Oral antiemetics such as odansetron (Zofran) and promethazine (Phenergan) may be tried. Often 5% dextrose with lactated Ringer's solution and multivitamins are initiated via peripheral line, with potassium chloride added as needed. IV antiemetics have been used successfully when oral agents fail and may consist of a combination of different medications.[12]

Medication	FDA Pregnancy Risk Category
Antihistamine (diphenhydramine)	B
Phenothiazine (promethazine)	C
Promotility agent (meoclopramide)	B
H₂ antagonist (famotidine, ranitidine)	B
Vitamin (pyridoxine/B₆)	A
5-HT3 receptor antagonist (odansetron)	B
Corticosteroid	C

Aggressive use of pharmacologic antiemetics may prevent the need for long-term home or hospital parenteral nutrition. Alternative remedies, such as ginger, have also been reported to decrease nausea and vomiting, but the long-term effects in pregnancy are unknown.[12] Enteral nutrition, administered as intestinal tube feedings, has also been used successfully[12] and should be tried before parenteral nutrition. Enteral nutrition has been reported to decrease the incidence of nausea and vomiting.[12,18,19] At-home peripheral parenteral nutrition (PPN) and total parenteral nutrition (TPN) have also been used successfully during pregnancy.[12,20] Often a combination of antiemetics is used to relieve symptoms, and an oral diet as tolerated, tube feedings, or parenteral nutrition is administered to maintain nutritional status. The combined therapies may last several weeks, until adequate intake of fluids and solids is possible.[12] Oral intake may be improved with attention to individual preferences and tolerances, and the book *No More Morning Sickness* by Miriam Erick contains helpful food lists as women with HG progress to oral diets. Foods are grouped according to tastes and tolerance for salty, sweet, sour, earthy, and cold/crunchy foods.[21] Weight gain and close nutrition monitoring are essential to ensure a healthy outcome during HG.

26. How is food-borne illness avoided during pregnancy?

According to the U.S. Dietary Guidelines,[8] pregnant women should not consume unpasteurized juices and milk products and raw sprouts. They should also avoid raw or undercooked meat, poultry, eggs, fish, and shellfish. Leftovers and ready-to-eat foods such as hot dogs should be cooked until steaming hot to avoid listerosis, caused by *Listeria monocytogenes*. Listerosis can cause premature delivery, stillbirth, or infection in the newborn. Other possible food sources of listerosis to be avoided are Mexican soft cheeses, homemade cheese, cheese purchased from street vendors, and other soft cheeses such as brie, feta, blue, and camembert.[11]

27. Are there any special dietary considerations for lactating women?[11]

Encouragement and education about lactation should be provided in both prenatal and postpartum settings. Nutrition information includes following the Recommended Dietary Allowances[9] to include an additional 500 kcal/day and the following:

- Continue a well-balanced diet[8] and multivitamin mineral supplement.
- Increase consumption of liquids to at least 2 quarts per day. Suggest drinking a glass of water, juice, or milk each time the baby nurses and at mealtimes. Avoid caffeinated beverages and alcohol.
- Foods with strong or spicy flavors may alter the taste of breast milk. If the food causes the infant discomfort, it can be eliminated from the diet.
- Check with your physician before taking any medications.
- Avoid any illegal drug use.
- Avoid breastfeeding if HIV-positive.
- Avoid smoking; passive exposure to tobacco smoke may also reduce infant growth.

REFERENCES

1. Medical Research Council Vitamin Study Research Group. Prevention of neural tube defects: Results of the Medical Research Council Vitamin Study. Lancet 338:131–137, 1991.
2. Brown AS, Fernhoff PM, Waisbren SE, et al: Barriers to successful dietary control among pregnant women with phenylketonuira. Genet Med 4:84–89, 2002.
3. Korenbort CC, Steinberg A, Bender C, Newberry S: Preconception care: A systematic review. Matern Child Health J 6(2):75–88, 2002.
4. Institute of Medicine: Nutrition during Pregnancy. Part I: Weight. Gain Part II: Supplements. Washington, DC, National Academy Press, 1990.
5. Foote J, Rengers B: Maternal use of herbal supplements. Nutr Complement Care 1:2000.
6. Institute of Medicine: Dietary Reference Intakes for Thiamin, Riboflavin, Niacin, Vitamin B6, Folate, Vitamin B12, Pantothenic Acid, Biotin and Choline. Washington, DC, National Academy Press, 1998.
7. Institute of Medicine: Dietary Reference Intakes for Vitamin A, Vitamin K, Arsenic, Boron, Chromium, Copper, Iodine, Iron, Manganese, Molbydenum, Nickel, Silicon, Vanadium and Zinc. Washington, DC, National Academy Press, 2001.
8. Food Guide Pyramid. Washington, DC, US Department of Agriculture Center for Nutrition Policy and Promotion. Home and Garden Bulletin No. 252, 1996.
9. Food and Nutrition Board. Recommended Dietary Allowances, 10th ed. Washington, DC, National Academy Press, 1989.
10. Gutierrez Y, King JC: Nutrition during teenage pregnancy. Pediatr Ann 22:99–108, 1993.
11. Kaiser L, Allen L: Position of the American Dietetic Association: Nutrition and lifestyle for a healthy pregnancy outcome. J Am Diet Assoc 102:1479–1490, 2002.
12. Wagner BA, Worthington P, Russo-Stieglitz KE, et al: Nutritional management of hyperemesis gravidarum. Nutr Clin Pract 15:65–76, 2000.
13. Centers for Disease Control: Recommendations to prevent and control iron deficiency in the United States. MMWR 47: 1–36, 1998.
14. American Diabetes Association: Preconception care of women with diabetes. Diabetes Care 24:S66–S687, 2001.
15. American Diabetes Association: Gestational diabetes mellitus. Diabetes Care 24:S77–S79, 2001.
16. Gadsby R, Barnie-Ashdead AM, Jagger C: A prospective study of nausea and vomiting during pregnancy. Br J Gen Pract 43:245–248, 1993.
17. Hsu JJ, Clark-Gena R, Nelson DK, et al: Nasogastric enteral feedings in the management of hyperemesis gravidarum. Obstet Gynecol 88:343–346, 1996.
18. Gulley RM, Pleog NV, Gulley J: Treatment of hyperemsis gravidarum with nasogastric feeding. Nutr Clin Pract 8:33–35, 1993.
19. Serrano P, Velloso A, Garcia-Luna PP, et al: Enteral nutrition by percutaneous endoscopic gastrojejunostomy in severe hyperemesis gravidarum, a report of two. Clin Nutr 17:135–139, 1998.
20. Chevreau N, Anthony PS, Kessinger K: Managing hyperemesis gravidarum with home parenteral nutrition: Treatment parameters and clinical outcomes. Infusion 65:22–28, 1999.
21. Erick M: No More Morning Sickness: A Survival Guide for Pregnant Women. New York, Plume, 1993.

IV. Nutrition for Promoting Health and Preventing Disease

14. SPORTS NUTRITION

Ann C. Grandjean, EdD, FACN, CNS, and Jaime S. Ruud, MS, RD

1. Can nutrition really make a difference in sports performance?
Definitely yes. An athlete's accomplishments in competitive sport are determined by a variety of behavioral, socioeconomic, cultural, and environmental factors. While a number of these are not within the control of the individual, nutrition can be controlled by the athlete to a large extent. All other factors being equal, diet can make a significant difference in performance.

2. Are the nutritional needs of athletes different from those of nonathletes?
Somewhat surprisingly, no. There is nothing exotic about the nutritional requirements of athletes. Who are athletes? They may be grade-school wrestlers or professional baseball players. Many are adolescents, but others are the parents of adolescents. They range from 4 feet to 7 feet tall and from under 100 to over 300 pounds. Their training may be an hour two days a week with the fast-pitch softball team in the city league or 400 bicycle miles a week. Age, gender, body size, and training schedule determine the athlete's dietary needs. They need the same nutrients as nonathletes. The consequences of poor nutrition may be more immediately apparent in athletes than in nonathletes. While variations exist in nutrient requirements, the variance in energy requirement is even greater.

3. How many calories does an athlete need?
Calorie requirements vary from person to person and depend on body size, age, sport, and intensity of the training program. An estimation of energy needs can be obtained by multiplying the athlete's weight in pounds by one of the following factors.

Activity Level	Male	Female
Light	17	16
Moderate	19	17
Heavy	23	20
Very Heavy	26	23

But these rules of thumb are only estimates of "average" requirements. Exact requirements will vary greatly. An athlete weighing 125 pounds may expend 140–240 calories in 30 minutes of volleyball. But the same person would burn up 350 calories in 30 minutes of rowing or sculling. And a 200-pound person would expend over 500 calories during the same 30 minutes of rowing.

According to the above chart, a male putting in long hours of very heavy training would need 26 calories per pound, or 58 calories per kg per day. Energy needs for a male weighing 175 pounds would be (175×26) or 4550 calories per day. Some male triathletes have been measured to expend as much as 68 calories per kg per day, emphasizing that individual variation is significant.

4. How do you determine if an athlete's caloric intake is adequate?
Look at daily weights. Maintaining ideal competitive weight is the best indicator of adequate calorie intake. Athletes who consistently maintain their weight are in energy balance. While the table above can provide a rough estimate, the exact number of calories needed will vary greatly between athletes. Thus, maintaining weight is the best guide for determining adequate calorie intake.

5. If maintaining body weight is the indicator for calorie intake, how do you determine if an athlete is getting the required nutrients?

Indicators of inadequate nutrition in athletes are frequent illness, chronic fatigue, inability to complete workouts or training sessions, and reports of inadequate strength or endurance. Obviously, factors other than diet can also cause these symptoms. A computerized dietary analysis is the most exact method for determining adequate intakes but may not take individual variation into account.

6. How does one determine adequate hydration?

The most accurate method is nude weights taken before and after practice or competition. That's why there are scales in locker rooms. A one-pound weight loss is equivalent to 480 ml (16 ozs) of fluid. As a general rule, a moderate exercise regimen will cause a one-to-two-pound weight loss during the session. If the athlete is losing more than that, then fluid intake is too low.

7. What if weighing is not possible?

Urine output and frequency of urination must be monitored. The body continuously produces waste products, some of which are eliminated in urine. Since this is an essential bodily function, the kidneys will "take" the water they need to produce urine, even when the body is dehydrated. However, the kidneys will concentrate the urine as much as possible, which makes the urine appear dark yellow and have a strong odor. Light colored, non-odorous urine is a fairly reliable indicator that the athlete is hydrated. The frequency and character of urine output are especially important to monitor in hot weather. Outdoors, with an ambient temperature of 85 degrees or higher, it is surprisingly easy to become dehydrated.

Diuretics can cause the urine to be light yellow, regardless of hydration status. Some vitamin pills can make the urine bright yellow, although concentration and frequency will still reflect hydration.

8. What recommendations can be given to an athlete regarding fluid intake?

Athletes need to make a conscious effort to consume fluids regularly and in sufficient amounts to ensure normal body functions and thermal regulation. The American College of Sports Medicine recommends 500 ml (17 oz) of fluid about 2 hours before exercise. During exercise, athletes should start drinking early and at regular intervals at a rate sufficient to replace fluid loss. Again, the ambient temperature and humidity will affect fluid needs. Most people drink too little water during a period of exercise. The athlete should take a mandatory "water break" every half-hour or even more often in hot or dry weather. Thirst, under condition of exercise in a hot environment, is unreliable as a guide to hydration.

9. Athletes often report that drinking water causes a side ache frequently referred to as "stitch." Is this true?

Not at all. In fact, just the opposite may be true. The exact cause of stitch is not known, but not drinking enough fluids is thought to be one of the causes. Other causes include abnormal contractions of the diaphragm, muscle spasm, indigestion, incorrect breathing, or being out of shape. Too much training has also been suggested as a cause. Whatever the etiology of stitch, drinking water is most certainly not the culprit.

10. What's the harm in not replacing lost fluid?

Dehydration. A modest fluid loss of only 1% of body weight—1–2 pounds—impairs thermoregulation. Even this much dehydration can lead to a decrease in performance. Somewhat larger deficits of 2–3% of body weight can have adverse effects on performance by raising the heart rate, reducing the sweat rate, and increasing the body core temperature. Moderate dehydration, in hot weather, can lead to heat exhaustion or heat stroke. Severe dehydration can kill (see Table).

Adverse Effects of Dehydration

PERCENT OF BODY WEIGHT LOSS	SYMPTOMS
0	None
1	Thirst threshold, impaired thermoregulation, decreased exercise capacity
2	Stronger thirst, vague discomfort, sense of oppression, loss of appetite
3	Dry mouth, reduction in urinary output, hemoconcentration
4	Decrement of 20–30% in physical work capacity
5	Difficulty in concentrating, headache, impatience, sleepiness
6	Severe impairment in temperature regulation, increased respirations leading to tingling and numbness of extremities
7	Stupor and collapse, especially if combined with heat and continued exercise

11. I've always heard that it is important for athletes to eat lots of carbohydrate. Now I'm hearing that protein is more important. Which is correct?

Both protein and carbohydrates can affect performance. The energy for muscles to perform work is provided by carbohydrates, protein, and fat. However, unlike protein and fat, carbohydrate stores in the body are severely limited. There is enough glycogen to last for 12–16 hours at normal levels of activity. Glycogen rapidly becomes depleted with intense activity and the ability to exercise at a relatively high intensity is impaired. The athlete who does not consume adequate carbohydrate can experience fatigue and reduced exercise capacity.

12. How much carbohydrate do athletes need?

Recommended carbohydrate intake varies depending on training program and type of sport. Endurance athletes and athletes who train for more than 90 minutes daily need approximately 8–10 grams of carbohydrate per kilogram of body weight each day to restore muscle glycogen levels. This is equivalent to 600–750 grams of carbohydrate per day for an athlete weighing 75 kg (165 lbs). For athletes involved in intermittent power or sprint activities, 5 grams of carbohydrate per kilogram of body weight is adequate to support training. For the same 165-lb athlete, this would be 375 grams.

13. How much protein do athletes need?

Research shows that athletes have increased protein requirements compared to nonathletes. The recommended dietary allowance for the sedentary adult is 0.8 grams per kilogram per day. Endurance athletes require 1.2–1.4 g/kg/day and strength athletes, 1.4–1.8 g/kg/day.

14. Why do athletes need more protein?

Two factors cause an increased protein requirement. The first factor is energy. As energy intake decreases, protein requirements increase. Athletes who reduce food intake to control body weight frequently do not consume adequate calories and as a result have higher protein requirements. They must compensate for the body's tendency to burn protein for energy if caloric intake is limited. The second factor is increase in muscle mass. Training in general, and weight training specifically, increases protein requirements. Both of these factors affect the percentage of protein in the diet. Where a sedentary individual may require only 15% protein in the diet, an athlete training every day may require 20% or even as much as 25%.

15. Athletes often report they're not getting the increases in weight or muscle mass they desire. Will more protein help?

Not usually. The most common cause of inadequate muscle gains is an inadequate weight training program. If it is clear that the athlete's resistance training program is adequate, then inadequate calorie intake may be the problem. It takes approximately 2500 calories over normal requirements for every pound of muscle gained and only part of this must be protein. Only if the training program and overall caloric intake are both adequate will there be a substantial benefit to increasing the amount of protein in the diet.

16. Is it true that liquid meal-replacements can help in weight gain?
The primary purpose of a liquid supplement is to supply calories. There are several liquid supplements on the market today. The best drink is simply a matter of choice. Although liquid supplements will not build muscle without a resistance training program or take the place of an adequate diet, they can boost calorie and nutrient intake. While they provide a convenient source of calories, it must be remembered that excess calories from any source will be converted to body fat.

17. Athletes want to gain muscle, not fat. What is the best way to determine if an athlete's weight gain is muscle gain?
Hydrostatic (underwater) weighing is the gold-standard measurement but very often is not available or practical. Skinfold measurements can be a simple, reliable, and reasonably accurate option for determining body composition. It is essential to have a trained individual conduct the assessment to ensure accuracy. Body impedance measurement can give a fairly reliable indication of body fat and lean body mass; however, it is better at tracking changes than it is at determining absolute values.

18. I've heard that creatine is being used by athletes to increase muscle mass and improve performance. What is creatine?
Creatine is a compound made by the liver, kidney, and pancreas. It is found in meat and fish. Creatine is stored mainly in skeletal muscle as free creatine or bound to a phosphate molecule (creatine phosphate, PCr). The creatine phosphate molecule is the immediate source of energy for muscle contraction. Theoretically, supplementing with creatine should increase the immediate sources of energy. The level of creatine phosphate is regulated by the body so that simply supplying more creatine will not change the resting levels of chemical energy in the muscle. However, it may increase the body's ability to synthesize creatine phosphate and to respond to stress. Creatine is relatively nontoxic and is harmless in small amounts (see below).

19. Who should take creatine and how much should they take?
Creatine is used by athletes participating in a wide range of sports including power sports such as weight lifting and wrestling, team sports like football and volleyball, and sports requiring short, explosive action such as the 100-meter dash and the discus. Recommended doses and regimens vary but the standard loading dose is a total of 20–30 grams a day (divided into 4 equal doses) for 5–7 days followed by a maintenance dose of 2 grams a day. Common recommendations are to take creatine with a carbohydrate drink to increase uptake.

20. Does creatine actually improve performance or increase muscle gain?
Studies show that creatine supplementation may increase intramuscular concentrations of PCr, enhance anaerobic power, speed recovery from intermittent high-intensity exercise, enhance muscular strength, and increase lean body mass. However, not all studies have reported significant changes and creatine has not been tested in young athletes. Experience shows that some athletes have positive results while others do not. Research indicates that vegetarians respond more positively than meat eaters.

21. What are the potential effects or risks associated with creatine use?
Gut cramping and diarrhea are sometimes reported, especially during the loading phase. Muscle cramping and weight gain have been reported by athletes using creatine long term. Creatine is metabolized into uric acid; elevated uric acid levels could result in gouty arthritis in susceptible athletes. The long-term effects of taking recommended doses of supplemental creatine or consuming doses above recommended levels have yet to be determined.

BIBLIOGRAPHY

1. American College of Sports Medicine: Position stand on exercise and fluid replacement. Med Sci Sports Exerc 28:i–vii, 1996.
2. American College of Sports Medicine: Position stand on the female athlete triad.Med Sci Sports Exerc 29:i–ix, 1997.
3. Greenleaf JE, Harrison MH: Water and electrolytes. In Layman DK (ed): Nutrition and Aerobic Exercise. Washington, D.C., American Chemical Society, 1986.
4. Reimers KJ, Ruud JS, Grandjean AC: Sports Nutrition. In Mellion MB (ed): Office Sports Medicine, 2nd ed. Philadelphia, Hanley & Belfus, 1996.

15. NUTRITION AND THE HEART

William S. Harris, PhD, and Charles W. Van Way III, MD

1. What is the effect of nutrition on the heart?

There is good scientific evidence that nutrition has a profound effect on the development of heart disease. This evidence has been incorporated into daily life. For example, many restaurants have a menu section devoted to "heart healthy" choices, which are supposed to prevent the development of heart disease. Of course, this implies that all of the other choices promote the development of heart disease, which is probably not the intent of the restaurateur. Unfortunately, a "heart healthy" designation can also be the kiss of death for a menu selection in some restaurants! But we digress.

The evidence is fairly strong that nutrition can help to prevent hypertension (see chapter 22, Hypertension). Hypertension is a systemic disease which, if untreated, ends in congestive heart failure. So in that sense, nutrition can protect the heart.

But there is more direct effect of nutrition. Appropriate nutrient intake can change both the incidence and severity of coronary heart disease (CHD).

2. How much impact can dietary change have on CHD?

There are several studies in the literature showing that patients who make specific dietary changes can change their risk for heart attacks very significantly.

In two of these, the Oslo Diet Study and the St. Thomas Atherosclerosis Regression Study (STARS), patients were given relatively minor changes in diet patterns, similar to the National Cholesterol Education Program Step 1 diet (see below). In the Oslo study, CHD rates were cut nearly in half after about 10 years of adherence to the test diet. In the STARS study, plaque size was measurably decreased in less than 2 years. These two studies showed that relatively modest changes in diet may produce real benefits.

The Lifestyle Heart Study used a very strict low-fat, low-cholesterol program (similar to the Pritikin diet) in conjunction with increased exercise and stress-reduction training to achieve clear plaque regression within only one year in patients with known disease.

The evidence for a cardioprotective effect of fish and fish oils is rapidly accumulating. The omega-3 faty acids in these foods may be the most potent cardioprotective factors in the diet. (See Chapter 35, Omega-3 Fatty Acids and Heart Disease.) In short, people at increased risk for CHD can alter their future at the dinner table without retreating to the medicine cabinet.

3. What are the recommendations for dietary lowering of high blood cholesterol?

The recommendations of the National Cholesterol Education Program (NCEP) for control of elevated blood cholesterol are outlined below. They assume a diet based on total energy needs appropriate for the individual, together with limitations on cholesterol and saturated fat. Soluble fiber and margarines containing plant sterol/stanol esters are now recommended by the NCEP as additional strategies for lowering cholesterol.

Diet Therapy for High Blood Cholesterol: Recommendations from the NCEP

NUTRIENTS	LEVEL
Total fat (% energy intake)	25–35%
Saturated Fat (% en)	< 7%
Monounsaturated Fat (% en)	Up to 20%
Polyunsaturated Fat (% en)	Up to 10%
Carbohydrate (% en)	50–60%
Cholesterol (mg/day)	< 200

en = energy intake or kilocalories.

4. What are the effects of diet upon the major etiologic factors for coronary heart disease?
The major etiologic factors in coronary artery disease are blood lipids, thrombosis, cigarette smoking, hypertension, and diabetes. Diet has an effect on some of these but not others. The major effects of diet appear to be on blood lipids, hypertension, and diabetes. Thrombosis is probably not affected by diet, although omega-3 fatty acids can mildly inhibit platelet aggregation. The desire to smoke cigarettes is not known to be affected by diet.

5. How does diet affect blood lipids?
The most clearly documented connection between dietary patterns and CHD risk is the effects on blood lipids and lipoprotein levels. Saturated fatty acids, particularly those found in animal fats (palmitic, lauric and myristic), will alter hepatic metabolism in such a way as to decrease the removal of low density lipoproteins (LDL) from the blood. This elevates blood LDL levels. Since LDL particles are the richest in cholesterol, blood cholesterol rises as well as blood LDL. There is virtual unanimity in the medical community that reductions in dietary levels of these fatty acids will reduce serum LDL levels and thereby reduce CHD risk. Reduction in total fat (not just the saturated fatty acids) is much more controversial and will be discussed below.

6. What effect does the dietary management of hypertension have on the risk of coronary heart disease?
Dietary measures to reduce blood pressure are relatively simple (see Chapter 22, Hypertension) and have been clearly shown to reduce the risk of hypertension. These measures include weight reduction, modest sodium restriction, and modest alcohol restriction. The usual recommendations include reducing weight to normal, keeping sodium intake at 2–4 g/day, and keeping alcohol intake to 2 drinks per day or less. Interestingly, there appears to be a benefit to modest alcohol intake of 1–2 drinks per day, and an additional benefit to drinking red wine. These are associated with a somewhat lower incidence of CHD than zero alcohol intake. The mechanism by which moderate alcohol intake reduces CHD risk is not clear, however.
Since hypertension is a known risk factor for CHD, dietary measures which reduce hypertension should reduce CHD risk. However, no studies have yet shown that these changes actually reduce heart attacks.

7. Is there an effect of diet upon endothelial dysfunction and lipid peroxidation?
This is one of the newest and most exciting areas in nutrition. Atherosclerosis is basically a disease of the vascular endothelium. Endothelial "health" plays a significant role in CHD risk. When it is stressed, normal endothelium secretes a variety of compounds that cause the vessels to relax. Vessels in patients at risk for CHD do not relax as they should. While the mechanisms causing this involve alterations in nitric oxide metabolism, the details are not clear. It is known, however, that dietary factors can improve endothelial responsiveness. Any intervention that lowers serum cholesterol levels or increases antioxidant status will help normalize endothelium reactivity. The former can be accomplished by decreasing saturated fat and cholesterol intakes, and the latter by increasing the consumption of antioxidant vitamins, notably vitamins C and E (there is more evidence for vitamin E than C). These vitamins seem to work by preventing LDL oxidation which is known to contribute to decreased endothelial responsiveness. Intakes needed to achieve meaningful reductions in oxidation potential are approximately 400–800 mg of vitamin E and about 1 g of vitamin C.

8. What is the role of homocysteine in CHD?
Homocysteine is an amino acid formed in the body, an intermediate in the metabolic pathway of methionine, an essential, sulfur-containing amino acid. When plasma levels of homocysteine are markedly increased, the risk for thrombosis and premature cardiovascular disease are high. Those with mildly increased levels often have a genetic defect in one of the enzymes that controls homocysteine levels, together with a B-vitamin deficiency. The three vitamins which serve as cofactors in homocysteine metabolism are folic acid, pyridoxine (B_6) and cobalamin

(B_{12}). Until recently, mild elevation of plasma homocysteine was thought to be harmless. But studies have now clearly linked increased homocysteine levels with heightened risk for vascular disease. It is especially important that CHD patients consume adequate amounts of these vitamins, preferably from natural foods (fruits, vegetables, grains) or else from supplements. Commonly recommended amounts are folic acid (800–1,000 µg), B_6 (50 mg) and B_{12} (50 µg).

9. Do antioxidant vitamins reduce CHD risk?

Although a large body of epidemiologic, animal, and biochemical evidence points to a cardioprotective effect of antioxidant vitamins (especially E and C), several recent randomized, controlled trials have not. In particular, the Heart Protection Study examined the effects of an antioxidant "cocktail" including 600 mg of E, 250 mg of C, and 20 mg of beta-carotene in over 20,000 subjects at increased risk for CHD. After 5 years, there was no difference whatever in CHD event rates between the placebo and the cocktail groups. Thus, megadoses of vitamins E or C are not currently recommended for CHD prevention.

10. What is the best diet for prevention of CHD?

A diet emphasizing grains, fruits, vegetables, and low-fat dairy products; containing fish; and low in saturated fatty acid-containing animal products, would be the ideal CHD prevention diet. This is similar to the NCEP recommended diet and emphasizes lowering the total fat intake by reducing saturated fat intake. But what should replace them—carbohydrates or monounsaturated or polyunsaturated fatty acids?

The arguments for reducing total fat (i.e., substituting carbohydrates for saturated fats) are fairly strong. First, obesity will be reduced, since it's easier to lose weight eating carbohydrates than fat. Second, less fat means lower postprandial lipemia, which should be antiatherogenic. Third, a low-fat diet provides a degree of cancer prevention. On the other hand, there is a case for substituting monounsaturated fats for saturated fats, sometimes known as the "olive oil" strategy. There is a low rate of CHD among Mediterranean populations consuming large amounts of olive oil (among other "heart-healthy" foods). Low-fat, high-carbohydrate diets usually raise serum triglyceride and lower HDL cholesterol (so-called "good cholesterol"). In addition, recent experience has shown that obesity isn't really reduced by low-fat diets, since most such diets today are richer than ever in sugar. Sugar and other carbohydrates are a prominent component of "low-fat" or "fat-free" foods. This controversy will likely continue for some time, because the only way to settle it would be a large randomized clinical trial with "hard" cardiac endpoints and such a trial would be far too costly in today's fiscal environment.

BIBLIOGRAPHY

1. Connor WE, Connor SL: The case for a low-fat, high-carbohydrate diet. N Engl J Med 337:562–563, 1997.
2. Expert Panel on Detection, Evaluation, And Treatment of High Blood Cholesterol in Adults (Adult Treatment Panel III): Executive Summary of The Third Report of The National Cholesterol Education Program (NCEP). JAMA 285:2486–2497, 2001
3. Gaziano JM, Manson JE: Diet and heart disease: The role of fat, alcohol and antioxidants. Cardiol Clin 14:69–83, 1996.
4. Hallikainen MA, Uusitupa MI: Effects of 2 low-fat stanol ester-containing margarines on serum cholesterol concentrations as part of a low-fat diet in hypercholesterolemic subjects. Am J Clin Nutr 69:403–410, 1999.
5. Heart Protection Study Collaborative Group: MRC/BHF Heart Protection Study of cholesterol lowering with simvastatin in 20,536 high-risk individuals: A randomised placebo-controlled trial. Lancet 350:7–22, 2002.
6. Katan MB, Grundy SM, Willett WC: Beyond low fat diets. N Engl J Med 337:563–566, 1997. Letter by Ornish D. Low-fat diets, N Engl J Med 338, 127, 1998.
7. Krummel D: Nutrition in Cardiovascular Disease. Chapter 23 in Mahan LK, Escott-Stump S (eds): Krause's Food, Nutrition, and Diet Therapy. 9th ed. Philadelphia, W.B. Saunders, 1996.
8. Simon HB: Patient-directed, non-prescription approaches to cardiovascular disease. Arch Intern Med 154:2283–2296, 1994.
Website Healthy People 2010: http://www.health.gov/healthypeople/About/

16. DIET AND CANCER

Mary Ann Kaylor, RD, MMSc, Alan B. Marr, MD,
and Charles W. Van Way III, MD

1. Are there foods known to cause cancer?

There are no known individual foods that are carcinogenic. Some chemicals, pesticides, and food additives, however, have been identified as potentially hazardous. The Food and Drug Administration enforces strict controls with these agents. Higher associations of esophageal and gastric cancers occurs in areas where large amounts of salt-cured, smoked, and nitrite-cured foods are consumed. High salt and nitrate intake are considered risk factors for these cancers but little is known about the mechanisms by which they may cause cancer.

Obesity, a sedentary life-style, and a diet low in vegetables, fruits, whole grains, fish, and poultry seems to be associated with both breast and colorectal cancer. Despite conflicts in epidemiologic studies, there seems to be general agreement. However, it is not known whether prudent dietary habits (e.g., fruits, vegetables) prevent cancer, or whether less prudent habits (high fat, high processed food, high red meat) cause cancer. Much is unknown in this area.

2. Can some foods prevent cancer?

Antioxidants, which come from a variety of food sources, may be protective against cancer. Antioxidants work to reduce free radicals in the body. Free radicals are highly reactive, short-lasting chemical species which contain one or more unpaired electrons. The endogenous sources of oxidants include normal respiration, phagocytosis, cytochrome P450 enzymes, and peroxisomes. Fatty acid oxidation causes release of peroxisomes which may cause oxidative exercise.

Antioxidants act as a natural defense mechanism to block excessive oxidation and free radical damage. Substances currently being studied for their antioxidant properties include selenium, carotenoids, tocopherols, and ascorbic acid. Carotenoids are thought to act in a chemoprotective role in their link to cancer. One carotenoid may capture up to four free radicals, rendering them inactive. Tocopherols represent a group of compounds generally referred to as Vitamin E. Vitamin E is a biologic antioxidant that also acts as a scavenger of oxygen radicals and terminates free-radical chain reactions at the cellular membrane level. Ascorbic acid, or Vitamin C, appears to be an important antioxidant in plasma, extracellular fluids, intracellular space, and the cellular membrane. Epidemiologic studies indicate that Vitamin C, independent of its antioxidant properties, has an anticarcinogenic action which involves its ability to detoxify carcinogens. The antioxidant role of selenium is believed to be related to superoxide dismutase.

Food sources of these vitamins include carrots, tomatoes, oranges, orange juice, cantaloupe, and green vegetables, such as broccoli, spinach, and green beans. Meat and animal products are the most reliable food sources of selenium. Selenium may be present in fruits and vegetables. The content varies with the soil content in which the vegetables are grown.

3. Is fiber important in decreasing cancer risk?

High-fiber diets have been associated with lowering cancer risks, particularly colorectal cancer. Plant-based diets low in calories from fat, high in fiber, and rich in legumes, whole grain foods, vegetables, and fruits reduce the risk of endometrial cancer. Fiber increases intestinal transit time, allowing less time for intestinal flora to produce carcinogens or for carcinogens to act on intestinal cells. Fiber may also act as an anticarcinogenic agent by binding fecal bile acids, which may have carcinogenic properties in increased amounts.

Dietary fiber is divided into two categories. These are soluble and insoluble fiber. Soluble fibers include gums, pectins, mucilages, and some hemicelluloses. Insoluble fiber include cellulose, lignin, and some hemicelluloses. The recommendation for fiber intake is 20–35 grams a day with an insoluble:soluble ratio of 3:1 which is the ratio that is found in plant foods.

High fiber foods include whole grain crackers and breads, whole wheat flour, and vegetables such as carrots, corn, peas, and beans. Also high in fiber are fruits such as peaches, figs, raisins, apples, berries, and apricots. Examples of grains high in fiber are bran and barley. Consumption of 6–11 servings of grains and 5–9 servings of fruits and vegetables will provide a variety of those recommended amounts.

4. Would taking supplements be as good as eating foods?

No. Vitamins should not be used to replace food. Supplementation is typically not necessary if the diet is well-balanced. According to the American Dietetic Association, the best nutritional strategy for promoting optional health and reducing the risk of chronic disease is to obtain adequate nutrients from a wide variety of sources. Vitamin and mineral supplementation is appropriate when well-accepted, peer-reviewed, scientific evidence shows safety and effectiveness.

Food sources provide many additional benefits, such as fiber. Other benefits of food sources is that many more elements may yet be undiscovered. For example, beta-carotene is only one of more than the 400 carotenoids that have been identified. Plant foods also contain natural pesticides that have anticarcinogenic properties in small amounts but may not be safe in larger amounts. In addition, nutritional supplements can cause problems that are related to nutrient imbalances and toxicities.

5. Is dietary fat related to cancer?

There are indications that high-fat intake may be associated with higher risks of prostate, renal cell, colorectal, and breast cancers. Fat sources particularly implicated with this higher risk are from animal sources such as red meat, eggs, and dairy foods. But the specific role of dietary fat in breast cancer remains highly controversial. Two controlled clinical trials are now underway to research this issue further, the Women's Health Initiative and the Women's Intervention Nutrition Study. Some studies suggest a link between dietary fat and breast cancer, particularly in postmenopausal women. Fish oil consumption may protect against the promotion of cancer by animal fat in colorectal and breast cancer. Other epidemiologic studies suggest that the consumption of monounsaturated fat, particularly olive oil, may reduce the risk of breast cancer.

6. How does diet affect other cancers?

Dietary factors may influence several types of cancer. Generally, an increase in cholesterol intake has been associated with elevated cancer risk, while increased consumption of fruits and vegetables has been associated with lower risks. Diets high in animal products, such as red meats, eggs, and dairy foods may encourage the development of prostate cancer. Lycopene, a carotenoid present in tomatoes, may protect against prostate cancer. Salivary gland cancer may be partially prevented by a high vitamin C intake (more than 200 mg/day). It has even been suggested that some nutrients may inhibit the carcinogenic effects of tobacco in head and neck cancer. Frequent intake of fried or sauteed meat increased the risk of renal cell cancer by approximately 60%. A significant protective effect was observed with an increased consumption of fruit. In 1991, the National Cancer Institute began the program, "5 A Day for Better Health." This program was to encourage Americans to eat five or more servings of fruits and vegetables every day. This initiative was based on data suggesting that 35% or more of all cancer deaths may be attributable to unhealthy dietary practices, or at least may be preventable by improved nutrition.

7. Does alcohol cause cancer?

Most clinicians would say that excessive alcohol intake can, indeed, lead to cancer. Alcoholics seem to be more likely to have have cancer of the esophagus, pancreas, and oral cavity, and possibly the breast. The studies that confirm this association are somewhat controversial, and studies in the literature often conflict with one another. There is some epidemiologic evidence that even a high alcohol intake does not increase the risk of pancreatic cancer. Alcohol does increase estrogen levels in women, which may, in turn, be related to the development of certain types of breast tumors. There is evidence to indicate that alcohol has adverse effects on serum carotenoids, which have a protective effect against cancer. Plasma concentrations of selenium and vitamin E are decreased in alcoholics. Alcohol may increase the risk of developing cancer by removing or opposing some of the protective factors in the diet.

8. Is there a higher risk of cancer with obesity?
Epidemiologic studies have not been consistent in demonstrating a causal relationship between obesity and cancer. There is increased mortality from all causes in individuals with a body mass index (BMI) more than 30, and there appears to be an increase in certain disease states, including some cancers. Specifically, there has been evidence that supports a relationship between breast cancer and obesity. Inadequate exercise is also a factor in the cancer risk. Exercise appears to protect against cancers of the breast, reproductive tract, and colon. These include increased colonic transit time, suppression of sex hormone secretion, and reduction of body fat deposits, where androgens are converted to toxic estrogen derivatives. Insulin resistance, associated with obesity and concomitant hyperinsulinemia, may play a role in development of breast tumors through the synergistic elevation of estrogen.

9. Is green tea protective against cancer?
Astoundingly, Chinese green tea may be a protective agent. Chinese green tea has some potentially anticarcinogenic properties. It is produced with a process that retains its polyphenols. Polyphenols are considered antioxidants, and these polyphenols inhibited tumor formation and growth when fed to animals. They inhibit metabolic activation of dietary carcinogens and block carcinogen DNA adduct formation. The specific protective agent or agents are uncertain, but epigallocatechin-3-gallate specifically and green tea catechins in general have been shown to have antitumor effects.

Although clinical studies have been limited, some suggestive studies have been published. A study by Gao, et al., demonstrated a protective effect of green tea by showing a decreased incidence of esophageal cancer. Wu et al. found that breast cancer in Asian-American women was inversely related to green tea consumption.

BIBLIOGRAPHY

1. Albanes D, Virtamo J, Taylor PR, et al: Effects of supplemental beta-carotene, cigarette smoking, and alcohol consumption on serum carotenoids in the Alpha-Tocopheral, Beta-carotene Cancer Prevention Study. Am J Clin Nutr 66:366–372, 1997.
2. Bosaeus J, Daneryd P, Lundholm K: Dietary intake, resting energy expenditure, weight loss, and survival in cancer patients. J Nutr 132(Suppl 11):3465S–3466S, 2002.
3. Blackburn GL, Copeland T, Khaodhiar L, Buckley RB: Diet and breast cancer. J Womens Health (Larchmt) 12:183–192, 2003.
4. Braga M, Gianotti L, Nespoli L, et al: Nutritional approach in malnourished surgical patients: A prospective randomized study. Arch Surg 137:174–180, 2002.
5. Braga M, Gianotti L, Radaelli G, et al: Perioperative immunonutrition in patients undergoing cancer surgery: A prospective randomized study.
6. Brusselmans K, De Schrijver E, Heyns W, et al: Epigallocatechin-3-gallate is a potent natural inhibitor of fatty acid synthase in intact cells and selectively induced apoptosis in prostate cancer cells. Int J Cancer 106:856–862, 2003.
7. Caygill CP, Dharlett A, Hill MJ: Fat, fish, fish oil, and cancer. Br J Cancer 74:159–164, 1996.
8. Copeland EM, Copeland EM III: Historical perspective on nutritional support of cancer patients. CA Cancer J Clin 48(2):67–68, 1998.
9. Dietary Fiber. An analysis of the role of fiber in proper nutrition. From the Advances in Fiber Symposium, December 11, 1989, Atlanta, Georgia.
10. Fung T, Hu FB, Fuchs C, et al: Major dietary patterns and the risk of colorectal cancer in women. Arch Intern Med 163:309–314, 2003.
11. Gao YT, McLaughlin JK, Blot WJ, et al: Reduced risk of esophageal cancer associated with green tea consumption. J Natl Cancer Inst 86:855–858, 1994.
12. Giles G, Ireland F: Diet, Nutrition, and Prostate Cancer. Int J Cancer S10:13–17, 1997.

13. Ginbsurg ES, Mello NK, Mendelson JH, et al: Effects of alcohol ingestion on estrogens in post-menopausal women. JAMA 276:1747–1751, 1996.
14. Goodman MT, Wilkens LR, Hankin JH, et al: Association of soy and fiber consumption with the risk of endometrial cancer. Am J Epidemiol 146:294–306, 1997.
15. Goodwin PJ, Ennis M, Pritchard KI, et al: Diet and breast cancer: Evidence that extremes in diet are associated with poor survival. J Clin Oncol 21:2500–2507, 2003.
16. Greenwald P, Sherwood K, Mcdonald SS: Fat, caloric intake and obesity: lifestyle risk factors for breast cancer. J Am Diet Assoc 97:S24–S30, 1997.
17. Heys SD, Walker LG, Smith I, Eremin O: Enteral nutritional supplementation with key nutrients in patients with critical illness and cancer: A meta-analysis of randomized controlled trials. Ann Surg 229:467–477, 1999.
18. Horn-Ross PL, Morrow M, Ljung BM: Diet and the risk of salivary gland cancer. Am J Epidemiol 146:171–176, 1997.
19. Joossens JV, Hill MJ, Elliot P, et al: Dietary salt, nitrate and stomach cancer mortality in 24 countries. European Cancer Prevention (ECP) and INTERSALT Cooperative Research Group. Int J Epidemiol 25:494–504, 1996.
20. Lindbald P, Wolk A, Bergstrom R, et al: Diet and risk of renal cell cancer: A population-based case-control study. Cancer Epidemiol Biomarkers Prev 6:215–223, 1997.
21. Position of the American Dietetic Association: Vitamin and mineral supplementation. J Am Diet Assoc 96:73, 1996.
22. Rivadeneira DE, Evoy D, Fahey TJ, et al: Nutritional support of the cancer patient. CA Cancer J Clin 48(2):69–80, 1998.
23. Rock CL, Jacob RA, Bowen PE: Update on the biological characteristics of the antioxidant micronutrients: Vitamin C, Vitamin E, and the carotenoids. J Am Diet Assoc. 96:693–702, 1996.
24. Schattner M: Enteral nutritional support of the patient with cancer: Route and role. J Clin Gastroenterol 36:297–302, 2003.
25. Shephard RJ: Exercise and cancer: Linkages with obesity? Crit Rev Food Sci Nutr 36:321–339, 1996.
26. Snyderman CH: Nutrition and head and neck cancer. Curr Oncol Rep 5:158–163, 2003.
27. Stoll BA: Obesity and breast cancer. Int J Obes Relat Metab Disord 20:389–392, 1996.
28. Tang FY, Nguyen N, Meydani M: Green tea catechins inhibit VEGF-induced angiogenes in vitro through suppression of VE-cadherin phosphorylation and inactivation of Akt molecule. Int J Cancer 106:871–878, 2003.
29. Tavani A, Pregnolato A, Negri E, et al: Alcohol consumption and risk of pancreatic cancer. Nutr Cancer 27:157–161, 1997.
30. Van Bokhorst-De Van Der Schueren MA, Quak JJ, von Blomberg-van der Fleir BM, et al: Effect of perioperative nutrition, with and without arginine supplementation, on nutritional status, immune function, postoperative morbidity, and survival in severely malnourished head and neck cancer patients. Am J Clin Nutr 73:323–332, 2001.
31. Wu AH, Yu MC, Tsent CC, et al: Green tea and risk of breast cancer in Asian Americans. Int J Cancer 106:574–579, 2003.

17. VEGETARIAN DIETS

Peter L. Beyer, MS, RD

1. What is a vegetarian diet?

A vegetarian diet can take several forms, and the degree of adherence to the dietary pattern may vary greatly among individuals. The categories listed below are just a few forms of the vegetarian diet. Other versions from religious, cultural, and faddist groups may result in further modifications. The definitions below are not necessarily "official" or exclusive terms but are used to help describe types of food groups typically included/excluded. Some individuals may be "casual" vegetarians in that they may only occasionally restrict specific types of meat (e.g., beef or beef and pork); some persons may limit their diet more than the most restrictive category described below. When nutrition adequacy is of concern, it is appropriate to inquire into actual dietary practices, the degree to which they are followed, and the duration of the dietary patterns.

- Vegan: usually the strictest of vegetarian categories; includes fruits, vegetables, grains, nuts, and legumes. In a small percent of individuals, only raw foods are consumed.
- Lacto-ovo vegetarian: includes fruits, vegetables, grains, nuts and legumes, milk and milk products, eggs (may also be only lacto or only ovo).
- Pesco vegetarian: like lacto-ovo but adds fish.
- Semi- or pseudo-vegetarian: poultry and fish or fowl may be consumed in addition to the lacto-ovo or pesco diet. Some individuals, when asked if they practice vegetarianism, simply mean that they eat some vegetables.

2. How do the vegetarians' diets differ from the typical Western diet in terms of nutrient content?

The typical Western diet is high in protein and sugars and fairly high in saturated fatty acids, n-6 fatty acids, trans fatty acids, total fat, and total calories. Meat consumption and protein intake are fairly high, and fruit and vegetable intake is only about half the 5 or more servings recommended from the combined group daily. Our diets are typically low in fiber and low in omega-3 fatty acids. Western dietary habits translate to low-to-marginal intakes of calcium, vitamin D, folate, vitamin B_6, potassium, magnesium, copper, zinc, and iron. The groups most commonly lacking adequate nutrient intake include infants, teen-age girls, women, and the elderly.

Removing animal products (meats, fishes, eggs, and dairy products) from the American diet decreases protein but also removes a major source of fat, calories, iron, calcium, and vitamin B_{12}. Vegetarian diets tend to be lower in protein, saturated fat, N-3 fatty acids, cholesterol, and calories. Vegetarian diets are normally higher in omega-6 fatty acids and dietary fiber than the typical Western diet. Nutrient content may vary greatly, however, depending on the individual's dietary practices. Vegan diets tend to be lower in total fat and calories than lacto-ovo diets, and meeting micronutrient needs is more difficult. On the positive side, intake of fruit and vegetables, whole grains, legumes, and nuts tends to be greater in all types of vegetarian patterns than standard Western diets.

3. Are vegetarian diets healthier than the typical American diet?

The answer is a qualified yes. Epidemiologic and case-control studies in vegetarian groups show lower rates of all-cause morbidity and mortality. In prospective studies, carefully selected vegetarian diets usually result in several positive health outcomes compared with traditional eating habits. The benefits include decreased risk of coronary artery disease and hypertension, lower body mass index, fewer deaths from type II diabetes, decreased morbidity from renal disease, and decreased risk of several types of cancers. Vegetarian diets or high fruit and vegetable intake is associated with lower risk for lung, oral, pharyngeal, laryngeal, esophageal, colorectal, breast and endometrial cancers.

4. What is it about the vegetarian diet that improves health risks?

The lower risk of coronary artery disease and hypertension may be due to lower intake of saturated fat and cholesterol and greater intake of dietary fiber, potassium, antioxidants, nutrients, certain vitamins, plant sterols, and other protective phytochemicals. Lower risk of several forms of cancer may also be related to the protective effects of phytochemicals, antioxidants, and fiber as well as lower fat and protein consumption in the vegetarian diet. Consumption of fruits, vegetables, nuts, and whole grains appears to be among the strongest protective factors for many health issues. Consumption of small amounts of low-fat animal foods, however, along with an abundance of fruits and vegetables, does not increase health risks. In countries where a wide variety of plant foods is not always available, eating meats probably adds to the population's well-being.

5. Do lifestyle patterns of vegetarians (other than diet) influence health risks?

Yes. Vegetarians tend to smoke less, consume more fiber and less alcohol, and exercise more. The vegetarian-type diet, however, still tends to be protective when the lifestyle risk factors are controlled for. In other words, smoking, excessive alcohol consumption, and a sedentary lifestyle are risk factors for both vegetarians and omnivores. Vegetarians may suffer the consequences of adverse lifestyles somewhat less than omnivores.

6. Can one assume that people will improve their diet by eating a vegetarian diet?

No. Compared with most Western diets any type of vegetarian diet tends to result in a better diet and improved health. In some persons, however, a vegetarian diet simply translates to a bad diet without meat. Many vegetarians know little about nutrition or health and may not improve health at all. Vegan diets lack several nutrients (see below) and require more planning to meet nutrient requirements. Some lacto-ovo vegetarians may consume rather large amounts of high-fat dairy products and choose high-calorie, high-fat forms of other foods—somewhat negating the benefits of reducing meats in the diet. In a small percent of adolescent males and females, vegetarian diets also may signal disordered eating practices as well as other health concerns.

7. Can one meet all nutrient requirements with a vegetarian diet?

Yes. But the more restrictive the form of vegetarian diet, the more care is required to meet nutrient needs. A well-selected lacto-ovo diet can meet the needs of most individuals with perhaps the exception of vitamin B_{12}. Incidence of low serum B_{12} and elevated homocysteine levels have been reported in some vegetarian groups, which may negate some cardioprotective value of vegetarian diets. Vitamin B_{12} is found in eggs and dairy products, but serum B_{12} levels of lacto-ovo vegetarians are not as high as in omnivores. Most cow milk is fortified with vitamin D, but not all dairy products are fortified. If the person's sunlight exposure is not adequate, vitamin D may need to be added. Zinc is another nutrient that may be lacking in some vegetarian diets. Many cereals, juices, milk, and meat substitutes have supplemental nutrients to increase the nutrient content. Non-heme iron from plant foods is not well absorbed, but the increased levels of ascorbic acid in the vegetarian diets may facilitate the absorption.

Vegan diets do not provide sufficient iron or calcium for pregnant women and infants. Premenopausal women may have low iron stores but may not be iron-deficient unless they are multiparous, have unusual blood losses, or participate in strenuous athletic events. Fortified foods or vitamin mineral supplements can be recommended to complete nutrient needs.

Nutrients That May Be Lacking in Vegetarian Diets

TYPE OF DIET	ALL GENDERS, AGES	PREGNANT FEMALES, INFANTS
Lacto-ovo	Vitamins B_{12} and D	+ Iron
Vegan	Vitamins B_{12} and D, calcium, zinc	+ Iron, calcium, zinc, calories

8. Does one have to combine foods on vegan diets in a certain way to get all of the essential amino acids?

No. Older recommendations were to combine plant foods that were lacking in specific amino acids with other foods that provided them at each meal. More recent studies show that if the diet is adequate in total protein and includes a mixture of foods consumed in a 24-hour period, the amino acid needs for protein synthesis can be met. However, consumption of higher-quality plant proteins, such as legumes and soy products, is normally recommended to provide sufficient protein in vegan diets.

9. How can one assure that nutrient needs are being met when consuming a vegetarian diet?

For a **lacto-ovo vegetarian** diet nutritional needs can generally be met with the following combination of foods:
• Breads, grains, cereals (primarily whole grain): 6–11 servings
• Legumes: 1–2 servings
• Vegetables (including dark green leafy): 3–5 servings
• Fruits: 2–4 servings
• Nuts and seeds: 1–2 servings
• Milk, yogurt, or cheese: 1–3 servings
• Eggs: 1–2 servings

For a vegan diet:
• Breads, grains, cereals (primarily whole grain): 8–12 servings
• Legumes: 1–3 servings
• Vegetables (including dark green leafy): 4–6 servings
• Fruits: 2–5 servings
• Nuts and seeds: 1–2 servings
• Fortified soy products: 1–3 servings

In each case, the number of servings required depends on the calorie and protein requirements of the individual. For especially the higher calorie ranges for the vegan diet, additional fats and carbohydrates may be required to meet calorie requirements. For vegans, several plant-based foods and beverages are fortified with calcium and other nutrients.

BIBLIOGRAPHY

1. Donaldson MS: Metabolic vitamin B_{12} status on a mostly raw vegan diet with follow-up using tablets, nutritional yeast, or probiotic supplements. Ann Nutr Metab 44:229–234, 2000.
2. Frazer GE: Associations between diet and cancer, ischemic heart disease and all-cause mortality in non-hispanic white California Seventh-day Adventists. Am J Clin Nutr 70S:532–538, 1999.
3. Haddad EH, Sabate J, Whitten CG: Vegetarian food guide pyramid: A conceptual framework. Am J Clin Nutr 70S:616S–619S, 1999.
4. Messina VK, Burke KI: Position of the American Dietetic Association: Vegetarian diets. J Am Dietet Assoc 97:1317–1321, 1997.
5. Nestle M: Animal v. plant foods in human diets and health: Is the historical record unequivocal? Proc Nutr Soc 58:211–218, 1999.
6. Perry CL, Mcquire MT, Neumark-Sztainer D, Story M: Characteristics of vegetarian adolescents in a multiethnic urban population. J Adolesc Health 29:406–416, 2001.
7. Potter JD: Cancer prevention: Epidemiology and experiment. Lancer Lett 114:283–286, 1997.
8. Walter P: Effects of vegetarian diets on aging and longevity. Nutr Rev 55S:S61–S68, 1997.
9. Willett WC: Convergence of philosophy and science: The Third International Congress on Vegetarian Nutrition. Am J Clin Nutr 70S:434S–438S, 1999.

18. HEALTH FOOD AND NUTRITIONAL SUPPLEMENTS

Stanley M. Augustin, MD, and Charles W. Van Way III, MD

1. What is the difference between health foods, nutritional supplements, and herbal medicines?

The use of alternative medicines is increasingly widespread in the world. Surveys report that at least one-third of Americans used herbal medicines in a year. In Germany millions of prescriptions for herbal medicines are written each year. This chapter deals with some of the most commonly used nutritional supplements not discussed elsewhere in the book.

Health foods are foods that serve a health purpose, such as protein supplements used by body builders. Nutritional supplements provide concentrated amounts of specific nutrients or other active ingredients such as vitamins and fiber. Herbal medicines are the leaves, flowers, bark, roots, seeds, or berries of plants and are used for the treatment of diseases. There is overlap between herbal medicines and nutritional supplements. For example, garlic can be classified as health food, nutritional supplement, or medicinal herb.

Herbal medicines include a wide spectrum of substances ranging from homemade teas prepared from collected herbs to regulated medicinal products. At least 122 distinct chemical substances derived from plants are important pharmaceutical agents. In the pharmacopoeias of developed countries, 25% of the drugs are substances first isolated from plants and another 25% are modifications of chemical first found in plants. A standard textbook in the field lists more than 100 separate medicinal herbs; one catalog lists over 200 items, some of which are combinations. The *Materia Medica Pharmacopoeia*, a 400-year-old book of Chinese herbal, mineral, and animal medicines, lists 1900 preparations.

2. How are health foods and nutritional supplements regulated?

The U.S. Food and Drug Administration is charged with regulating food, nutritional supplements, and pharmaceuticals. The 1994 Dietary Supplement Health and Education Act set up a new framework for FDA regulation of dietary supplements. The FDA oversees safety, manufacturing, and product information such as claims in labeling, package inserts, and accompanying literature. The Federal Trade Commission regulates the advertising of dietary supplements.

Anything that is sold as a food or nutritional supplement has to be accurately labeled and should contain the product advertised and should be pure and free of harmful substances. The FDA has a greater authority over pharmaceutics than foods or nutritional supplements. Pharmaceutical agents must be tested extensively to determine their precise dosage and effect and cannot be sold to treat a disease until clinical trials have been done. Nutritional supplements or herbal medicines do not have to meet such strict requirements as long as no specific medical claims are made for them. Such products can be sold under "structure and function claims," such as "improves blood flow." The FDA does not authorize or test dietary supplements before they go to the market. Once a dietary supplement is marketed, the FDA has to prove that it is unsafe before it can take action to restrict its use.

3. What is echinacea?

Echinacea is currently a top-selling herbal product in the U.S. It is derived from the above-ground parts of the echinacea plant. There are three species of echinacea: *Echinacea angustifolia*, *Echinacea pallida*, and *Echinacea purpurea*. It has suggested that echinacea enhances phagocytosis, modulates cytokines, and activates both macrophages and natural killer cells, increasing nonspecific immunity. Echinacea is used for the prevention and treatment of upper respiratory infections as well as treatment of chronic wounds, chronic arthritis, and the adverse effects of chemotherapeutic agents.

4. What is garlic?

Garlic is a member of the onion family. It has been claimed to be beneficial in infections, tumors, diabetes, hypertension, hyperlipidemia, and arteriosclerosis. The sulphur-rich compounds in garlic that contain cysteine mediate its medicinal properties. The thiosulphate allicin is formed when the garlic bulb is crushed. Allicin has been shown to inhibit 3-hydroxy-3-methyl-glutaryl co-enzyme A reductase (HMG-CoA), an important enzyme in cholesterol biosynthesis. It also inhibits platelet aggregation.

5. What is ginseng?

Ginseng has been used in Eastern medicine as a stimulant, tonic, and diuretic. This root is one of the most popular herbs in the world. Of three main species of ginseng, *Panax ginseng* is the most commonly used. The active ingredient is ginenoside, a glycosylated steroid. Its benefits include immunomodulation, mood elevation, increased vitality, and hypoglycemia.

6. What is ginkgo biloba?

Ginkgo biloba is grown worldwide as an ornamental tree. Its extract is used as an herbal medicine. The extract is believed to act as a free radical to protect vascular walls and nerve cells. It also decreases platelet aggregation, erythrocyte aggregation, and blood viscosity to increase blood flow. Additionally, ginkgo is used in Germany to treat cognitive deficits in Alzheimer's disease and multi-infarct dementia.

7. What are pine bark extract and grape seed extract?

Pine bark extract, best known under the brand name Pycnogenol, and grape seed extract appear to have antioxidant activity. The active ingredients are flavonols, which are known as *oligomeric proanthocyanidins*. The compounds are supposedly more potent than vitamin E. Grape seed extract has been said to have the cardioprotective effects of red wine but without the alcohol. Pine bark extract appears to reduce platelet aggregation. All in all, they appear to be comparable to taking vitamin E. The clinical studies showing benefit from vitamin E are more convincing than the claims made for these two extracts.

8. What is St. John's wort?

St. John's wort (*Hypericum perforatum*) is extracted from several flowers and leaves. It contains at least ten pharmacologically active compounds. It has been used for centuries for depression and anxiety. Crude extracts of St. John's wort have a high affinity for gamma-aminobutyic acid (GABA) receptors. One isolated compound, hypericin, inhibits multiple chemicals in biologic depression models. It inhibits norepinephrine and dopamine and serotonin reuptake into the synapse; it also weakly inhibits monoamine oxidases A and B.

9. What is alfalfa?

Alfalfa has been widely promoted as a mineral supplement. It contains calcium, magnesium, phosphorus, potassium, and vitamins. Besides that, it is one of a number of supplements containing chlorophyll, which is thought to have beneficial effects on the gastrointestinal tract, as well as on other organs. There is not a great deal of evidence that chlorophyll ingestion is beneficial.

10. What is valerian?

Valerian is derived from the perennial *Valerina officinalis*. It is used in Europe as an anxiolytic and sleeping aid. It inhibits the degradation and reuptake of GABA.

11. What is glucosamine?

Glucosamine, an amino sugar, is synthesized in the body from glucose and glutamine. It is a precursor of collagen synthesis. It is one of the standard food supplements. People have recommended it for asthma, bursitis, food allergies, osteoporosis, tendinitis, and skin problems. It is sold under a number of brand names and is also available as the similar compound, N-acetyl glucosamine (NAG).

12. What is hongqu?
Hongqu is a traditional Chinese herbal medicine derived from a red yeast grown on rice. Among its 15–20 ingredients is lovastatin, which is a pharmaceutical used to lower cholesterol.

13. Is honey a health food?
Interestingly enough, honey is not just a sugar syrup. It contains 20–35% protein and has some vitamin content. For that reason, many health food advocates and vegetarians favor it over other sugars. Its popularity as a health food is not new. It was quite widely used during the 1960s, especially in the counterculture. There was, and is, a general feeling that the "natural" sweetness of honey is superior to processed sugar.

14. What is the benefit of yeast?
Brewer's yeast, otherwise known as nutritional yeast, is grown on hops, much as in beermaking, then harvested and killed. The resultant product is about half protein and contains a large amount of B-complex vitamins and minerals. It serves basically as a protein supplement and is thought to boost energy. It also is thought to enhance the immune system.

15. What is wheat germ?
Wheat germ is perhaps the most widely-known health food. It is formed from the embryo of the wheat berry. It contains vitamin E, the B-complex vitamins, and a number of minerals. It is thought by its advocates to be without equal as a breakfast food, providing energy during the entire day. It is used as a general nutritional supplement.

16. What about corn germ?
Corn germ is very analogous to wheat germ. Made from the embryo of the corn plant, it contains especially high values of zinc. It is used in a similar fashion to wheat germ.

17. Does the average individual need supplemental fiber?
The typical diet in America, and indeed throughout the Western world, is high in processed foods and relatively low in fiber. For that reason, such high-fiber foods as whole-grain cereals, brown rice, bran, dried and fresh fruit, nuts, seeds, lentils, peas, and fresh vegetables should be a part of the normal diet.

Fiber can be divided into no less than seven categories: bran, cellulose, gum, hemicellulose, lignin, mucilages, and pectin. Nearly all are found in whole grains. Bran, gums, and mucilages are related. They are found in oatmeal, oat bran, and such supplements as fennel seed, glucomannan, guar gum, and psyllium seed. Cellulose is a component of most vegetables and such fruits as apples and pears. Hemicellulose is another indigestible carbohydrate which absorbs water and is therefore good for adding bulk to the diet. It controls constipation and promotes weight loss. It is found in green leafy vegetables, apples, bananas, pears, beets, and cabbage. Lignin, found in carrots, green beans, peaches, strawberries, peas, and tomatoes, supposedly helps to lower cholesterol. Pectin, found in grapefruits, oranges, apples, bananas, beets, peas, and okra, is another fiber which slows food absorption after meals. It supposedly helps to prevent the post-prandial hyperglycemia seen in diabetics, lowers cholesterol, and reduces the risk of heart attacks and gallstones. Grapefruit pectin has actually been put to therapeutic trial as a cardioprotective and cholesterol-lowering agent. As might be expected, there are a number of combination supplements on the market.

18. What is the benefit of grapefruit?
The juice of the grapefruit contains compounds that may decrease atherosclerotic plaque formation and inhibit cancer cell proliferation.

19. What is ginger?

The tuberous part of the ginger plant is used for the treatment of headaches, colds, indigestion, and rheumatologic conditions. Gingerol is the active component of ginger, but its mechanism is unclear. It seems to stimulate the GI tract either centrally or via serotonin. Its anti-inflammatory effect is via inhibiting arachidonic acid metabolism.

20. What is Ma Huang?

Ephedra or *ma huang* is a popular and controversial medicine. It is obtained from the roots and branches of a shrub native to central Asia. Traditionally it is used for asthma and bronchitis. It has appetite-suppression properties and is popular as a weight loss agent. Ma huang contains numerous alkaloids such as ephedrine, pseudoephedrine, methyl ephedrine, and norpseudoephedrine. The ephedrine is a noncatecholamine sympathomimetic agent that acts indirectly as the alpha- and beta-adrenergic receptors, causing increased blood pressure and heart rate. There are numerous reports of adverse reactions, such as seizures, hypertensive emergencies, myocardial infarctions, strokes, and multiple deaths related to ephedra. It has recently been restricted in the U.S.

21. Does the use of nutritional supplements give any athletic advantage?

Recent analysis of the available studies of the most popular nutritional supplements (androstenedione, creatine, chromium, ephedra, and protein and amino acid supplements) have shown that only creatine may be marginally beneficial. The benefit was found to be only marginal in professional athletes. Since most of the products have side effects, the authors have cautioned against their use.

BIBLIOGRAPHY

1. Food and Drug Administration: Dietary Supplements Containing Ephedrine Alkaloids. Washington, DC, FDA, 1997.
2. Food and Drug Administration: Overview of Dietary Supplements. Washington, DC, Center for Food Safety and Applied Nutrition, 2001.
3. Gershwin ME, German JB, Keen C: Nutrition and Immunology: Principles and Practice. Humana Press, 1999.
4. Lawrence ME, Kirby DF: Nutrition and sports supplements: Fact or fiction? J Clin Gastroenterol 35(4):299–306, 2002.

V. Nutrition and Weight

19. NUTRITIONAL MANAGEMENT OF WEIGHT LOSS

Paul G. Cuddy, PharmD, Theresa A. Fessler, MS, RD, CNSD,
Cheryl A. Gibson, PhD, and L. Beaty Pemberton, MD

1. What is the difference between the terms overweight and obese?
Overweight implies more weight than desirable for a given frame size and gender. Many people are overweight without being obese. **Obese** refers to a specific excess of body fat. It is theoretically possible for a patient to be obese but not overweight. However, most clinicians define obesity as the next step beyond overweight.

The exact classification of a given patient is sometimes arbitrary. Many clinicians base the determination of obesity on published tables of weight, according to age, gender, height, and body build. The Metropolitan Height and Weight Tables of 1983 are a good reference. One often-used definition of obesity is 20% above the upper limit of the normal range. In the United States, overweight is presently defined as a body mass index (BMI) between 25 and 29.9 kg/m², whereas obesity is defined as a BMI of 30 kg/m² or greater.

2. How many overweight adults exist in the United States? Do high-risk groups exist?
The age-adjusted prevalence of obesity was recently reported (1999–2000) at 30.5%, up from 22.9% in NHANES III. The prevalence of overweight also increased to 64.5% from 55.9%. The prevalence of extreme obesity also increased from 2.9% to 4.7%. The NHANES III study identified a much higher overweight prevalence in black, non-Hispanic women (52.3%) and Mexican-American women (50.1%). Mexican-American males (36.4%) demonstrated a higher overweight prevalence than other male subgroups. The NHANES study also found that roughly 14% of children and 12% of adolescents were overweight.

3. What is the body mass index (BMI)? How is it calculated?
The BMI (or Quetelet index) is the most commonly recommended method for classifying body weight. It is easily calculated by dividing the patient's weight in kilograms by the square of the patient's height in meters.

Example: What is the BMI for a 70-inch-tall patient weighing 220 pounds?

Converting inches and pounds to meters and kilograms, this patient is 1.78 m tall and weighs 100 kg. Therefore:

$$BMI = 100 \text{ kg}/(1.78 \text{ m})^2 = 31.6 \text{ kg/m}^2$$

4. How should BMI be used to classify body weight in patients?

	OBESITY CLASS	BMI (kg/m²)
Underweight		< 18.5
Normal		18.5–24.9
Overweight		25.0–29.9

(Table continued on next page.)

	OBESITY CLASS	BMI (kg/m^2)
Obesity		
Class I	I	30.0–34.9
Class II	II	35.0–39.9
Extreme obesity	III	≥ 40.0

5. What are the major consequences of obesity in adults?
Conditions associated with increased morbidity in overweight and obese patients include coronary heart disease, hypertension, type 2 diabetes, osteoarthritis, sleep apnea, stroke, gallstones, and cancer (endometrial, postmenopausal breast, and colon).

6. What essential issues should be addressed in assessing an overweight patient?
There are six steps to the *Shape Up America* treatment model:
1. Weigh the patient, and calculate the BMI
2. Identify the existence of any co-morbidities of obesity
3. Identify other risk factors (e.g., waist/hip ratio > 1.0 in males, and 0.8 in females)
4. Determine the patient's health-related risk (based on BMI and existence of co-morbidities)
5. Determine any weight reduction exclusions (e.g., pregnancy, anorexia nervosa)
6. Determine the patient's readiness to lose weight
The table in the following question can be used to identify health risk based solely on BMI or to identify the adjusted risk (based on BMI and the presence of 1 or more comorbidities).

7. What are the main treatment modalities for weight reduction? When are they indicated?
According to the *Shape Up America* treatment protocol, the following approach is reasonable:

BMI CATEGORY	HEALTH RISK	ADJUSTED RISK
< 25	Minimal	Low
25–27	Low	Moderate
27–30	Moderate	High
30–35	High	Very high
35–40	Very high	Extremely high
> 40 (morbid obesity)	Extremely high	Extremely high

For people at minimal or low health risk, a healthy diet, increased physical activity, and lifestyle changes are appropriate. People at moderate health risk should follow the same principles and restrict calories. People at high or very high risk become candidates for pharmacotherapy following measures for those at minimal-to-moderate risk. For people at extremely high health risk, surgical interventions may be warranted.

8. What major types of weight loss programs are available? For whom is each type appropriate?
In *Weighing the Options*, three major types of weight loss programs are identified: self-help, nonclinical, and clinical. A person may be appropriate for a **self-help type of plan** if he or she is educated in wise food choices and understands potential risks involved. People or small groups may utilize self-help books, videos, or other weight loss products when conducting their own weight loss plans.

Nonclinical programs are often commercialized and are supervised by layperson counselors who are trained in the use of certain food products and/or behavior modification techniques. These counselors might have no formal educational background in weight loss, but their training should be approved by health professionals. Nonclinical programs may be appropriate for the generally healthy patient who lacks sufficient motivation or knowledge in the area of weight loss and who requires frequent reinforcement for behavior modification. Nonclinical plans should be avoided by patients who have diseases for which specific dietary restrictions are necessary or who have other physical or mental health problems that require medical monitoring. **Clinical weight loss programs** are run by one or a group of licensed professionals and may or may not be part of a commercial business. Some clinical programs involve a multidisciplinary team, including physicians, dietitians, psychologists, and exercise physiologists. Multidisciplinary clinical programs are useful for severely obese patients who have failed with other weight loss approaches or for any patient who requires frequent medical follow-up. In addition to more formalized weight loss programs, many hospitals provide outpatient weight loss counseling for either individuals or groups that are facilitated by registered dietitians. Participation in these programs usually requires physician's orders. Clinical programs are useful for patients who have specific dietary needs or restrictions and for those who desire individual rather than group counseling.

9. How much weight loss is necessary to achieve reductions in the comorbidities of obesity?

Surprisingly little. The ultimate goal is a sustained reduction in weight. It is far more sensible to set modest but realistic weight loss targets initially than to set unrealistic goals. A weight loss of as little as 10–15 pounds, for example, can be associated with meaningful reductions in blood pressure, glycosylated hemoglobin, and cholesterol. In most overweight adults, a reduction of 15 pounds of excess body weight translates to a loss of 2–3 BMI units. Once the patient is trained in a more productive but sustainable eating style and lifestyle, it becomes practical to look at continuing modest weight loss over a 1- to 2-year period.

10. What are very low calorie diets (VLCDs)? What are some important considerations?

VLCDs provide 400–800 kilocalories and 45–100 gms of protein per day in the form of regular foods or as liquid formulas. These diets are intended to produce 18–20 kg weight loss in 12 weeks. Another definition for VLCD is a diet that provides less than or equal to 10 kCal/kg. VLCDs were popular in the mid 1970s and early and late 1980s. VLCDs should last for no more than 3 months. In practical use, they are often preceded by a 1200–1500 kilocalorie balanced diet. VLCDs are designed to provide adequate complete protein, vitamins, and minerals, with severe restriction of fat and carbohydrate. If regular foods are used, a vitamin/mineral supplement should be included. Patients should also drink 2 liters of a noncaloric fluid daily. After the VLCD, patients return to a gradual refeeding period, followed by a balanced calorie-restricted diet to prevent weight regain.

11. Describe the evaluation and monitoring of patients on very low calorie diets.

Initial evaluation of patients for VLCDs should consist of physical examination and history, including diet and weight history, medications, and laboratory tests. During the diet period, patients should be carefully monitored by a physician and dietitian and provided with counseling for proper eating behaviors. Nutrient deficiencies, electrolyte imbalance, development of gallstones, and excessive loss of lean body mass are risks. Patients are likely to regain the weight after completion of the VLCD. A long-term maintenance plan, specifically designed with behavior modification techniques in relation to maintaining a healthy diet and engaging in physical activity, is essential for success.

12. Which types of patients are suitable for very low calorie diets?

VLCDs have been recommended for patients who are at least 30% overweight and who do not have cancer, type 1 diabetes mellitus, hepatic or renal disease, cardiac dysfunction, or severe psychological problems. VLCDs should not be used by pregnant or lactating women, children, adolescents, or the elderly. Patients opting for VLCDs should have failed at other more conventional methods of weight loss or have a medical reason for rapid weight loss. Patients must be willing to change their eating behaviors and levels of physical activity for long-term maintenance of weight loss.

13. What is the benefit of exercise along with diet in achieving weight loss?
Physical activity may minimize the decline in basal metabolic rate that occurs with caloric restriction, thus promoting continued weight loss. Physical exercise helps prevent loss of lean body mass that can occur during weight loss diets while enhancing loss of body fat. Exercise enhances psychological well-being and suppresses appetite. Exercise is beneficial to the heart, improves sensitivity to insulin, reduces hypertension, and improves serum lipid profiles.

The increased energy expenditure of physical activity might increase the dieter's need for protein to avoid negative nitrogen balance. Severely obese patients should exercise with caution, because they have lower tolerance for physical activity. The American Heart Association stresses the importance of including an exercise component in weight management programs. Regular exercise also appears to help maintain long-term weight maintenance and prevent weight gain, which frequently accompanies aging.

14. Why are several popular diets high in protein and very low in carbohydrate?
High protein diets, in a variety of forms, are a perennial in the popular diet industry. They are effective for a number of reasons. Lowering the carbohydrate intake does lower the overall calories. The diet is intended to change the body's metabolism toward the utilization of fat stores. Plasma insulin levels are lower in a low-carbohydrate diet, thus promoting ketosis and the use of fat for energy. Carbohydrate is needed to fuel the Krebs cycle; thus ketosis occurs with the absence of carbohydrate. Protein produces more diet-induced thermogenesis than does carbohydrate or fat; theoretically, therefore, it can increase energy expenditure. Finally, the dieter may be pleasantly impressed with the large initial loss of weight, which is in part due to diuresis.

In any diet, adequate protein is necessary to help spare lean body mass, which is at risk for being lost with caloric restriction. Weight loss diets should provide at least 0.8–1.5 grams of protein per kg of ideal body weight per day.

15. What amount of caloric restriction is recommended in a conventional weight loss diet?
Five hundred kilocalories per day deficit promotes a theoretical loss of 1 lb of body fat per week (3500 kcal per 1 lb of fat). When prescribing caloric levels for weight loss, dietitians typically subtract 500 kcal from estimated energy need calculations. Patients should be reminded that if weight loss is too rapid and extreme, loss of lean body mass can occur.

An "acceptable" weight loss, consisting of 75% fat and 25% lean body mass can be achieved by a deficit of 3500 kcal per lb. Thus an energy deficit of 1000 kcal per day can result in 1 pound of weight loss in 3.2 days, or 2 pounds per week. Increasing the rate of weight loss beyond 2 lb per week will lower the "acceptability" of weight loss because a greater percentage of lean tissue will be lost.

16. Is the proportion of fat and carbohydrate calories in a diet plan important, or is appropriate weight loss dependent only on total amount of calories?
A balanced diet in which most nonprotein calories come from carbohydrate is recommended over a diet that contains a high percentage of fat. Dietary carbohydrate is more effective at sparing body proteins than is fat. Fat in the diet may also be converted to body fat more efficiently than carbohydrate. Carbohydrates produce more diet-induced thermogenesis than fats. In addition, fat is much more calorie-dense; thus, if a diet contains a high proportion of fat calories, the overall quantity of food would need to be more severely restricted.

17. How are diet drinks useful for weight loss? Are they always beneficial?
Diet drinks are useful as nutritionally balanced meal replacements for dieters who have difficulty making proper food choices or for whom conventional foods may cause temptation to overeat. These drinks are low in fat and provide protein, carbohydrate, fiber, and vitamins and minerals. When used properly, these supplements can assist in weight loss; however, they do not assure long-term weight control. Use of diet drinks should be combined with counseling for

behavior modification and education for better eating habits. Patients should be cautioned that the drinks themselves do not promote weight loss and are an additional source of calories if merely added to their current diet.

18. Which nutrients may require supplementation or are of particular importance for patients on weight loss diets?

Aside from calorie restriction, a person on a weight loss diet should pay specific attention to water, vitamins, minerals, and protein foods.

19. Why is additional water recommended?

Additional water is always recommended for patients on low-calorie diets to aid in excretion of ketones, to prevent dehydration, and to provide a feeling of fullness to help avoid overeating. If fiber intake has been increased, additional water is necessary to avoid fecal impaction. Water is not only energy-free, but also it costs energy to raise it to body temperature. Theoretically, it takes 10 kilocalories to raise a 12-ounce glass of cold water to body temperature. In addition, if the patient is drinking extra water, it is unlikely that he or she will be drinking excessive calorie-containing fluids.

20. Why is a multivitamin and/or mineral supplement necessary?

A multivitamin and/or mineral supplement is necessary for patients on calorie levels of 1200 or below, because the amount of food is usually inadequate to provide all nutrient requirements. Loss of sodium and potassium can take place along with the diuresis that occurs with rapid weight loss. Inadequate vitamins and minerals can be a problem if excess sugars, fats, or alcoholic beverages are used in a diet plan. For example, on a calorie-restricted diet, a woman may not eat an adequate amount of dairy foods and thus requires a calcium supplement.

For a patient who is in the refeeding stages after a very low calorie diet, potassium, magnesium, and phosphorus may need to be supplemented. These minerals can be driven intercellularly because of carbohydrate metabolism, insulin secretion, and anabolism, causing plasma levels to drop dangerously low.

21. How is adequate intake of high-quality protein ensured?

Adequate high-quality protein is also important during caloric restriction. High-quality protein can be gained from eating lean meats, poultry, fish, eggs, and nonfat dairy products. Lack of protein can lead to malnutrition, excessive loss of lean body mass, and depressed immune function.

22. Why are dieters encouraged to eat 3 meals per day instead of just 1 large meal?

Cholesterol, triglyceride, and insulin levels will be lower if calories are spaced throughout the day rather than eaten all at once. Eating at three separate times each day increases the likelihood that a person receives a variety of foods and therefore a more balanced nutrient intake. Eating breakfast and lunch should also decrease the likelihood that a person overeats in the evening.

23. What drugs facilitate weight loss?

Presently, drugs carrying FDA-approved labeling for weight loss work through the central nervous system on either the adrenergic or serotonin systems or by interfering with fat absorption within the gastrointestinal tract. The most widely used drugs for weight loss includes sibutramine and orlistat. The once popular Fen-Phen weight loss product was a combination of phentermine and fenfluramine but has been removed from the market because of its association with pulmonary hypertension and valvular heart disease. Dexfenfluramine alone has been abandoned for the same reason. Sibutramine (class IV controlled substance) works systemically. It inhibits serotonin and norepinephrine reuptake primarily and exerts weak inhibition of dopamine uptake. Orlistat works within the GI tract and inhibits gastric and pancreatic lipases, thereby inhibiting the breakdown of triglycerides; fat absorption is inhibited by approximately 30%.

24. Do drugs work for weight loss?
Yes. Sibutramine is recommended at a starting dose of 10 mg daily with subsequent titration to 15 mg per day as needed. Studies lasting from 6 months to 1 year reveal weight loss of 5–7 kg, with most loss occurring early in therapy. Up to 35% of patients lose approximately 10% of baseline weight. Orlistat should be administered with meals in a dose of 120 mg 3 times daily. Studies report that patients taking orlistat for up to 1 year lost an average of 6.1 kg of weight.

25. When is surgery indicated for weight loss?
Since the majority of overweight adults in the United States are at low-to-moderate health risk, they are not candidates for surgical weight loss therapy. However, surgery may be considered in appropriately selected patients with severe obesity defined as a BMI ≥ 40 kg/m^2 or those with a BMI of ≥ 35 mg kg/m^2 who possess a high risk for obesity-associated morbidity or mortality. Since the typical long-term weight loss from diet, exercise, and drug therapy is generally limited to 20% of baseline weight, people who need to lose 40% or 50% of body weight, such as patients with morbid obesity, are unlikely to be successful with less aggressive interventions. But even with surgery, the maximum weight loss is rarely enough to restore patients to normal body weight. A responsible patient sincerely interested in long-term weight loss may be counseled and evaluated for surgery.

26. What is the best surgical operation to facilitate weight loss?
Several operations have succeeded one another in popularity over the past 35 years since obesity surgery was first begun. The Mason shunt or gastric bypass was popularized in 1967. A small gastric pouch was created, to which a segment of jejunum was connected. The current best choice is a variant of this procedure in which the stomach is connected to a long roux-en-y loop of jejunum. This operation combines gastric restriction with partial jejunal bypass. There are many complications, ranging from mild to fatal. About one patient in 60, for example, suffers a gastric leak from the staple lines that are placed across the stomach.

A variety of jejunoileal bypass procedures were attempted. They limited nutrient absorption from the intestinal tract and created a partial malabsorption syndrome. Long-term complications include a variety of vitamin and electrolyte disturbances, biliary tract and liver malfunctions, and mechanical complications from the procedure. Most surgeons today believe the jejunoileal bypass operation is contraindicated for the treatment of morbid obesity due to the frequency of serious and sometimes life-threatening complications.

BIBLIOGRAPHY

1. American Dietetic Association: Timely statement of the American Dietetic Association: Very low calorie weight loss diets. J Am Diet Assoc 89:975–976, 1989.
2. Atkinson RL: Role of nutrition planning in the treatment for obesity. Endocrinol Metab Clin North Am 25:955–964, 1996.
3. Blackburn G: Effect of degree of weight loss on health benefits. Obesity Res 3:211–216S, 1995.
4. Bray GA, Ryan DH, Gordon D, et al: A double-blind randomized placebo-controlled trial of sibutramine. Obesity Res 4:263–270, 1996.
5. Clinical Guidelines on the Identification, Evaluation, and Treatment of Overweight and Obesity in Adults—The Evidence Report. National Institutes of Health. Obesity Res 6 (Suppl 2):51S–209S, 1998.
6. Committee to Develop Criteria for Evaluating the Outcomes of Approaches to Prevent and Treat Obesity, Food and Nutrition Board. Thomas PR (ed): Weighing the Options. Criteria for Evaluating Weight Management Programs. Washington, DC, National Academy Press, 1995.
7. Davidson MH, et al: Weight control and risk factor reduction in obese subjects treated for two years with orlistat: A randomized controlled trial. JAMA 281:235–242, 1999.
8. Flegal KM, et al: Prevalence and trends in obesity among US adults, 1999–2000. JAMA 288:1723–1727, 2002.
9. James WPT, et al: Effect of sibutramine on weight maintenance after weight loss: A randomized trial. Lancet 356:2119–2125, 2000.
10. National Task Force on the Prevention and Treatment of Obesity: Long-term pharmacotherapy of obesity. JAMA 276:1907–1915, 1996.

11. PiSunyer FX: Short term medical benefits and adverse effects of weight loss. Ann Intern Med 119:722–726, 1993.
12. Shape up America and American Obesity Association: Guidance for the treatment of obesity. 1996.
13. Sjostrong L, et al: Randomized placebo-controlled trial of orlistat for weight loss and prevention of weight regain in obese patients. Lancet 352:167–173, 1998.
14. Update: Prevalence of overweight among children, adolescents, and adults—United States, 1988–1994. MMWR 46(9):199–202, 1997.
15. Wadden TA, Vanitallie T (eds): Treatment of the Seriously Obese Patient. New York, Guilford Press, 1992.

20. EATING DISORDERS

Monique Ryan, MS, RD, CNSD

1. What is an eating disorder?

Eating disorders are psychiatric disorders. There are several types of eating disorders, but generally they are distinguished by abnormal eating patterns and cognitive distortions regarding food, weight, and body image. Currently the *Diagnostic and Statistical Manual of Mental Disorders IV* (DSM-IV) defines three eating disorders: anorexia nervosa, bulimia nervosa, and eating disorder not otherwise specified (EDNOS). Binge-eating disorder is classified under the EDNOS grouping. Anorexia athletica is a subclincal eating disorder. Despite being psychiatric disorders, eating disorders are markedly characterized by significant medical and nutrition-related complications that often impair health and can be life-threatening. Eating disorders usually begin before age 30 and affect more females than males.

2. How prevalent are eating disorders in both women and men?

Five to 10 million people in the United States are affected by eating disorders, with 5% of females and 1% of males having anorexia nervosa, bulimia nervosa, and binge-eating disorder. The lifetime occurrence of anorexia nervosa in women ranges from 0.5% to 3.7% and from 1.1% and 4.2% for bulimia nervosa. Although health care professionals are often more familiar with the diagnosis of anorexia nervosa and bulimia nervosa, patients with EDNOS account for 50% of the population with eating disorders.

3. Describe the tools available for assessing eating disorders.

Because eating disorders are complex, often hidden, and involve self-reports of eating-related behaviors, they can be difficult to assess and diagnose. The DSM-IV diagnostic criteria for eating disorders are outlined in Table 1, along with some of the physical characteristics of eating disorders. Instruments designed as diagnostic tools include the Eating Attitudes Test (EAT) and the Eating Disorder Inventory (EDI). The EAT-26 contains 26 items on which individuals self-report how statements apply to them and is the most commonly used questionnaire. The newest version of the EDI contains 91 items that focus on eleven subscales. EAT and EDI were not designed to make a clinical diagnosis of an eating disorder, but to assess the attitudes and behaviors of individuals who meet the clinical criteria for anorexia nervosa and bulimia nervosa. These instruments appear to be reliable and valid in the nonathletic population. Because most patients with an eating disorder are first assessed by a primary care physician, a list of questions as outlined in Table 2 can help detect an eating disorder.

Table 1. Eating Disorders: Physical Characteristics and Diagnostic Criteria

Anorexia Nervosa	Bulimia Nervosa
Physical characteristics	Physical characteristics
Hair loss and growth of fine body hair	Frequent weight fluctuations
Low pulse rate	Difficulty swallowing and throat damage
Sensitivity to cold	Swollen glands
Stress fractures, osteopenia, or osteoporosis	Damaged tooth enamel from gastric acid
Overuse injuries	Electrolyte imbalances and dehydration
Abnormal fatigue	Menstrual irregularities
Gastrointestinal problems	Diarrhea or constipation

(Table continued on next page.)

Table 1.   Eating Disorders: Physical Characteristics and Diagnostic Criteria (Continued)

Anorexia Nervosa (*cont.*)

Diagnostic criteria

Resistance to maintaining body weight at or
above a minimally normal weight

Intense fear of gaining weight or becoming fat
even though underweight

Distortion in the way in which one's body
weight or shape is experienced, denial of the
seriousness of current low body weight

Infrequent or absent menstrual periods in
females who have reached puberty

Bulimia Nervosa (*cont.*)

Diagnostic criteria

Recurrent episodes of binge eating, characterized by a sense of lack of control and by an
excessive amount of food within a short period

Purging behavior such as self-induced vomiting,
misuse of laxatives, diuretics, enemas, or other
medications

Binge eating and purging behavior occur on
average at least twice weekly for 3 months

Self-esteem is inappropriately influenced by
body shape and weight

Eating Disorder Not Otherwise Specified

Diagnostic criteria

Binge-eating disorder and episodes of binge
eating without the use of compensatory
behavior as seen in bulimia nervosa.

Repeatedly chewing and spitting out, but not
swallowing large amounts of food.

The criteria for anorexia nervosa are met, except
that body mass is in the normal range despite
significant weight loss.

The criteria for bulimia nervosa are met except
that the frequency of binge eating and purging
behavior occur less than twice weekly and less
than three months.

All the criteria for anorexia nervosa are met
except that the individual has regular menstrual
periods.

Regular purging behaviors occur after
consuming small amounts of food.

Binge Eating Disorder

Diagnostic criteria

Recurrent episodes of binge eating characterized by eating in a dsicrete period of time any
amount of food that is large than most people
would eat under similar circumstances, and a
sense of a lack of control.

The binge episodes are associated with three or
more of the following:

  Eating more rapidly than normal

  Eating until uncomfortably full

  Eating large amounts of food when not
  physically hungry

  Eating alone because of embarrassment of the
  volume of food

  Feeling disgusted, depressed or guilty after
  eating

There is marked distress regarding binge
eating.

The binge eating occurs on average at least
two days a week for 6 months.

The binge eating is not associated with
regular use of inappropriate compensatory
behaviors.

Anorexia Athletica

This term has been used to describe a subclinical eating disorder. It is characterized by disordered
eating and compulsive exercising. There is an intense fear of weight gain despite weighing below the
expected normal weight for age and height. Weight loss is achieved by food restrictions and extensive compulsive exercise; there may also be use of self-induced vomiting and abuse of laxatives and
diuretics

Table 2. Questions for Detecting an Eating Disorder

1. Has there been a change in your weight?
2. What did you eat yesterday?
3. Do you ever binge?
4. Have you ever used self-induced vomiting, laxatives, diuretics, or enemas to lose weight or compensate for overeating?
5. How much do you exercise in a typical week?
6. How do you feel about how you look?
7. Are your periods regular?

Adapted from Powers P, Santana C: Eating disorders: A guide for the primary care physician. Primary Care 29:81–98, 2002.

4. What are the characteristics of anorexia nervosa?

Anorexia nervosa was first described on 1874. Although it was once thought to affect mainly Caucasian women from the middle and upper socioeconomic classes, more recent data suggest that it is just as prevalent in all ethnic groups and socioeconomic classes. For African-Americans, integration into mainstream culture has resulted in greater body image dissatisfaction. Hispanics may also over-control food and exercise behaviors to achieve the culturally desirable norm. Eating disorders are also on the rise in the Asian population. Anorexics are typically 15–20% below normal weight and practice marked food avoidance. Despite being below normal weight, they exhibit an extreme fear of becoming fat and a distorted body image, and often describe themselves as ugly and fat. A body mass index (BMI) < 18.5 is considered underwieght, and a BMI < 17.5 is diagnostic for anorexia nervosa. A characteristic often shared by anorexics is perfectionism and an obsessive need for order. Anorexia is the most common cause of significant weight loss in adolescent girls. There are two subsets of anorexia nervosa. Patients with the restrictive type typically eliminate foods that contain fat and often exercise to lose weight. The binge-and-purge subset of anorexia involves bingeing and purging through self-induced vomiting, laxatives, diuretics, and enemas. About 50% of patients with anorexia nervosa eventually develop bulimia nervosa. One decade after initial diagnosis, one-third of anorexics continue to meet the criteria for diagnosis. Many of these patients also have other psychiatric disorders, such as obsessive-compulsive disorders, personality disorders, anxiety disorders, affective disorders, and substance use disorders. Abuse and trauma may precede the eating disorder in some patients.

5. What are some of the physical consequences of anorexia nervosa?

A high level of morbidity and mortality is associated with eating disorders. Without treatment, mortality has been estimated at 18–20% of anorexic patients (though 10% may be more accurate), accounting for the highest premature mortality rate of any psychiatric disorder. Cardiac-related complications, renal failure, and suicide are the most common causes of death. Physical symptoms include lanugo hair formation on the face and trunk, brittle and dry hair, dry skin, cyanosis of hands and feet, cardiac arrhythmia, bradycardia, hypothermia, orthostatic hypotension, arrested growth and development, and reduced heart mass. The starvation of anorexia nervosa can lead to delayed gastric emptying, decreased gut motility, and severe constipation. Amenorrhea, hypothalamic dysfunction, weight loss, and decreased body fat are seen in anorexia nervosa. Osteopenia and osteoporosis are potential medical complications, as are structural brain abnormalities. Laboratory values in such patients may be normal but masked by chronic dehydration. Some abnormal lab values may include electrolyte disturbances, leukopenia, thrombocytopenia, and low serum glucose. Elevated cholesterol and abnormal lipid profiles related to mild hepatic dysfunction, decreased bile acid secretion, and erratic eating patterns are often seen.

6. Is there any place for intensive nutritional support in anorexia nervosa?

Aggressive nutritional supports is indicated, if at all, for the patient who is at high risk for dying of malnutrition. Nutritional support with enteral nutrition using a nasogastric or nasoenteric tube is possible. The patient may resist this treatment, pull out the tube, or induce vomiting. Patients with anorexia nervosa can also be treated with total parenteral nutrition (TPN) and may be more accepting of this therapy than of enteral nutrition. Although TPN does not correct the psychiatric issues or abnormal dietary patterns, it does correct malnutrition and buy some time to allow the patient to undergo psychiatric and therapy designed to correct the underlying problem.

7. What is bulimia nervosa?

Bulimic patients are of normal weight or overweight and experience episodes of binge eating that is followed by purging or other inappropriate compensatory behaviors. Patients with this disorder are distinguished from people who are 15% or more below ideal body weight (IBW) and binge and purge; such people are diagnosed with the binge/purge subtype of anorexia nervosa. As in anorexia nervosa, there are also two subtypes of bulimia nervosa, the purging and nonpurging types. In all bulimics, the cycle of bingeing and inappropriate compensatory behavior must occur twice weekly for at least 3 months. Binge eaters are characterized by a lack of self-control, body image dissatisfaction, and a tendency to see themselves as fatter than they are. Self-induced vomiting and use of laxatives and diuretics characterize the purging subtype of bulimia. In the nonpurging subtype, patients fast or over-exercise. Although not a diagnostic criterion, menstrual disturbances are fairly common in bulimia nervosa. In contrast to the anorectic patient who demonstrates rigidly controlled behavior, the bulimic is often impulsive and emotionally unstable. The family situation is often chaotic, and there may be a biologic vulnerability to depression. Bulimia typically develops between mid adolescence and the late 20s and appears across the socioeconomic spectrum. Dieting to conform to societal norms of thinness may lead to bingeing, and the cycle of bingeing and compensatory behavior begins. Much of the time, the bulimic patient restricts her diet, and this restriction is a subsequent trigger for out-of-control binge eating. Purging often provides initial relief, followed by guilt and shame. These patients often have rules regarding what constitutes good and bad food. Twenty percent of patients continue to meet diagnostic criteria for bulimia nervosa 5–10 years after initial diagnosis. About 30–40% of patients with bulimia nervosa develop anorexia.

8. What are the physical consequences of bulimia nervosa?

The mortality rate of bulimia nervosa is estimated at 5% 10 years after initial diagnosis. Patients must be closely assessed for medical conditions and complications related to purging, such as gastric-esophageal reflux disease (GERD), sore throat, esophagitis, swelling of the salivary glands, and dental decay. Rupture of the esophagus at or just above the esophagogastric junction may occur. Partial esophageal tearing may produce life-threatening bleeding. Treating these medical conditions may result in reduced vomiting and allow treatment to become more focused. Depending on the extent of food restriction during the non-binge cycle, varying degrees of nutritional abnormalities can result. Purging behaviors usually do not prevent absorption and utilization of calories, with an average retention of 1200 calories from various size binges. Patients with bulimia nervosa can also suffer from cardiac arrhythmia, dehydration, electrolyte imbalance, electrocardiograph changes, cardiomyopathy, and congestive heart failure. Other symptoms include muscle weakness and fatigue.

9. Describe the diagnostic criteria for eating disorder not otherwise specified.

Many patients who present with EDNOS are subacute cases of anorexia nervosa and bulimia nervosa. Females may meet all of the criteria for anorexia nervosa except absence of menses or have a weight within the normal range despite significant weight loss. Binge eating and compensatory mechanisms may occur less frequently than twice weekly, but there is regular use of inappropriate compensatory behavior. Table 1 outlines some behavioral examples of EDNOS. The patient can also present with medical concerns, although they are not as severe as the complications in anorexia nervosa or bulimia nervosa.

10. Are there any other types of eating disorders?

EDNOS also includes binge-eating disorder (BED), which is characterized by bingeing behavior without any type of compensatory behavior. It includes consumption of a large amount of food in a discrete period of time and a sense of lack of control during the eating episode. Other characteristics include eating very rapidly, feeling uncomfortably full, eating large amounts when not hungry, and eating alone to hide the quantity of food consumed. Most patients with BED are overweight or obese and suffer from related medical complications such as diabetes, hypertension, elevated blood lipids, and gallbladder disease. Such patients often seek weight management treatment rather than eating disorder treatment. BED is listed in the Appendix of the DSM-IV but should be an official diagnostic entity in the next edition.

11. What is the most effective way to treat an eating disorder?

The most effective treatment of an eating disorder involves an interdisciplinary health care team. Psychiatric treatment is the foundation of treating these disorders, with management of medical and nutritional complications playing important roles. It is preferable that the patient be referred to a physician familiar with eating disorders for a thorough physical exam and ongoing monitoring and medication management. Psychotherapy is the responsibility of a social worker, psychologist, psychiatrist, or licensed counselor. The registered dietitian assesses the patient's nutritional status, nutrition knowledge and beliefs, and current eating patterns and implements the nutrition treatment plan. Like the psychotherapist and physician, the dietitian should have ongoing contact with the patient. Treatment may range from hospitalization on a medical or psychiatric floor to inpatient programs, outpatient day programs, and regular weekly contact with treatment team members, depending on the severity of medical and behavioral components of the eating disorder. No single professional can provide the medical, psychiatric, and nutritional care that these patients require. The team of professionals who provide this care should communicate regularly. In anorexia nervosa, some of treatment goals are attaining a healthy weight, improvement in eating behaviors, and improved psychological state. Weight restoration alone does not indicate recovery, and weight gain should not proceed without psychological support and counseling. In bulimia nervosa, it is incompatible to diet and lose weight and to recover from the eating disorder at the same time. The primary intervention goal is to normalize eating patterns and eliminate bingeing. Cognitive-behavioral therapy and medication management are highly effective in treating bulimia nervosa.

12. What groups of people are at risk for developing an eating disorder?

Groups at high risk for developing eating disorders include female adolescents, female athletes, and insulin-dependent diabetics. Eating disorders are the third most common chronic illness in adolescent females, with an incidence as high as 5%. Large numbers of adolescents may have disordered eating without meeting the strict criteria for eating disorders and can be classified as EDNOS.

Another group at high risk for developing an eating disorder is athletes. The eating disorder often results from the belief that weight loss and body fat reduction result in improved performance. Athletes also share the traits of perfectionism and compulsiveness seen in anorexia nervosa. The term *anorexia athletica* has been used to describe subclinical eating disorders in athletes and is characterized by disordered eating and compulsive exercising. The athlete may also engage in bingeing, self-induced vomiting, and laxative or diuretic use. Secondary eating disorders may develop in athletes participating in a sport where low body fat or low body mass is emphasized. Eating disorder behaviors often resolve when the athlete's career is over. Other athletes may be more susceptible to development of a full-blown clinical eating disorder.

There is some indication that eating disorders may be more common in adolescent females with type I diabetes than in their nondiabetic peers. Insulin is manipulated to induce weight loss in response to bingeing, and a cycle of dietary control and bingeing can develop. Other risk factors for developing an eating disorder include a family history of eating disorders or obesity, conflicting family dynamics, and societal pressures. It is estimated that 5–10% of all men with eating disorders have full-blown anorexia nervosa or bulimia nervosa. Such men are often members of groups that emphasize weight loss such as dancers, athletes, models, and performers. Male anorexics often have a history of obesity.

BIBLIOGRAPHY

1. American Dietetic Association: Position statement: Nutrition intervention in the treatment of anorexia nervosa, bulimia nervosa, and eating disorders not otherwise specified (EDNOS). J Am Diet Assoc 101:810–819, 2001.
2. American Psychiatric Association: Diagnostic and Statistical Manual of Mental Disorders, 4th ed. Washington, DC, American Psychiatric Association, 1994.
3. BoLinn GW, Morawski SG, Fordtran JS: Purging and calorie absorption in bulimic patients and normal women. Ann Intern Med 99:14–17, 1983.
4. Houtkooper L: Eating disorders and disordered eating in athletes. In Burke L, Deakin V (eds): Clinical Sports Nutrition, 2nd ed. New York, McGraw-Hill, 2000, pp 210–240.
5. Jones JM, Lawson ML, Daneman D, et al: Eating disorders in adolescent females with and without type I diabetes: Cross-sectional study. BMJ 320:1563–1566, 2000.
6. Kaye WH, Weltzin TE, Hsu LK, et al: Amount of calories retained after binge eating and vomiting. Am J Psychol 150:969–971, 1993.
7. Mehler PS: Diagnosis and care of patients with anorexia nervosa in primary care settings. Ann Intern Med 134:1048–1059, 2001.
8. Powers PS: Initial assessment and early treatment options for anorexia nervosa and bulimia nervosa. Psychiatr Clin North Am 19:639–655, 1996.
9. Powers P, Santana C: Eating disorders: A guide for the primary care physician. Primary Care 29:81–98, 2002.
10. Wells LA, Sadowski CA: Bulimia nervosa: An update and treatment recommendations. Curr Opin Pediatr 13:591–597, 2001.

IV. Nutrition in Specific Diseases

21. DIABETES MELLITUS

Kudakwashe M. Mushaninga, MS, RD, LD, and John M. Miles, MD

1. What is diabetes mellitus?

Diabetes mellitus is a group of metabolic diseases characterized by hyperglycemia due to defects in insulin secretion, insulin action, or both. The chronic hyperglycemia of diabetes is associated with long-term damage, dysfunction, and failure of various organs, especially the eyes, kidneys, nerves, heart, and blood vessels. Pathogenic processes involved in the development of diabetes range from autoimmune destruction of the β-cells of the pancreas with consequent insulin deficiency (common in type 1) to abnormalities that result in resistance to insulin action (common in type 2). According to the International Diabetes Federation and the American Diabetes Association, diabetes is present when fasting plasma glucose is ≥ 126 mg/dl (7 mmol/L) or greater on two occasions or 2-hour plasma glucose ≥ 200 mg/dl (11.1 mmol/l) during an oral glucose tolerance test or symptoms of diabetes and casual plasma glucose ≥ 200 mg/dl.

2. What is the prevalence of diabetes?

An estimated 17 million people have diabetes (6.2% of the American population). Approximately 11.1 million people are diagnosed, whereas 5.9 million people are undiagnosed. Clinic-based reports and regional studies indicate that type 2 diabetes is becoming more common among Native American, African American, and Hispanic and Latino children and adolescents. The risk for death among people with diabetes is about 2 times that of people without diabetes.

3. What are the most common forms of diabetes?

Type 1 diabetes (due to lack of insulin production by beta cells of the pancreas) has two forms: immune-mediated diabetes mellitus and idiopathic diabetes mellitus. Immune-mediated diabetes results from a cell-mediated autoimmune destruction of the beta cells of the pancreas. Idiopathic diabetes has an unknown etiology. Autoimmune destruction of β-cells has multiple genetic predispositions and is also related to environmental factors that are still poorly defined. Although patients are rarely obese when they present with this type of diabetes, the presence of obesity is not incompatible with the diagnosis.

Type 2 diabetes, also referred to as non–insulin-dependent diabetes or adult-onset diabetes, is a term used for people who have insulin resistance and usually relative (rather than absolute) insulin deficiency. At least initially, and often throughout their lifetime, these patients do not need insulin treatment to survive. There are probably many different causes of this form of diabetes. Identification of specific pathogenic processes and genetic defects will permit better differentiation in the future. Most patients with this form of diabetes are obese, and obesity itself causes some degree of insulin resistance.

Gestational diabetes mellitus (GDM) is defined as any degree of glucose intolerance with onset or first recognition during pregnancy. The definition applies regardless of whether insulin or only diet modification is used for treatment or whether the condition persists after pregnancy. It does not exclude the possibility that unrecognized glucose intolerance may have antedated or begun concomitantly with the pregnancy. GDM complicates 4% of all pregnancies in the U.S., resulting in 135,000 cases annually. The prevalence may range from 1% to 14% of pregnancies, depending on the population studied. Clinical recognition of GDM is important because therapy, including medical nutrition therapy, insulin when necessary, and antepartum fetal surveillance, can reduce the well-described GDM-associated perinatal morbidity and mortality. Maternal complications related to GDM also include an increased rate of cesarean delivery and chronic hypertension. GDM increases the risk of developing diabetes later in life, although not all women with GDM will develop diabetes.

4. What are the long-term complications of diabetes?

Long-term complications of diabetes include retinopathy with potential loss of vision; nephropathy leading to renal failure; peripheral neuropathy with risk of foot ulcers, amputation, and Charcot joints; and autonomic neuropathy causing gastrointestinal, genitourinary, and cardiovascular symptoms and sexual dysfunction. Glycation of tissue proteins and other macromolecules and excess production of polyol compounds from glucose are among the mechanisms thought to produce tissue damage from chronic hyperglycemia. Patients with diabetes have an increased incidence of atherosclerotic cardiovascular, peripheral vascular, and cerebrovascular disease. Hypertension, abnormalities of lipoprotein metabolism, and periodontal disease are often found in people with diabetes. The emotional and social impact of diabetes and the demands of therapy may cause significant psychosocial dysfunction in patients and their families.

5. What is the effect of weight loss on type 2 diabetes?

Almost 90% of all people with newly diagnosed type 2 diabetes are overweight. Being overweight or obese is a leading risk factor for type 2 diabetes. The recently completed Diabetes Prevention Program (DPP) proved that type 2 diabetes can be prevented or delayed by reducing weight and increasing physical activity. The DPP participants were adults who were at increased risk of developing type 2 diabetes. The study found that the participants who increased physical activity and lost 5–7% of body weight (10–15 pounds) reduced progression to diabetes by 58% during the course of the study. Weight loss has been shown to lower plasma glucose, triglycerides, and very-low-density lipoprotein (VLDL) concentrations in a high proportion of people with type 2 diabetes. Weight loss also reduces blood pressure.

6. What are the recommendations for physical activity for patients with diabetes?

The recent Surgeon General's Report on Physical Activity and Health underscores the pivotal role of physical activity in health promotion and disease prevention. It recommends that people accumulate 30 min of moderate physical activity on most days of the week. It is becoming increasingly clear that the epidemic of type 2 diabetes sweeping the globe is associated with decreasing levels of activity and an increasing prevalence of obesity. Thus, the importance of promoting physical activity as a vital component of the prevention as well as management of type 2 diabetes must be viewed as a high priority. For people with type 1 diabetes, the emphasis must be on adjusting the therapeutic regimen to allow safe participation in all forms of physical activity consistent with an individual's desires and goals. Ultimately, all patients with diabetes should have the opportunity to benefit from the many valuable effects of physical activity.

7. What are the goals of medical nutrition therapy for diabetes?

1. Attain and maintain optimal metabolic outcomes, including the following:
   - Blood glucose levels in the normal range or as close to normal as is safely possible to prevent or reduce the risk for complications of diabetes
   - A lipid and lipoprotein profile that reduces the risk for macrovascular disease
   - Blood pressure levels that reduce the risk for vascular disease
2. Prevent and treat the chronic complications of diabetes. Modify nutrient intake and lifestyle as appropriate for the prevention and treatment of obesity, dyslipidemia, cardiovascular disease, hypertension, and nephropathy.
3. Improve health through healthy food choices and physical activity.
4. Address individual nutritional needs, taking into consideration personal and cultural preferences and lifestyle while respecting the individual wishes and willingness to change.

8. Do very-low-calorie diets have a place in the management of type 2 diabetes?

Very-low-calorie diets (VLCDs) have been used to achieve short-term weight reduction in patients with diabetes. These diets are appealing because of initial dramatic improvements in the metabolic profile. However, weight regain occurs in a high proportion of individuals. The long-term benefits of VLCDs are uncertain, and they should not be recommended for the long-term management of type 2 diabetes.

9. Should simple sugars be avoided in patients with diabetes?

For many years, the official position of the American Diabetes Association (ADA) was that diabetic people should avoid simple sugars. Several studies have shown that simple sugars in the context of a mixed meal have the same effect on blood glucose levels as complex carbohydrates. Sugar is an acceptable component in the meal plan. It is not necessary to restrict milk or fruit intake in patients with diabetes. It is important to take into account the energy content of sugar-containing foods, although concentrated sweets should be discouraged. Total calorie intake is more important than macronutrient composition of a meal.

10. Should people with diabetes be on a low-fat diet?

It is interesting that this controversy arises in the diabetic more than in the nondiabetic population; a low-fat diet is still strongly recommended for the prevention and treatment of coronary artery disease. Several studies have shown that when an isocaloric high-carbohydrate, low-fat diet is compared with a diet higher in fat and lower in carbohydrate, the high-carbohydrate tends to result in hypertriglyceridemia. Because of this observation, the most recent dietary guidelines published by the ADA hedge on the subject of fat content and state that diets moderately high in monosaturated fat may be acceptable as long as saturated fat is restricted. The studies that show hypertriglyceridemia as a result of ingestion of a high-carbohydrate diet were conducted in clinical research centers and may not be relevant to free-living individuals, who tend to consume fewer calories on a low-fat diet than on a diet higher in fat. Therefore, it is probably still best to recommend a high-carbohydrate (50–60% of calories), low-fat (20–30% of calories) diet for people with type 2 diabetes.

11. What are the dietary protein requirements in diabetes?

Diabetic patients should strive for a moderate protein intake. Although it is true that protein turnover is increased in poorly controlled diabetes, this should not influence recommendations on dietary protein intake. When diabetes is controlled, protein metabolism becomes normal. The average dietary protein intake in the U.S. is 1.5 gm/kg, which is in excess of the recommended daily allowance and may contribute to nephrosclerosis and osteoporosis. Studies have shown that restricting protein in patients with diabetic nephropathy reduces proteinuria. It is, therefore, prudent for diabetic patients with renal disease or poorly controlled diabetes to avoid high-protein diets. The diabetic diet should contain moderate amounts of protein, usually 15–20% of total energy.

12. Can people with diabetes drink alcohol?

Yes, but there are certain dangers specific to diabetes. Alcohol is a potent inhibitor of gluconeogenesis. Alcohol, especially when consumed separately from a meal and without a carbohydrate (e.g., dry wine, whiskey and water), can induce hypoglycemia. This is a practical concern in patients who are taking hypoglycemic agents such as insulin and sulfonylureas. The hypoglycemic effect of alcohol is less important when it is consumed with food. Diabetic patients obtain the same salutary effects of moderate alcohol intake as anyone else, such as increased HDL cholesterol and reduced coagulability. Alcohol in moderation is acceptable in most people with diabetes provided that it does not add excessive caloric content to the meal (e.g., 1–2 glasses of wine). If diabetics choose to drink alcohol, daily intake should be limited to one drink for adult women and two drinks for adult men. One drink is defined as 12 oz of beer, 5 oz of wine, or 1.5 oz of distilled spirits. An exception is the patient with severe hypertriglyceridemia, because alcohol can worsen this condition.

13. Is micronutrient supplementation important in diabetes?
Supplementation of micronutrients is not recommended in diabetes. Physicians are often asked about chromium picolinate, which has been touted as a treatment for diabetes. Chromium is a cofactor of insulin. When rats are given a synthetic diet that does not contain chromium, they develop diabetes. There is no reliable clinical test for chromium deficiency in humans. Studies of tissue levels of chromium have suggested that subclinical chromium deficiency may occur in the elderly American population. It has been suggested that chromium deficiency may be a cause of adult onset diabetes. However it is difficult for a human on a normal diet to become deficient in chromium, and studies in which RDA levels of chromium have been given to diabetic patients have failed to show benefit, although higher levels (1000 mg) have proved beneficial. Therefore, chromium supplementation is not currently recommended. Magnesium and zinc have been suggested as supplements but are also not generally indicated. A patient with poorly controlled diabetes, especially one who is taking diuretics, may become deficient in magnesium, but no benefit has been shown from magnesium therapy in diabetics who are not magnesium-deficient. It has been suggested that zinc supplementation might aid in the healing of leg ulcers, but evidence is lacking. Zinc deficiency can retard wound healing, but zinc deficiency is extremely rare.

14. What is the best general advice to give a patient with diabetes?
Diet and exercise recommendations for diabetic patients should be similar to those for the general population, although it is more important for a diabetic patient to maintain physical fitness. A diet high in complex carbohydrate (with emphasis on fiber) and low in fat with some limitations on simple sugar and alcohol content is recommended for everyone, but especially for diabetics. Consistency of food intake is also important, to avoid episodes of hyperglycemia. Exercise, which is important for everyone, is especially important for the diabetic patient. The goal should be 5–10% body weight loss, which can reduce progression of diabetes and improve glycemic control.

BIBLIOGRAPHY

1. American Diabetes Association: Report of the Expert Committee on the Diagnosis and Classification of Diabetes Mellitus. Diabetes Care 26:S5–20, 2003.
2. American Diabetes Association: Evidence-based nutrition principles and recommendations for the treatment and prevention of diabetes and related complications. Diabetes Care 26:S51–61, 2003.
3. American Diabetes Association: Physical activity/exercise and diabetes mellitus. Diabetes Care 26:S73–77, 2003.
4. American Diabetes Association: Diabetes and your weight. Available at <http://www.diabetes.org/main/weightloss/diabetes.jsp>.
5. American Diabetes Association: National Diabetes Fact Sheet. Available at <http:www.diabetes.org/main/info/facts/facts/_natl.jsp>.
6. American Diabetes Association: Nutrition recommendations and principles for people with diabetes mellitus. Diabetes Care 17:519–522, 1994.
7. Garg A, Bonanome A, Grundy SM, et al: Comparison of a high carbohydrate diet with a high monounsaturated fat diet in patients with non–insulin-dependent diabetes mellitus. N Engl J Med 319:829–834, 1988.
8. Henry RR, Wiest-Kent TA, Schaeffer L, et al: Metabolic consequences of very low-calorie diet therapy in obese non–insulin-dependent diabetic and diabetic subjects. Diabetes 35:155–164, 1986.
9. Mahan K, Escott-Stump S (eds): Krause's Food, Nutrition and Diet Therapy, 10th ed. Philadelphia, W.B. Saunders, 2000.
10. Nuttall FQ, Brunzell JD: Principles of nutrition and dietary recommendations for individuals with diabetes mellitus: 1979. Diabetes 28:1027–1030, 1979.
11. Peters AL, Davidson MB, Eisenberg K: Effect of isocaloric substitution of chocolate cake for potato in type 1 diabetic patients. Diabetes Care 13:888–892, 1990.
12. Rabinowitz MB, Gonick HC, Levin SR, Davidson MB: Effects of chromium and yeast supplementation on carbohydrate and lipid metabolism in diabetic men. Diabetes Care 6:319–327, 1983.

22. HYPERTENSION

Stanley M. Augustin, MD, and Charles W. Van Way III, MD

1. Why is the dietary management of hypertension important?

Hypertension is one of the most common diseases of adults. Between 40 and 50 million Americans have hypertension. Nutritional factors are as important as pharmacologic therapy in the management of hypertension. Up until the past three decades, patients with hypertension generally died early. But with modern pharmacologic, nutritional, and lifestyle management, patients with hypertension can live a normal life span. It is no exaggeration to say that the control of hypertension has been one of the great medical triumphs of the past 50 years. But because so many people have the disease and because all of them should receive life-long management, the sheer amount of work involved in management is a major challenge to our health care system. This challenge is not being especially well met. For example, it was found in 1993 that one-third of subjects were not even aware that they had hypertension. This figure had not changed substantially for thirty years. Despite all of the efforts that have been made, there are still a large number of people with untreated hypertension in the population. Furthermore, of those who have hypertension, it is estimated that 20–40% are not being adequately treated.

2. Can dietary measures prevent hypertension?

Somewhat, although not completely. The various risk factors involved in hypertension can be divided into two categories: nonmodifiable and modifiable. Nonmodifiable factors include race, gender, ethnicity, and family history. Modifiable factors include diet, physical activity, weight, and smoking. Recent trials have shown that careful attention to these factors can have a positive effect on blood pressure. The Dietary Approaches to Stop Hypertension Study showed that a diet high in fruit and vegetables with low-fat dairy products significantly lowered systolic and diastolic blood pressure. The Diet, Exercise and Weight Loss Intervention Trial has shown that lifestyle change, along with antihypertensive therapy, can result in substantially lower blood pressure and cholesterol levels.

3. What is the optimum weight for the management of hypertension?

There is a proven relationship between body mass and arterial pressure. At least 30% of Americans are obese, as defined by a body mass index (BMI) > 30. Recent trials showed that a reduction in body weight of as little as 4 kg resulted in a significant decrease in both systolic and diastolic pressure as well as the incidence of hypertension. The weight loss should be 5% of the patient's body weight.

4. Besides diet, what modifications should the hypertensive patient make?

Exercise is the first major change. The amount of exercise does not have to be great. Only 30 minutes of scheduled exercise three times a week can have a beneficial effect and the exercise needs to be no more elaborate than brisk walking. Of course, more is probably better. The minimal level provides little cardiovascular conditioning, although it does help the hypertension.

Exercise has three benefits. First, it appears to have a direct effect on the blood pressure. Even mild exercise will lower the blood pressure by 6 or 7 mmHg. Second, it is a very useful adjunct to the weight loss program which is almost always necessary. And third, it helps to break the cycle of physical inactivity, low self-image, and overeating which characterizes many of these patients—the "couch potato cycle."

The other major change—for some people—is elimination of smoking. Anyone with hypertension who still smokes is engaging in self-destruction. Counseling of such patients can be challenging. The basic technique used in counseling is to tell the patient with cardiovascular disease what will happen to them if they continue smoking. Many people think that smoking primarily damages the lungs and, as long as they can don't have lung cancer, they aren't in trouble. But the excess cardiovascular mortality related to smoking is three times as large as the excess mortality related to lung cancer. The importance of stopping smoking for the long-term health of the patient with known cardiovascular disease cannot be overemphasized. Smoking cessation by itself can significantly improve the hypertension.

5. How much sodium restriction is optimal in the treatment of hypertension?

More than 60 randomized studies have analyzed the benefit of sodium reduction on hypertension. Moderate salt restriction is defined as 6 grams of salt per day. The DASH-Sodium Trial showed that a combination of diet with sodium restriction (3–6 grams of salt per day) can be an effective replacement for drug therapy in the treatment of early stages of hypertension.

6. What is the difference between grams of sodium and grams of salt?

The sodium content in diets can be calculated in four different ways: sodium in milligrams or in grams, sodium in mEq, or salt (sodium chloride) in grams. The difference between them is often confusing. If a diet contains 6 grams per day of salt (NaCl), the amount of sodium is 2400 mg, or 2.4 grams, or 100 mEq. Putting it another way, 1 gram of salt contains 400 mg of sodium, or 16.7 mEq. A 500-mg sodium diet, probably the most restrictive diet in general use, is equivalent to 1.2 grams of salt and contains 21 mEq of sodium.

7. Explain the association between potassium and hypertension.

Most studies suggest an inverse relation between potassium intake and blood pressure and cerebral vascular events. The mechanisms include lowering of peripheral resistance and suppression of the renin-angiotensin mechanism. A recent meta-analysis showed a slight reduction in both systolic and diastolic blood pressure (systolic: 3.1–4.4 mmHg; diastolic: 1.9–2.5 mmHg) in both normotensive and hypertensive patients.

8. Describe the interaction between diuretics and diet.

Historically, the first treatments for hypertension was a rigid low-sodium diet combined with weight loss. As drug therapy for hypertension has progressively improved over the past 60 years, the necessity for severe sodium restriction has diminished. Diuretics have played a significant part in this progression. One of the reasons that hypertensive patients today can be treated with a diet in the range of 1800–2400 mg sodium is that the use of diuretics makes more rigid diets unnecessary.

At the same time, diuretic therapy has introduced its own set of problems. Diuretic therapy has profound effects upon the electrolyte composition of the body. After all, diuretics are intended to control hypertension by excreting sodium chloride and decreasing the size of the intracellular space. There are a number of diuretics, each with its own type of action. The commonly used thiazide diuretics and the loop diuretics cause excess secretion of potassium, which must be replaced. The so-called potassium-sparing diuretics, such as spironolactone, have less effect on potassium. All diuretics may increase the excretion of calcium and magnesium.

The diuretics can all produce gastrointestinal side effects in some patients. These are usually not severe, however, and rarely limit use of the drugs.

9. What are the major drug-nutrient interactions in hypertension?

Unfortunately, most of the drugs used to control blood pressure either interact with nutrients or have gastrointestinal side effects, or both. The following table summarizes this material (see also Chapter 42, Drug-Nutrient Interaction).

DRUG (CLASS AND NAME OF TYPICAL DRUG)	SIDE EFFECTS
β-blockers (propranolol)	Anorexia, dry mouth, nausea, diarrhea, abdominal pain
α- and β-blockers (labetalol)	Dry mouth, taste changes, nausea, diarrhea

(Table continued on next page.)

DRUG (CLASS AND NAME OF TYPICAL DRUG)	SIDE EFFECTS
α₁ receptor blockers (prazosin)	Dry mouth, nausea, diarrhea, constipation
ACE inhibitor (enalapril)	Anorexia, taste changes, dry mouth glossitis and stomatitis, nausea, abdominal pain, diarrhea, constipation
Calcium channel blockers (verapamil)	Nausea, constipation
Vasodilator (hydralazine)	Anorexia, dry mouth, taste changes, nausea, diarrhea, constipation

Given that the effects of adrenergic blockade are widespread, there is little surprise that adrenergic blockers might show gastrointestinal side effects. These are unpredictable and variable. One patient might have diarrhea, and another constipation and abdominal pain. These side effects are not usually limiting but can be troublesome in some patients.

10. How do calcium and magnesium affect hypertension?
Currently no studies show that calcium can prevent hypertension. There are reports of significant decreases in systolic pressure with calcium supplementation (1000–2000 mg/day) in hypertensive patients but not in normotensive patients. Other studies have not supported these results. Although magnesium can lower blood pressure, there are no specific recommendations for its use to treat or to prevent hypertension.

11. What is the effect of alcohol on hypertension?
Moderate consumption of alcohol, particularly red wine, shows a cardioprotective effect. The exact mechanism is unclear, but it is postulated that this effect is due to antioxidation and antithrombosis via platelet aggregation. However, numerous studies show a linear association between excessive alcohol consumption and hypertension. Patients who are hypertensive should avoid alcohol.

12. Discuss the association between fish oil and hypertension.
There are conflicting reports in regard to fish oil and hypertension. Fish oil can modestly reduce blood pressure in normotensive patients, but a recent study has shown no effect of omega-3 fatty acids on blood pressure. They do not seem to prevent hypertension in normal populations. Omega-3 fatty acids, however, seem to have cardioprotective effects through lowering cholesterol.

13. Does caffeine predispose to hypertension?
Drinking coffee has long been suspected as a risk factor for hypertension. Coffee has been shown to modestly raise systolic and diastolic blood pressure by 2.4 and 1.2 mmHg, respectively). There is an increase in incidence of hypertension in coffee drinkers vs. nondrinkers, but no causal relationship has been established.

14. What is the problem with licorice in hypertension?
Natural licorice contains a substance called *glycyrrhizic acid*. This appears to be capable of inducing a state of hypermineralocorticism by the inhibition of 11b-hydroxysteroid dehydrogenase. Licorice-induced hypertension has been reported clinically. Natural licorice should be specifically avoided in patients who are being treated for hypertension.

15. How should hypertension be managed in the elderly patient?
The systolic blood pressure rises as people age. However, diastolic hypertension is as abnormal in the elderly as it is in the young. Systolic hypertension is also harmful, although the range of normal is somewhat higher over 70 than in younger people. Hypertension is a major problem in the aging population. According to some estimates, up to half of elderly people have hypertension.

Management is the same as for younger patients. Weight reduction, sodium restriction, alcohol limitation, and exercise are all important components in the overall management of hypertension in the older adult. Exercise is a particularly important aspect, because the elderly often fail to maintain a regular exercise program. In one recent study, simply walking more than two miles per day was associated with an overall mortality rate half that seen in men who walked less than one mile per day. Of course, one has to be fairly healthy to begin with in order to walk two miles a day at age 70.

BIBLIOGRAPHY

1. Allender PS, Culter JA, Follmann D, et al: Dietary calcium and blood pressure: A meta-analysis of randomized clinical trials. Ann Intern Med 124:825–831, 1996.
2. Appel LJ, Moore TJ, Obarzanek E, et al: Clinical trial of the effects of dietary patterns on blood pressure. N Engl J Med 336:117–124, 1997.
3. Bucher HC, Cook RJ, Guyatt GH, et al: Effects of dietary calcium supplementation on blood pressure: A meta-analysis of randomized controlled trials. JAMA 275:1016–1022, 1996.
4. De Lorimer AA, Tompkins RK: Alcohol, wine and health. Am J Surg 180:357–361, 2000.
5. Desai BB: Handbook of Nutrition and Diet. New York, Marcel Dekker, 2000.
6. Dickey RA, Janick JJ: Lifestyle modification in the prevention and treatment of hypertension. Endocr Pract 7:392–399, 2001.
7. Goldber IJ, Mosca L, Piano MR, Fisher EA: Wine and your heart: A science advisory for health care professionals from the Nutrition Committee, Council on Epidemiology and Prevention and Council on Cardiovascular Nursing of the American Heart Association. Stroke 103:591–594, 2001.
8. Hakin AA, Perovitch H, Burchfiel CM, et al: Effects of walking on mortality among nonsmoking retired men. N Engl J Med 338:94–99, 1998.
9. Hardman JG, Limbird LE (eds): Goodman and Gillman's The Pharmacological Basis of Therapeutics, 9th ed. New York, McGraw-Hill, 1996.
10. Kotchen TA, McCarron DA: Dietary electrolytes and blood pressure: A statement for healthcare professionals from the American Heart Association Nutrition Committee. Circulation 98:613–617, 1998.
11. Kris-Etherton PM, Etherton TD, Carlson J, Gardner C: Recent discoveries in inclusive food-based approaches and dietary patterns for reduction in risk for cardiovascular diseases. Curr Opin Lipidol 13:397–407, 2002.
12. Miller ER, Erlinger TP, et al: Results of Diet, Exercise and Weight Loss Intervention Trial. Hypertension 40:612–618, 2002.
13. National High Blood Pressure Education Program Working Group: Report on hypertension in the elderly. Hypertension 23:275, 1994.
14. Shils M, Olsen J, Shike M, Ross C: Modern Nutrition in Health and Disease, 9th ed. Philadelphia, Lippincott Williams & Wilkins, 1999.
15. Slama M, Susic D, Frohlich ED: Prevention of hypertension. Curr Opin Cardiol 17:531–536, 2002.
16. Van Way CW (ed): Handbook of Surgical Nutrition. Philadelphia, Lippincott, 1992.
17. Whelton PK, He J, Culter JA, et al: Effects of oral potassium on blood pressure: Meta-analysis of randomized controlled clinical trials. JAMA 277:1624–1632, 1997.

23. RENAL FAILURE

Pamela Charney, MS, RD, LD, CNSD, David I. Charney, MD, FACP, and Charles W. Van Way III, MD

1. What are the major metabolic defects in renal failure?

In both acute and chronic renal failure the patient can have acidosis, oliguria, water retention, urea retention, sodium retention, and potassium retention. Metabolic acidosis can cause abnormalities of bone metabolism as well as protein metabolism. Calcium and phosphate metabolism is disordered due to abnormalities in renal phosphate excretion, vitamin D metabolism, and parathyroid gland responsiveness to serum calcium levels; in addition, each of these abnormalities interacts with the other. The net result can be hypocalcemia, hyperphosphatemia, ectopic calcification, and osteodystrophy. In chronic renal failure, both anemia and clotting abnormalities are seen.

2. How are the caloric needs calculated in renal failure?

In chronic renal failure as well as end-stage renal disease, caloric needs should be calculated in the usual way using predictive equations such as the Harris-Benedict equation (see Appendix I). If indirect calorimetry is available, a more accurate determination of needs is possible. The patient should be encouraged to consume adequate calories. Patients with renal failure often have suboptimal energy intake with resulting weight loss that is difficult to treat once dialysis is initiated. In general, most patients require about 30–35 calories/kg body weight. Patients who are very active may need more, whereas those who are elderly or sedentary may need less to maintain body weight and lean body mass.

Patients on peritoneal dialysis can absorb significant amounts of dextrose from dialysate solutions. Calculations of caloric requirements must take this into account because 500–1000 kcal can be absorbed per day, depending on dialysate dextrose concentration and peritoneal dwell time.

Acute renal failure may be associated with increased energy expenditure because of the underlying condition. Indirect calorimetry is most useful in this population, although predictive equations can be utilized with due caution to avoid over- and under-feeding.

3. What are the protein needs of patients in renal failure?

Use of protein restriction in patients with renal failure is controversial. Lower protein diets (0.6–0.8 gm protein/kg) may slow the progression of renal failure in some patients. Protein modifications are not necessary in patients with a glomerular filtration rate (GFR) greater than 40 ml/min. Lower protein diets may slow the build-up of uremic toxins, improve acidosis, and assist with control of phosphorus and potassium. However, if low protein diets are recommended, close monitoring by a registered dietitian is vital. Extremely low protein intake, with supplements of ketoacid analogs of amino acids, are extremely difficult to utilize without meticulous nutritional monitoring.

During acute renal failure hypermetabolism and protein catabolism can occur. Protein restriction is not indicated unless dialytic therapy is not available or rapid recovery is expected. Protein should be provided according to clinical condition and dialysis utilized to manage fluid electrolyte status. Most critically ill patients require from 1.5–2.0 gm protein/kg.

Patients on chronic hemodialysis have somewhat increased protein requirements secondary to the loss of some amino acids through the dialysis process. It is recommended that patients on hemodialysis receive approximately 1.2 gm protein/kg, with the majority coming from high biologic value protein. Peritoneal dialysis leads to even greater protein losses; thus the recommended intake of protein for such patients is higher, ranging from 1.3 to 1.5 gm/kg. It can be difficult for some patients to achieve these levels of protein intake; close monitoring is required. Because many foods high in protein are also high in phosphorous, choice of protein source can be problematic for patients with hyperphosphatemia. The assistance of a renal dietitian is needed in most cases.

4. What is the renal failure formula used in total parenteral nutrition (TPN) and enteral nutrition?

In the early 1970s it was thought that provision of a diet with only essential amino acids would reduce the need for dialysis by decreasing urea production. Some early studies did indeed show decreased reliance on dialysis in patients with both acute and chronic renal failure. However, most of these studies compared the essential amino acid solution with hypertonic dextrose alone and thus are difficult to interpret. Amino acid solutions became available for use in TPN for patients with acute renal failure; however, they have failed to improve outcomes compared with standard amino acid solutions. It is currently recommended that standard amino acid solutions be used for patients with acute and chronic renal failure who require TPN.

Enteral formulas containing only essential amino acids are no longer recommended for patients with renal failure who require enteral feeding. Special enteral formulas are now available with low and moderate protein content. Both of these formula types contain lower amounts of electrolytes, especially phosphorus and potassium. The lower protein formula is designed for patients with chronic renal failure and is not indicated for patients who are acutely ill. As stated above, patients who are acutely ill do not require protein restriction unless there is a contraindication to dialytic therapy. Patients who are acutely ill and receiving an enteral formula with lower electrolyte levels should be closely monitored because refeeding syndrome (acute hypophosphatemia, hypokalemia, and hypomagnesemia) is not unheard of in this population. In addition, electrolyte status can be tenuous in some patients.

5. What are the electrolyte needs of patients with renal failure? How are they calculated?

Sodium. As renal failure progresses, the kidney losses the ability to excrete sodium. In the presence of edema, weight gain, and hypertension, dietary sodium should be restricted to 2–4 gm/day, depending on fluid status. Patients on hemodialysis may require further restriction of sodium. Along with restriction of sodium is often restriction of fluid intake, particularly for patients on hemodialysis. It has been recommended that hemodialysis patients be restricted to fluid intake equal to urine output of plus 500 ml/day.

Potassium. Severe hyperkalemia can lead to cardiac arrhythmia and death. As renal failure progresses, dietary potassium restriction is indicated in most patients once GFR falls below 10 ml/min. Once hemodialysis is initiated, potassium intakes of less than 2–3 gm are usually well tolerated. Patients on peritoneal dialysis often do not require such strict restriction of dietary potassium. Patients with acute renal failure require close monitoring and potassium restriction initiated if hyperkalemia occurs.

Calcium and phosphorus. Renal failure is often associated with hyperphosphatemia and hypocalcemia. Hyperphosphatemia may not become problematic until GFR is less than 35–40 ml/min. Restriction of dietary phosphorus should be initiated; phosphate-binding medications are also utilized to prevent absorption of dietary phosphorus. Supplemental calcium may also be needed.

Vitamin D. Because the final hydroxylation of vitamin D occurs in the kidney, alterations in vitamin D metabolism are common in patients with chronic renal failure. Inadequate vitamin D production leads to the hypocalcemia described above as well as a loss of inhibition of parathyroid hormone production, increasing PTH levels already stimulated by the hyperphosphatemia and hypocalcemia.

6. Why should fat-soluble vitamins be avoided in patients with renal failure?

Patients on dialysis tend to lose the water-soluble vitamins during dialysis and often need supplemental amounts of these vitamins. Excessive vitamin C intake should be avoided due to the risk for hyperoxalosis. There is a risk for hypervitaminosis A if excessive supplements of vitamin A are provided. A specially formulated oral vitamin supplement is available for patients with renal failure. No such preparation exists for patients with renal failure who are receiving TPN. There is probably no adverse effect with short-term use of standard parenteral vitamin preparations in patients with renal failure. If long-term TPN is needed, levels should be monitored and consideration given to lowering the vitamin A content, if possible.

7. Do the requirements for trace elements change in renal failure?

Patients with renal failure often have some degree of anemia, caused by increased red cell destruction as well as decreased erythropoietin production in the kidney. Synthetic erythropoietin can successfully treat the anemia associated with renal failure along with supplemental iron, if needed. Iron can be given either orally or parenterally. If given orally, it should not be taken with phosphate binders. Transferrin saturation is a good indicator of the need for iron supplementation, along with ferritin levels. A transferrin saturation of less than 20% along with ferritin of less than 100 ng/dl may indicate the need for iron.

Aluminum toxicity has been noted in the past due to the use of aluminum-based phosphate binders, along with aluminum content of dialysate. Currently used phosphate binders do not contain aluminum, and aluminum is removed from water supplies used for dialysis.

There is currently not enough evidence to support increased requirements for other trace elements such as selenium, zinc, or chromium.

8. How do nutrient requirements change for patients with acute renal failure who are receiving continuous renal replacement therapy?

Various dialytic modalities are available for treatment in the intensive care unit (ICU). The development of continuous renal replacement therapy (CRRT) has improved provision of nutritional support to patients with acute renal failure. CRRT is provided continuously over 24 hours in the ICU, particularly for patients unable to tolerate the severe fluid shifts associated with intermittent hemodialysis. Peritoneal dialysis is not typically utilized in the ICU. The use of continuous dialysis therapy allows easing of both fluid and protein restrictions that may be necessary in patients on intermittent therapy. However, losses of water-soluble vitamins and amino acids may be exacerbated. In addition, the use of glucose-containing dialysate solutions results in glucose absorption and a decrease in caloric requirements delivered through other routes.

BIBLIOGRAPHY

1. Goldstein-Fuchs DJ, McQuiston B: Renal failure. In Matarese LM, Gottschlich MM (eds): Contemporary Nutrition Support Practice: A Clinical Guide. Philadelphia, W.B. Saunders, 2003.
2. Klahr S: Effects of renal insufficiency on nutrient metabolism and endocrine function. In Mitch WE, Klahr S (eds): Handbook of Nutrition and the Kidney. Philadelphia, Lippincott-Raven, 1998.
3. Klahr S, Levey AS, Beck GJ, et al: The effects of dietary protein restriction and blood pressure control on the progression of chronic renal disease. Modification of Diet in Renal Disease Study Group. N Engl J Med 330:877–884, 1994.
4. Laville M, Foque D: Nutritional aspects in hemodialysis. Kidney Int 58:S133–S139, 2000.
5. National Kidney Foundation: Clinical practice guidelines for nutrition in chronic renal failure. Am J Kidney Dis 35(6; Suppl 2):S17–S88, 2000.
6. Wolk R: Nutrition in renal failure. In Gottschlich MM (ed): The Science and Practice of Nutrition Support: A Case-Based Core Curriculum. Dubuque, IA, Kendall/Hunt, 2001.

24. NUTRITION IN RESPIRATORY DISEASE

Diana S. Dark, MD

1. Why is it important to feed malnourished patients who have respiratory disease?

Malnutrition can increase morbidity of respiratory disease, especially respiratory failure, by several mechanisms, most notably impairment of respiratory muscle function, decreased ventilatory drive, and changes in immune function. The adverse effects of malnutrition occur independently of the presence or absence of primary lung disease. However, malnutrition frequently occurs in advanced chronic obstructive pulmonary disease (COPD), and may contribute to the respiratory failure in some patients.

2. Are patients with respiratory disease at particular risk for malnutrition?

Patients with chronic respiratory problems are prone to the development of malnutrition. Investigators in the late 1960s first noted the association between weight loss and increased mortality in COPD. A later study demonstrated that weight loss was found in 70% of patients hospitalized with COPD. Abnormal anthropomorphic measurements were documented in half of these patients.

3. How are lung defense mechanisms altered by malnutrition?

Malnutrition has been shown to alter immune function and is a common cause of acquired immunodeficiency in humans. Although death from starvation is frequently accompanied by pneumonia, it is unclear whether the cause is an immune deficit or an alteration in pulmonary function which prediposes the patient to infection. Lung defense mechanisms are altered by effects on the antioxidant defense system and surfactant production and by changes in immunologic competence. The relationship between nutritional status and bacterial binding to the respiratory tract has been studied as well. Patients with permanent tracheostomy and profound nutritional depletion had a significantly higher tracheal cell adherence of bacteria when compared with controls or well-nourished patients with permanent tracheostomy. Compromised nutritional status may contribute to the high prevalence of gram-negative pneumonia in this patient population.

4. Are there mechanical problems in ventilation which result from malnutrition?

There may be. Malnourished patients appear to have a marked decrease in "sighing," and reduced tidal volume, V_{O2} and V_{CO2}. Studies of patients with chest wall weakness due to muscle disease have demonstrated a decrease in functional residual capacity. These depressions in depth of breathing (tidal volume, sighs) among nutritionally-depleted patients may predispose the patient to atelectasis and infection, providing one possible mechanism for the increased respiratory morbidity associated with starvation.

In COPD, primary abnormalities of decreased inspiratory pressure and increased work of breathing are common. Inspiratory muscle weakness, as assessed by maximal inspiratory pressure, results from both a mechanical disadvantage to inspiratory muscles consequent to hyperinflation as well as generalized muscle weakness. However, inspiratory muscle weakness must be severe for hypercapnia to occur.

5. How are respiratory muscles affected by malnutrition?

Weakness of respiratory muscles may occur with malnutrition. In simple starvation or undernutrition, fat and protein are lost, but the loss of protein is minimized. Nitrogen loss is spared by mobilization of fat. Enhanced fat oxidation is the principal source of energy in a starving but otherwise normal individual. Some protein wasting does occur despite the availability of fat as a source of energy, and protein wasting accelerates when fat stores are depleted. In patients with many critical illnesses, as opposed to simple fasting or starvation, protein catabolism, is used to provide energy. If caloric intake is inadequate, skeletal muscle protein is broken down to serve gluconeogenesis. Inspiratory and expiratory respiratory muscles, primarily the diaphragm and intercostal muscles, are skeletal muscles and are susceptible to catabolic wasting. Malnutrition reduces diaphragmatic muscle mass in health and disease. Low diaphragmatic weight has been shown to correlate with low body weight in patients with emphysema.

6. Can malnutrition affect the function of the respiratory muscles?
Respiratory muscle strength is related to muscle size and fuel supply, both of which are decreased in nutritional depletion. Few studies have directly examined respiratory muscle function and malnutrition. Maximum inspiratory pressure has been shown to be decreased in malnutrition, as have maximal inspiratory mouth pressures. This was demonstrated in malnourished patients with anorexia nervosa, a group of patients without other systemic diseases. Isolated mineral and electrolyte deficiencies, which occur with malnutrition, can also impair respiratory muscle function. Hypophosphatemia reduces diaphragmatic contractile strength as measured by transdiaphragmatic pressure (Pdi) in mechanically ventilated patients with acute respiratory failure. Hypocalcemia has been shown to decrease diaphragmatic contractile strength. Hypomagnesemia can also cause a decrease in respiratory muscle strength; repletion of magnesium can improve respiratory muscle function.

7. How does malnutrition adversely affect patients with respiratory disease?
Diminution in respiratory muscle function, from any cause, can certainly worsen or precipitate respiratory failure. The development of some electrolyte imbalances, most notably hypophosphatemia, has been shown to precipitate acute respiratory failure. In addition, low diaphragmatic contractile strength could potentially increase morbidity in patients with lung disease, adversely affecting weaning efforts in mechanically ventilated patients.

8. How is ventilatory drive altered by malnutrition?
Ventilatory drive is altered by malnutrition in several ways. Any condition that reduces the metabolic rate will also reduce the ventilatory drive, if only by decreasing CO_2 production. A decrease in metabolic rate has been shown to occur with starvation. Zwillich suggested that the interaction of nutrition and ventilatory drive was a function of the influence of nutrition on the metabolic rate. But Doekel has shown that the hypoxic ventilatory response falls during fasting, independent of, but parallel to, the fall in the metabolic rate. There appears to be a relationship between caloric restriction and hypoxemia, based on the lowered hypoxic threshold.

9. Are there other effects of malnutrition on the lungs?
The impact of malnutrition on the pulmonary parenchyma is less clear. Certainly there appear to be parenchymal effects independent of those of the respiratory muscles, including changes in surfactant production, protein synthesis, and proteolysis. Most of the limited data come from animal experiments using subacute and chronic food deprivation. Starvation appears to decrease production of surfactant, a substance that increases lung compliance and decreases the work of breathing. However, in these deprivation experiments lung function appears to be well preserved despite decreased surfactant production, suggesting that surfactant levels are still adequate despite undernutrition. Protracted starvation decreases protein and collagen production and increases proteolysis. These changes will decrease tissue elasticity and may possibly contribute to the morphologic similarities in the lung tissue between emphysema and starvation. The clinical importance of these changes is not yet well established.

10. How do the nutritional needs of patients with respiratory disease differ from the needs of other patients?
They are frequently less than other patients. The most common method used to calculate energy needs in patients is to determine the patient's basal energy expenditure (BEE), perhaps by

using the Harris-Benedict equations and then multiply the BEE by stress and activity factors to determine the total energy expenditure (TEE). But this method may result in an inaccurate determination of energy needs in patients with respiratory disease. There is a fairly common misconception that mechanical ventilation increases the patient's TEE. If anything, it decreases the TEE, by eliminating most of the work of breathing and by enforcing bed rest. In any case, the underlying disease state has the most influence on the energy expenditure. Simple respiratory failure is not usually hypermetabolic. The more complex adult respiratory distress syndrome (ARDS) seen in patients with sepsis or other infections, on the other hand, is usually associated with hypermetabolism. Estimation of energy needs by using the metabolic cart is more important in patients with respiratory disease than with other patients, because the predictive equations appear to be less reliable and because the consequences of overfeeding may be more severe (see below). The most accurate determination of energy expenditure is done by using indirect calorimetry. This can be done with the patient breathing room air, on supplemental oxygen, or mechanically ventilated.

There is some controversy surrounding the proportions of nutritional supplementation given to carbohydrates vs fat in patients with respiratory disease, particularly concerning the effects on the respiratory system. Carbohydrates have traditionally been considered a more efficient source of energy in acute illness of any kind. However, seriously ill patients may have a decreased ability to utilize carbohydrates. Because of this, it has been suggested that fat may be a preferable source of energy in critically ill patients including those with respiratory diseases. The current recommendation is for patients with lung disease to receive a caloric intake that matches estimated energy expenditure. Mixed carbohydrate-fat diets in which fat comprises 20–40% of the total calories should be used preferentially.

One of the goals of nutritional support is to maintain or replenish lean body mass. The average person stores approximately 20,000 kcal as protein, 1000 as carbohydrates, and over 140,000 as fats. A malnourished patient with chronic lung disease may have decreased stores. It takes only a short time in acute illness of any kind with inadequate nutrition to begin depletion of these stores. Because of the possible adverse effects of malnutrition on respiratory muscles, it is advised to maintain a positive nitrogen balance to avoid loss of body protein.

11. What are the consequences of overfeeding a patient who has respiratory disease?

Basically, excess CO_2 production. The respiratory quotient (RQ) is the ratio of carbon dioxide production to oxygen consumption. Different substrates produce different amounts of CO_2. Proteins yield 4 kcal/g, and have an RQ of approximately 0.8. Metabolism of carbohydrates yields approximately 4 kcal/g with an RQ of approximately 1. Fats yield 9 kcal/g with an RQ of 0.7. When excess food is given to the patient, the energy is stored as fat. The conversion of other substrates to fat, or lipogenesis, is accompanied by a high RQ (5 to 8) and results in higher production of CO_2. This in turn may cause increased work of breathing and may lead to hypercapnia, particularly in patients with fixed minute ventilation and limited pulmonary reserves. It is more important to monitor the total caloric intake and to maintain it at an appropriate level, than it is to increase the ratio of fat calories to carbohydrate calories being given.

12. What are the consequences of underfeeding a patient who has respiratory disease?

Most important are the changes in respiratory muscle function, ventilatory drive, and immune function, as detailed above. Much depends on whether the patient is depleted to begin with. A well-nourished patient will tolerate a period of underfeeding relatively well, but a patient who is malnourished to start with is at serious risk for respiratory failure and pneumonia.

13. Are there demonstrated benefits of feeding malnourished patients who have respiratory disease?

The goals of nutritional support include reversing or improving the alterations that may occur as a result of malnutrition. Ventilatory drive has been shown to return to normal with refeeding of a malnourished patient. Immune deficits can be corrected, at least in part, by correction of the malnutrition. Nutritional repletion has been shown to improve diminished respiratory muscle strength, although few studies address the effects of refeeding on respiratory muscle function in nutritionally depleted patients with respiratory disease. For example, one small study of 10 undernourished patients with COPD showed clearly that the addition of 1000 kcal/day resulted in significant increases in body weight, improved respiratory muscle strength, and endurance.

14. Are there particular concerns about refeeding in patients with respiratory disease?
The refeeding syndrome has been reported in patients who are too-rapidly repleted after a period of starvation (see chapter 38, Central TPN). Respiratory failure is the most serious manifestation of the refeeding syndrome. Hypophosphatemia, which may be a consequence of refeeding, can alter respiratory muscle function. Abnormalities in calcium and magnesium may also occur. In the malnourished patient with limited respiratory reserve, the refeeding syndrome can precipitate respiratory failure. It should be avoided by advancing to full feedings over a period of several days.

One study of hospitalized patients suffering from long-term semistarvation (greater than 15% weight loss) who received total parenteral nutrition (TPN) demonstrated a marked effect of protein intake on the ventilatory drive. While this is good from the standpoint of treating pulmonary disease, it can increase the work of breathing in a patient with limited pulmonary reserve.

15. Is there a preferred method of delivering nutritional support to patients with respiratory disease?
It is always preferable to use the enteral route **if at all possible** when providing nutritional support. If unable to use the gastrointestinal tract, nutritional support may be delivered either by the peripheral parenteral route or the central parenteral route. Patients with tracheostomy may be able to swallow adequately enough to preclude the use of another route. Swallowing disorders secondary to prolonged orotracheal intubation or tracheostomy have been reported and are not uncommon. Specifically, delayed triggering of the swallow response and pharyngeal pooling were observed universally in a small series of eleven patients with prolonged orotracheal intubation. If a patient has severe reflux or chronic aspiration, a parenteral route is preferred to ensure that respiratory function is not further impaired.

16. Are some methods of delivery contraindicated in patients with respiratory disease?
No method of nutritional support, when administered judiciously, is contraindicated because of the presence of respiratory disease. Just the opposite is true. Patients with respiratory disease, especially if combined with malnutrition, may benefit from aggressive nutritional support more than patients with other diseases.

BIBLIOGRAPHY

1. Arora NS, Rochester DF: Respiratory muscle strength and maximal voluntary ventilation in undernourished patients. Am Rev Respir Dis 52:64–70, 1982.
2. Askanazi J, Rosenbaum SH, Hyman AI, et al: Effects of parenteral nutrition on ventilatory drive. Anesthesiology 53(suppl 1):185, 1980.
3. Aubier M, Maurciano D, Lecoguic Y, et al: Effects of Hypophosphatemia on diaphragmatic contractility in patients with acute respiratory failure. N Engl J Med 313:420–424, 1985.
4. Burdet L, de Muralt B, Schutz Y, et al: Administration of growth hormone to underweight patients with chronic obstructive pulmonary disease. Am J Respir Crit Care Med 156:1800–1806, 1997.
5. De Troyer A, Bastenier-Geens J: Effects of neuromuscular blockade on respiratory mechanics in conscious man. J Appl Physiol 47:1162–1168, 1979.
6. DeVita MA, Spierer-Rudnback L: Swallowing disorders in patients with prolonged orotracheal intubation or tracheostomy tubes. Crit Care Med 18:1328–1330, 1990.
7. Doekel RC Jr, Zwillich CW, Scoggin CH: Clinical semi-starvation: Depression of hypoxic ventilatory response. N Engl J Med 295:358–361, 1976.
8. Gibson GJ, Pride NB, Newsom DJ: Pulmonary mechanics in patients with respiratory muscle weakness. Am Rev Respir Dis 118:373, 1978.
9. Halliwell B, Gutteridge JMC: Oxygen toxicity, oxygen radicals, transition metals and disease. Biochem J 219:1–14, 1984.

10. Long CL, Birkham RH, Geiger JW: Contribution of skeletal muscle protein in elevated rates of whole body protein catabolism in trauma patients. Am J Clin Nutr 34:1087–1092, 1981.

11. Marquis K, Debigare R, Lacasse Y, et al: Mid-thigh muscle cross-sectional area is a better predictor of mortality than body mass index in patients with chronic obstructive pulmonary disease. Am J Respir Crit Care Med 166:809–813, 2002.

12. Murciano D, Rigaud D, Pingleton S, et al: Diaphragmatic function in severely malnourished patients with anorexia nervosa. Am J Respir Crit Care Med 150:1569–1574, 1994.

13. Niederman MS, Merrill WW, Ferranti RD, et al: Nutritional status and bacterial binding in the lower respiratory tract in patients with chronic tracheostomy. Ann Intern Med 100:795–800, 1984.

14. Rosenbaum SH, Askanazi J, Hyman AI, et al: Respiratory patterns in profound nutritional depletion. Anesthesiology 51(suppl 1):366, 1979.

15. Thrulbeck WM: Diaphragm and body weight in emphysema. Thorax 33:438–487, 1978.

16. Whittaker JC, Ryan CF, Buckley P, et al: The effects of refeeding on peripheral and respiratory muscle function in malnourished chronic obstructive pulmonary disease patients. Am Rev Respir Dis 142:283–288, 1990.

17. Zwillich CW, Sahn SA, Weil JV: Effects of hypermetabolism on ventilation and chemosensitivity. J Clin Invest 60:900–906, 1977.

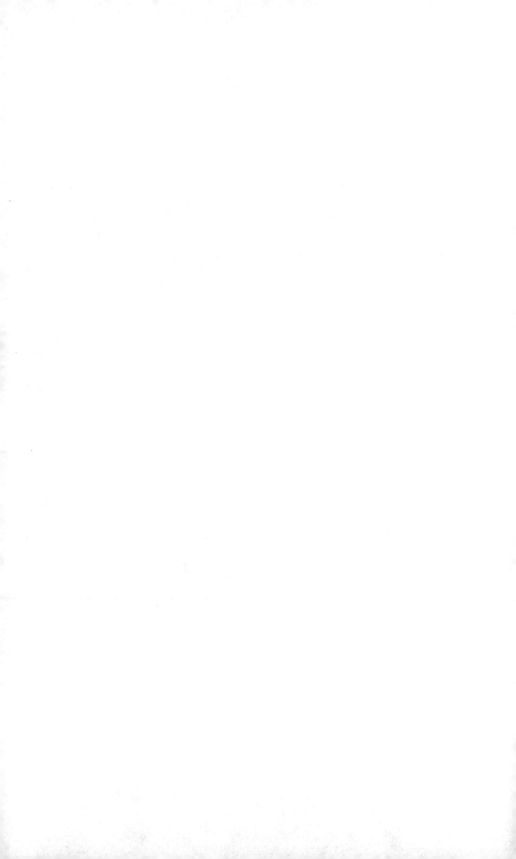

25. TRAUMA

Douglas M. Geehan, MD

1. Which trauma patients should receive nutritional support?

All patients who require admission for trauma-related problems should be evaluated for the adequacy of their prior nutritional status and current nutritional intake. The nature of injury predisposes these patients to both increased demands and inadequate intake. All trauma patients should be fed aggressively and as soon as possible after the injury.

A subset of trauma patients should be given intensive nutritional support in the form of enteral or parenteral nutrition. These include patients with burns, multiple injuries, major operation, and sepsis. Anyone with an injury severity score (ISS) of greater than 15 should receive intensive nutritional support. Although aggressive feeding may meet the needs of any of these, they will usually require intensive support.

2. Is all nutritional support equivalent in trauma patients?

Enteral nutrition is better than parenteral. It is always better to use the gut. In several studies, patients who received enteral nutrition had fewer septic complications such as pneumonia and wound infections than those receiving total parenteral nutrition. This was true whether the enteral nutrition was administered by nasogastric tube, nasojejunal tube, or jejunostomy. This difference was most pronounced in blunt trauma patients.

3. Does jejunostomy placement increase the complication rate after laparotomy for trauma?

Not generally, but it depends on the complication. In patients undergoing splenectomy for trauma, the incidence of abdominal abscess formation was not increased with the addition of a feeding jejunostomy. A catheter jejunostomy can be removed without the risk of intestinal fistula or leakage. On the other hand, there is a certain incidence of complications from jejunostomy placement itself, such as pneumatosis intestinalis, catheter displacement, and intestinal obstruction.

4. What can be done during a trauma laparotomy to facilitate enteral feeding?

Placement of a catheter jejunostomy at the time of laparotomy allows for delivery of postoperative enteral nutrition. In fact, enteral nutrition into the small intestine can be started immediately postoperatively. The small bowel does not show prolonged ileus like the stomach and the colon, and will even exhibit peristalsis with the abdomen open. If the patient will probably require long-term support, a larger jejunostomy or a gastrostomy can be created. For short-term feedings, the surgeon can simply place a soft nasoenteric tube through the stomach and pylorus during laparotomy. The tube can be manually guided into proper position. No surgical opening in the gastrointestinal tract is produced, and the tube can be removed easily if the patient recovers quickly. If the course is more protracted, the soft tube may remain in place and serve as a site of enteral access.

5. Does Injury Severity Score affect energy requirements? Are the Harris-Benedict equations accurate in estimating energy needs in trauma patients?

The ISS has not been shown to correlate with energy demands. Nonetheless, a high score means that the patient will probably need nutritional support, and the higher the score the longer it will be needed (see question 7).

The Harris-Benedict equations (HBE) are quite useful in estimating energy needs, if adjusted appropriately for the stress of the patient's injuries (see Appendix I). Trauma patients can be calculated with an activity factor of 1.2 (1.1 for ventilated patients) and a stress factor of 1.2–1.5. However, the HBE are only an estimate. Measurement of metabolic activity can be done with indirect calorimetry using the metabolic cart, which is especially useful if patients are on the ventilator. If the patient has a Swan-Ganz catheter, the caloric expenditure can be calculated from the oxygen consumption using the Fick principle (see Appendix I).

Frequent re-evaluation of energy and protein needs is necessary. Subsequent therapy can be guided by nitrogen balance to determine adequacy of protein intake. Caloric adequacy is difficult to determine, since the weight—usually the most reliable indicator—is unreliable in patients post-injury for a number of days.

Burn injury is a special case. Burned patients have marked hypermetabolism. A severe burn should be estimated using a stress factor of 1.8 or greater. The metabolic rate is not proportional to the amount of burn; while large burns show hypermetabolism, so do some smaller burns. For that reason, either indirect calorimetry or Fick principle measurement of oxygen consumption and energy expenditure is indicated.

6. If underfeeding trauma patients is harmful, why not overfeed to guarantee that all nutritional needs are met?

Overfeeding is also harmful. Both parenteral and enteral nutrition may generate significant complications. Overfeeding with total parenteral nutrition (TPN) may produce hyperglycemia, hypertriglyceridemia, overhydration, and electrolyte disturbances. Overfeeding with enteral nutrition may cause abdominal distention, cramping, or diarrhea. Diarrhea in particular can generate fluid and electrolyte derangements. Hyperglycemia and hypervolemia can complicate TPN. Trying to give too much enteral nutrition may result in enough intolerance to necessitate discontinuation of the feedings. Complications from nutritional support demand that a concerted effort to tailor the support to the patient's needs be carried out. The clinician must try to avoid both overfeeding and underfeeding.

7. Can patients at high risk for inadequate nutrition be identified prospectively?

This question has been studied in some detail. Patients were more likely to require nutritional support if they had an ISS greater than 26, an abdominal trauma index (ATI) greater than 10, if they required ICU care, and if they needed acute surgical intervention. Patients who had surgery with an ISS less than 6 (or no surgery and an ISS less than 12), an ATI less than 10, and were cared for on a regular nursing unit were able to eat a regular diet within 5 days. These criteria allow prospective identification of trauma patients most likely to benefit from early nutritional support.

8. Do patients with spinal cord injury require nutritional support?

Very much so. Such patients are frequently hypermetabolic, and require nutritional support in an amount appropriate for any victim of major injury (see question 5). But they may be difficult to feed. Loss of innervation of the abdominal cavity can complicate the clinical assessment of tolerance of enteral feeding. Many such patients have difficulty tolerating enteral feeding, and must be given TPN even though they have no gastrointestinal injury.

The denervation that results from a spinal cord injury leads to atrophy and muscle loss. There will usually be a negative nitrogen balance even in the face of acceptable nutritional support. The clinician must recognize this, or else efforts to create positive nitrogen balance may result in inappropriately high levels of support. Protein or amino acids should be given at the rate of 1–1.5 gm/kg/day, regardless of the nitrogen balance. The cord-injured patient will usually stabilize at a weight approximately 4.5 kg less than preinjury weight for paraplegia and 9.0 kg less for quadriplegia.

9. What is the best way to feed patients who have facial, oral, or jaw injuries?

The method will often depend on associated injuries. If the facial injuries are isolated, then the patient should be fed enterally. Blenderized food and/or supplemental formulas can be delivered to the patient via a syringe with a soft catheter into the mouth. This system allows for more palatable food to be used and prevents the associated problems that result from the accumulation of food in the teeth and hardware when patients try to eat or drink blenderized food directly.

10. Does short-term endotracheal intubation affect the patient's ability to swallow?

The presence of an endotracheal tube in direct contact with the oropharyngeal and laryngeal mucosa causes an injury that is transient and results in delayed swallowing reflex. In a study of patients who were intubated an average of 10 days, the swallowing reflex was delayed on the day of extubation and had returned to normal by one week. These findings suggest that patients should be assessed both early and late for evidence of swallowing dysfunction.

11. Can patients who have required prolonged ventilatory support be fed safely immediately after extubation?

Patients who have required ventilatory support for greater than three weeks have an incidence of abnormal swallowing of approximately 40%. These findings were demonstrated by bedside evaluation and, notably, were not associated with coughing or gagging.

12. Should trauma patients receive standard nutritional support, or do they have special requirements not seen in other patients?

Recent investigations have centered on enhancing specific agents of the nutritional milieu to improve patient outcome. This is true in trauma as well as in other conditions. Of specific interest has been administration of supplemental glutamine and arginine, use of omega-3 fatty acids to enhance immune responsiveness, and use of nucleic acids as a substrate for DNA and nucleotide synthesis. Decreased infectious complications and shortened ICU stay have been reported by various groups using such specialized formulas. They cost much more than standard formulations. Do they provide enough benefits to justify the increased cost? Advocates feel that the lower complication rate will produce lower overall costs. Studies are in progress.

Additional work investigating the role of growth hormone therapy has been undertaken. Small studies have shown improved nitrogen retention and, to a degree, shorter ventilator courses. Subsequent studies, with higher doses, showed increased mortality. Research continues to try to elucidate the proper role for growth hormone therapy.

BIBLIOGRAPHY

1. Barton RG: Nutritional support in critical illness. Nutr Clin Pract 9:127–139, 1994.
2. Boulanger BR, Brennemann FD, Rizoli SB, Nayman R: Insertion of a transpyloric feeding tube during laparotomy in the critically injured: rationale and plea for routine use. Injury 26:177–180, 1995.
3. Bower RH, Cerra FB, Bershadsky B, Licari JJ, Hoyt DB, Jensen GL, Van Buren CT, Rothkopf MM, Daly JM, Adelsberg BR: Early enteral administration of a formula (Impact) supplemented with arginine, nucleotides and fish oil in intensive care patients: Results of a multicenter, prospective, randomized, clinical trial. Crit Care Med 23:436–449, 1995.
4. Byers PM, Block EFJ, Albornoz JC, Pombo H, Kirton OC, Martin LC, Augenstein JS: The need for aggressive nutritional intervention in the injured patient: the development of a predictive model. J Trauma 39:1103–1109, 1995.
5. Dent D, Kudsk KA, Minard G, Fabian T, Nguyen T, Pritchard E, Pate L, Croce M: Risk of abdominal septic complications after feeding jejunostomy placement in patients undergoing splenectomy for trauma. Am J Surg 166:686–689, 1993.
6. de Larminat V, Montravers P, Dureuil B, Desmonts J: Alteration in swallowing reflex after extubation in intensive care unit patients. Crit Care Med 23:486–490, 1995.
7. Fischer JE: Metabolism in surgical patients: protein, carbohydrate and fat utilization by oral and parenteral routes. In Sabiston DC, Lyerly HK (eds): Textbook of Surgery: The Biological Basis of Modern Surgical Practice. Philadelphia, W.B. Saunders, 1996.
8. Fun-Chee L, Shanmuhasuntharam P: A simple method to enable feeding during maxillomandibular fixation of the jaws. Oral Surg Oral Med Oral Pathol 75:549–550, 1993.
9. Hammarqvist F, Sandgren A, Andersson K, et al: Growth hormone together with glutamine-containing total parenteral nutrition maintains muscle glutamine levels and results in a less negative nitrogen balance after surgical trauma. Surgery 129:576–586, 2001.
10. Kudsk KA, Croce MA, Fabian T, Minard G, Tolley EA, Poret A, Kuhl MR, Brown RO: Enteral versus parenteral feeding: Effects on septic morbidity after blunt and penetrating abdominal trauma. Ann Surg 215:503–513, 1992.
11. Rodriguez DJ, Sandoval W, Clevenger FW: Is measured energy expenditure correlated to injury severity score in major trauma patients? J Surg Res 59:455–459, 1995.

12. Ruokonen E, Takais J: Dangers of growth hormone therapy in critically ill patients. Ann Med 32:317–322, 2000.
13. Tolep K, Getch CL, Criner GJ: Swallowing dysfunction in patients receiving prolonged mechanical ventilation. Chest 109:167–172, 1997.
14. Zelby AS, McAllister WH: Complications of Spinal Cord Trauma. In Maull KI, Rodriguez A, Wiles CE (eds): Complications in Trauma and Critical Care. Philadelphia, W.B. Saunders, 1996.

26. PANCREATITIS

Wahid Wassef, MD, FACG

1. What is pancreatitis? How many types are there?

Pancreatitis is an inflammatory condition of the pancreas that develops as a result of inappropriate activation of pancreatic enzymes within the acinar cells.[1] This condition can result from hypertension in the pancreatic duct (i.e., stones, tumors, pancreas divisum), alteration of cellular membrane permeability (i.e., hypertriglyceridemia, hypercalcemia, alcohol), or hyperactive pancreatic enzymes (i.e., cationic trypsinogen mutations). Once the inflammation develops, it can result in the development of acute or chronic pancreatitis.

2. What are the similarities and differences between acute and chronic pancreatitis?

Acute and chronic pancreatitis are both inflammatory processes that develop in the pancreas. Both are also events that can occur once or more than once. Here is where the similarities end. In acute pancreatitis, the insult causes an injury that heals.[1] As a result, there is complete resolution of symptoms between attacks. In chronic pancreatitis, the insult occurs so often that the injury never heals.[2] In fact, it causes the development of a scarred, nonfunctioning pancreas. As a result, symptoms persist between attacks. Symptoms include pain, pancreatic exocrine insufficiency, and, in some cases, pancreatic endocrine insufficiency.

3. How does one approach the management of acute pancreatitis?

The management of acute pancreatitis is stage-dependent.[1] Patients with nonsevere pancreatitis are treated expectantly with pain medication and intravenous hydration. Patients with severe pancreatitis are fasted. They receive pain medication and antibiotics.[3] Occasionally, endoscopic retrograde cholangiopancreatography (ERCP) may be indicated.

The stage of acute pancreatitis can be determined in a number of ways.[4] The most clinically useful method is based on Ranson's criteria, a scoring system that depends on a number of specific lab values obtained on admission and 24 hours after admission. Patients with < 3 criteria are categorized as nonsevere pancreatitis; those with ≥ 3 are categorized as severe pancreatitis.

Ranson's Criteria

Criteria on admission
Age >50
White blood cell count > 16,000/cc
Blood glucose > 200 mg/dl
Lactate dehydrogenase > 350 IU/L
Aspartate aminotransferase > 250 IU/L

Criteria within 48 hours
Hematocrit decrease by > 10%
Blood urea nitrogen increase by > 5 mg/dl
Serum calcium < 8 mg/dl
Arterial oxygen < 60 mmHg
Base deficit > 4 MEq/L
Estimated fluid sequestration > 6L

4. What type of nutrition should patients with severe acute pancreatitis receive? How should it be monitored?

Patients with severe acute pancreatitis should be fasted since any oral intake would cause the release of cholecystokinin (CCK) and secretin, leading to acinar cell activation and an exacerbation of the pancreatitis.[5] They should be fed through total parenteral nutrition (TPN). This type of feeding bypasses the activation pathway, yet prevents starvation in this highly catabolic group of patients.[6] Due to the association between hyperlipidemia and acute pancreatitis, there used to be concern about the intravenous administration of lipids in this group of patients.[7] Currently, however, studies show that this approach is contraindicated only in patients with dyslipidemic pancreatitis (TRG > 400 mg/dl). Therefore, a triglyceride (TRG) level should be obtained in all patients with severe pancreatitis prior to the administration of TPN.

5. What type of nutrition should patients with nonsevere acute pancreatitis receive? How should it be monitored?

Patients with nonsevere acute pancreatitis could be fed orally.[8,9] However, since acute pancreatitis produces a paralytic ileus along with gastroparesis, the feeding must await clinical signs of improvement, such as flatus, bowel sounds, and resolution of pain.[10] Furthermore, since oral feedings may exacerbate the pancreatitis due to the release of CCK and secretin, patients should be fed gradually, starting with a clear liquid diet and slowly progressing to a low-fat diet. If the patient is unable to tolerate this type of a diet due to exacerbation of pancreatitis, TPN or an elemental diet should be considered.

6. How does one approach the management of chronic pancreatitis?

Chronic pancreatitis is a condition that results in persistent pain, pancreatic exocrine insufficiency, and pancreatic endocrine insufficiency.[2] The pain can develop as a result of pseudocysts, pancreatic duct hypertension, or the entrapment of afferent nerves near the pancreatic parenchyma. The pancreatic endocrine and exocrine insufficiencies are caused by recurrent episodes of pancreatitis that result in scarring and injury of more than 95% of the pancreatic parenchyma.

7. What type of nutrition should patients with chronic pancreatitis receive?

Patients with chronic pancreatitis need to be fed with nutrients that are low in fat and protein to minimize pancreatic stimulation and pain.[2] Limiting fat intake to 25–30 gm/day and protein intake to 1–1.5 gm/kg/day can accomplish these goals.[11] However, since this group of patients also suffers from pancreatic exocrine insufficiency, they need to receive pancreatic enzyme replacement therapy as well as fat-soluble vitamins.[12]

8. What is pancreatic enzyme replacement therapy? How should it be administered?

Pancreatic enzyme replacement therapy is used to supplement patients who have pancreatic insufficiency with enough pancreatic enzymes to absorb nutrients from food and avoid malnutrition.[13] On average, patients with pancreatic insufficiency need 28,000–30,000 IU of lipase for each 25 gm/fat.[14] This type of supplementation can be accomplished through the use of enteric- and non–enteric-coated pancreatic enzymes. Studies have demonstrated that the non-enteric pancreatic enzymes are superior to the enteric type.[15]

Pancreatic enzymes do not need to be used in all patients with chronic pancreatitis. Normally, one waits for the patient to develop signs and symptoms of malabsorption. Once these are demonstrated, patients are encouraged to decrease their fat content to 25 gm/day. If the symptoms persist, they are started on pancreatic enzyme replacement therapy. The recommended dose is concentration-dependent but should be split in half so that the patient receives half of the dose at the start of the meal and the other half at the end. Occasionally, acid suppressive therapy has been used in conjunction with the enzymes to improve efficacy if malabsorption persists.[16,17]

Pancreatic Enzyme Replacement Therapy

	NON–ENTERIC-COATED ENZYMES	ENTERIC-COATED ENZYMES
Types	Viokase, Cotazyme	Creon, Pancrease, Ultrase
Standard dosage	8 tabs/meal, in divided doses (4/preprandially and 4/post-prandially)	2–3 tabs/meal; they do not need to be given in divided doses

(Table continued on next page.)

Pancreatic Enzyme Replacement Therapy (Continued)

	NON–ENTERIC-COATED ENZYMES	ENTERIC-COATED ENZYMES
Contraindications	Hypersensitivity to pork protein	Hypersensitivity to pork protein
Drug interactions	None	None
Side-effects	Diarrhea, hyperuricemia and nausea	Diarrhea, hyperuricemia and nausea
Cost	Viokase: $0.34/tablet Cotazyme: $0.24/tablet	Creon: $0.42/tablet Pancrease: $0.42/tablet Ultrase: $0.40/tablet

9. How does management of diabetes differ in patients with pancreatitis and those without pancreatitis? How should this group of patients be monitored?
   Pancreatic endocrine insufficiency in patients with chronic pancreatitis should be treated in the same way as in those without pancreatitis. The goal is glycemic control. This goal can be accomplished through dietary modifications, oral hypoglycemic agents, insulin injection therapy, or, most commonly, combination therapy, depending on the severity of the condition. Such patients are at risk for the development of diabetic neuropathies and vasculopathies and should be closely screened for the development of these conditions.

BIBLIOGRAPHY

1. DiMagno EP, Go VLW, et al: Fate of orally ingested enzymes in pancreatic insufficiency: Comparison of two dosage schedules. N Engl J Med 296:1318–1322, 1977.
2. Dutta SD, Russell RM, et al: Deficiency of fat-soluble vitamins in treated patients with pancreatic insufficiency. Ann Intern Med 97:549–552, 1982.
3. Dutta SK: Comaparative evaluation of the therapeutic efficacy of a pH-sensitive enteric coated pancreatic enzyme preparation with conventional pancreatic enzyme therapy in the treatment of exocrine pancreatic insufficiency. Gastroenterology 84:476–482, 1983.
4. Heijerman HG: Omeprazole enhances the efficacy of pancreatin in cystic fibrosis. Ann Intern Med 114:200–201, 1991.
5. Kalfarentzos FE, Karatzas TM, Alevizatos BA, et al: Total parenteral nutrition in severe acute pancreatitis. J Am Coll Nutr 10:156–162, 1991.
6. Levy P, Pariente EA, et al: Frequency and risk factors of recurrent pain during re-feeding in patients with acute pancreatitis: A multi-variate multi-center prospective study of 116 patients. Gut 40:262–266, 1997.
7. Marulendra S: Nutrition support in pancreatitis. Nutr Clin Pract 10(2):45-53, 1995.
8. McClave SA, Snider HL, et al: Comparison of the safety of early enteral vs parenteral nutrition in mild acute pancreatitis. J Parent Enter Nutr 21:14–20, 1997.
9. NJ G: Enzymatic therapy in patients with chronic pancreatitis. Gastroenterol Clin North Am 28:687–693, 1999.
10. PA B: Practical guidelines in acute pancreatitis. Am J Gastroenterol 92:377–386, 1997.
11. Pederzoli P, Vesentini S, Campedelli A: A randomized multicenter clinical trial of antibiotic prophylaxis of septic complications in acute necrotizing pancreatitis with imipinem. Surg Gynecol Obstet 176:480, 1993.
12. Regan PT, DiMagno EP, et al: Comparative effects of antacids, cimetidine and enteric coating on the therapeutic response to oral enzymes in severe pancreatic insufficiency. N Engl J Med 297:854–858, 1977.
13. Scolapio JS: Nutrition supplementation in patients with acute and chronic pancreatitis. Gastroenterol Clin North Am 28:695–707, 1999.
14. Simpson WG: Enteral nutritional support in acute alcoholic pancreatitis. J Am Coll Nutr 14:662–665, 1995.
15. Stabile BE: Pancreatic secretion responses to intravenous hyperalimentation and intra-duodenal elemental full liquid diets. J Parent Enter Nutr 8:377–380, 1984.
16. Steinberg W: Acute pancreatitis. N Engl J Med 330:1198–1210, 1994.
17. Steer ML: Chronic pancreatitis. N Engl J Med 332:1482–1490, 1995.

27. LIVER AND GASTROINTESTINAL DISEASES

Kudakwashe M. Mushaninga, MS, RD, LD, and Stanley M. Augustin, MD

1. What is the most common carbohydrate intolerance?

Lactose intolerance affects persons of all age groups and is caused by an inability to digest significant amounts of lactose because of the genetically inadequate amount of the enzyme lactase. Lactose that is not hydrolyzed into glucose, and galactose remains in the gut and acts osmotically to draw water into the intestines. Fermentation of undigested lactose generates lactic acid, carbon dioxide, and hydrogen, resulting in bloating, flatulence, cramps, and diarrhea. Lactase deficiency is present in 15% of persons of Northern European descent, 80% of blacks and Latinos, and up to 100% of American Indians and Asians. The degree of lactose malabsorption varies greatly among patients; most people can tolerate up to 12 oz of milk without symptoms, especially when taken with meals rather than on an empty stomach. Omission of milk and lactose-containing foods alleviates symptoms of lactose intolerance. People can use milk and milk products treated with lactase enzyme as an effective way of alleviating symptoms of lactose intolerance.

2. Describe celiac disease and its nutritional care.

Celiac disease or gluten sensitive enteropathy is caused by a reaction to gliadin, the alcohol-soluble component of gluten. Damage to the villi of the intestinal mucosa results in malabsorption of nutrients. Clinical manifestations include diarrhea, weight loss, malaise, and malabsorption of vitamins D and K, calcium magnesium, albumin, and folic acid. A gliadin-free diet results in prompt clinical improvement. Vitamin, mineral, and extra protein supplementation should be included in the diet to help replenish depleted stores. A gluten-restricted diet omits all wheat, rye, oats, and barley. Label reading is very important because gluten-containing products may be used in food processing.

3. What are the common diseases of the large intestine?

Irritable bowel syndrome (IBS) is an abnormal stooling pattern associated with symptoms of intestinal dysfunction that persists for longer than 3 months. IBS is the most common disorder in gastrointestinal practice and affects 10% of adults, predominantly women. It is characterized by the presence of diarrhea, alternating with constipation, a sensation of incomplete evacuation, rectal pain, and mucus in the stool. The etiology of IBS is unknown but possible mechanisms are (1) exaggerated gastrocolic reflex, (2) abnormal colonic sensitivity to stretching, and (3) dietary intolerances. The goal of nutritional care in IBS is to relieve the condition, nourish the patient, and bring weight back to normal. A high-fiber diet with the exclusion of stimulants such as dairy products, chocolate, eggs, spices, caffeine, and wheat products is usually beneficial.

Diverticular disease is a collection of herniations of the colonic wall. Incidence of diverticulosis increases with aging; it is uncommon in children. Diverticulitis develops when accumulation of fecal matter in the diverticular pockets results in infection and inflammation, sometimes causing ulceration and perforation. In the past a low-fiber diet was prescribed, but a high-fiber diet promotes soft bulky stools that pass more swiftly and result in lower intercolonic pressures. For patients with an acute flare of diverticulitis, a low-residue or elemental diet is appropriate, followed by gradual return to a high-fiber diet.

4. What are the nutritional consequences of small bowel resection?

The severity of the symptoms of short bowel syndrome (SBS) is based on the extent of the resection and the specific level of resected small bowel. Resections of the small intestine usually do not cause significant problems unless 50% or more is removed. Extensive resection of the

129

small bowel results in impaired digestion of macronutrients and malabsorption of micronutrients and fluids. Dehydration, intractable diarrhea, steatorrhea, weight loss, and malnutrition are common characteristics. Secondary consequences of SBS include hypovolemia, hypoalbumenia, hypokalemia, hypomagnesemia, anemias, hyperoxaluria, and metabolic acidosis. Rare disorders such as essential fatty acid deficiency and d-lactic acidosis can also occur.

5. Describe the immediate and long-term nutritional care for SBS.

Postoperatively patients are very ill, and care must be taken to ensure proper wound healing. Patients require large volumes of isotonic fluid resuscitation for the first 24–48 hours. Total parenteral nutrition (TPN) is initiated after 48 hours as approximately 50% of needs and advanced to 100% of needs within 48–72 hours. Protein needs are 1.5–2 gm/kg average body weight, and fat calories are limited to less than 30% of nonprotein calories. Patients need 1.5 to 2 times their normal caloric requirements to meet needs and replace stool losses. Oral glutamine and human growth hormone injections may be administered to accelerate bowel adaptation. Gradual transition should be made from parenteral to enteral nutrition. Glutamine-enriched enteral feedings help with the adaptive process of the small intestine. The diet that has been most successful in weaning patients from home TPN is one that has complex carbohydrates, low fat, high fiber, 20% protein, 60% carbohydrate, and 20% fat in combination with growth hormone and glutamine. Oral diet promotes villus hyperplasia and optimizes bowel absorptive capacity; six small feedings are recommended as adaptation continues. Patients should avoid concentrated sweets, caffeine, and alcohol because they increase body fluid loss.

6. What is inflammatory bowel disease?

Inflammatory bowel disease (IBD) is an inflammatory process that involves the luminal gastrointestinal tract and is of unknown etiology. IBD most commonly includes Crohn's disease and ulcerative colitis. IBD occurs most often in patients between 15 and 25 years old. The incidence of Crohn's has been increasing in the past 30 years, whereas the incidence of ulcerative colitis has remained steady. Crohn's disease, also known as regional enteritis, is a chronic granulomatous inflammatory disease involving the small or large intestine with scarring and thickening of the bowel wall. Ulcerative colitis is chronic recurrent ulceration of the mucosa and submucosa of the colon and/or rectum.

7. Describe the nutritional care for IBD.

Patients with IBD develop an aversion to food, which results in malnutrition. The energy and protein content of the diet should be high, 40–50 kcals/kg ideal body weight (IBW) and 1–1.5 kg IBW. Small feedings are usually well tolerated. In the presence of steatorrhea, a low-fat diet and calcium, magnesium, and zinc supplementation are required. Use of medium-chain triglycerides and fish oil supplements with omega-3 fatty acids may be useful in treatment of Crohn's disease. During acute flare-up of Crohn's disease, bowel rest, TPN, and medical treatment can induce remission. The goal for nutritional management of Crohn's disease is to both lessen symptoms while maintaining nutritional adequacy.

8. What is end-stage liver disease?

The liver plays a key role in energy metabolism and bodily homeostasis. In essence, it is a filter for nutrients absorbed by the small intestine via the portal vein and for peripheral toxins via the hepatic artery. Within the liver nutrients are metabolized, stored, or distributed throughout the body, whereas toxins are metabolized and excreted through the blood or bile. Repeated toxic injury and regeneration to the hepatic epithelium eventually cause scar formation and fibrosis within the hepatic lobules. This process leads to loss of hepatic function and portal hypertension to maintain adequate perfusion. Portal hypertension leads to systemic shunting, thereby allowing toxins, nutrients, and microorganisms to bypass the hepatic filter. This causes the numerous derangements of liver failure.

Clinically, liver failure in not evident until 25–30% or less of total liver function remains. The etiologies for liver failure include chronic alcohol abuse, viral hepatitis, and medications.

Clinically, the duration and severity of the disease determine whether acute or chronic liver failure is present. Patients have a variety of derangements, as evidenced by malnutrition, jaundice, ascites, weight loss, secondary loss of visceral and somatic proteins, coagulopathy, neurologic derangements, and the stigmata of portal hypertension such as bleeding esophageal varices. The prognosis of end-stage liver disease worsens clinical outcome in total survival and infectious and perioperative complications. Therefore, it is important to address nutritional issues.

9. Why are there nutritional defects in liver disease?
Poor dietary intake is common in patients with liver disease. Alterations in craving for food, reduced ability to taste, early satiety, and malabsorption contribute to the poor intake. Current therapies for end-stage liver disease, such as medications (lactulose and neomycin), and sodium, fluid, and protein restriction, compound the problem. These factors, coupled with the multitude of metabolic abnormalities, worsen the nutritional defects. Such changes occur in both alcoholic and nonalcoholics with end-stage liver disease. The evaluation of the nutritional status of patients with liver disease can be difficult. Anthropometrical measurements are the most practical objective means of measurement. Other methods of assessing nutritional status such as total body weight, production of plasma proteins, and immune function are altered by the lack of protein production and accumulation of total body water that characterize end-stage liver disease.

10. What are the metabolic abnormalities of end-stage liver disease?
The cause of body wasting is unclear at this time, but there is evidence that end-stage liver disease results in increased catabolism. Carbohydrate and fat metabolism is clearly altered in liver disease; patients develop starvation-type metabolism more rapidly after overnight fasting. Significant insulin resistance occurs preventing peripheral glucose use. Additionally, there is a decrease in total glycogen stores within the liver and impaired glycogenolysis. These two factors cause an increased use of free fatty acids and protein for glucose production. Plasma levels of glucagon, epinephrine, cortisol, ammonia, and aromatic amino acids are elevated. End-stage liver disease also effects metabolism and storage of vitamins (B complex vitamins, vitamin A, vitamin K, folate, and thiamine) and micronutrients (zinc, copper, and iron), leading to additional complications due to deficiencies of these compounds.

11. What is hepatic encephalopathy? How is it affected by diet?
Hepatic encephalopathy is characterized by a variety of neurologic and behavioral disturbances associated with end-stage liver disease. The exact cause is unclear but is possibly related to impaired amino acid transport across the blood-brain barrier. Elevated levels of aromatic amino acids (phenylalanine, tyrosine, and tryptophan) and lower levels of the branched-chain amino acids (leucine, isoleucine, and valine) are found in the cerebrospinal fluid (CSF). This imbalance may contribute to elevation of false neurotransmitters, such as phenylethanolamine and gamma-amino butyric acid (GABA), which are also found in the CSF of patients with encephalopathy. The current treatment is to limit the amount of dietary protein to attempt to limit the amount of aromatic amino acids that patients receive and to decontaminate the gastrointestinal (GI) tract with lactulose and neomycin. Encephalopathy has been treated successfully by administering enteral or parenteral nutritional formulas with high amounts of branched-chain amino acids.

12. Describe the nutritional management of end-stage liver disease.
The nutritional therapy of liver failure is supportive in nature. The enteral route is preferred, but parenteral nutritional may be required if the GI tract is unavailable. The goal is to provide enough calories and protein to improve nutritional status without aggravating malabsorption or encephalopathy. The current recommendation from the 1997 ASPEN consensus group is to provide 1.3 times the resting energy expenditure or 25–30 kcal/ideal body weight. The current protein recommendation is 1.0–1.2 gm/kg protein. As hepatic encephalopathy worsens, protein replacement should be decreased accordingly. Nutritional formulas with enhanced amounts of

branched-chain amino acids seem to provide improved treatment of encephalopathy and short-term survival. Vitamin and micronutrient supplements should be given.

13. What is pancreatitis?

Pancreatitis is an inflammation of the pancreas and surrounding tissues caused by intrapancreatic activation of digestive enzymes and autodigestion of pancreatic acinar cells. Although there are many theories for the cause of the activation of digestive enzymes, the exact cause of the autoactivation of pancreatic enzymes is unclear. Direct cytotoxic injury from alcohol or medications, ductal obstruction, and duodenal reflux from gallstone passage are commonly cited causes. Acute inflammation of the pancreas can vary in severity. Patients present with epigastric abdominal pain that may radiate to the back with acute elevations of serum amylase and lipase. Although the majority of patients suffer from minimal pancreatic inflammation and organ dysfunction, a significant minority can progress to extensive tissue necrosis, sepsis, and multiorgan system failure. Patients who suffer prolonged inflammation with ductal disruption can lead to pseudocyst formation and chronic pain.

Chronic pancreatitis, however, primarily results from chronic injury to the pancreas. Progressive loss of pancreatic acinar cells and scarring produce chronic abdominal pain with periods of acute pain without elevation of amylase or lipase and malabsorption. Presenting symptoms are persistent abdominal pain, nausea, vomiting, and diarrhea in association with eating. Both acute and chronic cases of pancreatitis impair the production of pancreatic endocrine and exocrine function, resulting in malabsorption, glucose intolerance, and malnutrition.

14. Describe the nutritional and metabolic derangements in acute pancreatitis.

Acute pancreatitis commonly presents with systemic inflammatory response due to extensive release of proinflammatory mediators and cytokines such as interleukin-1 (IL-1), IL-6, IL-8, tumor necrosis factor, oxygen free radicals, and nitric oxide, and platelet-activating factor. This hypermetabolism leads to elevation of the resting energy expenditure as high as 1.5 times normal. Results include increased protein catabolism, increased gluconeogenesis with peripheral glucose intolerance, and increased lipolysis that can lead to rapid loss of lean body mass if increased nutritional needs are not replaced.

15. Describe the nutritional treatment for pancreatitis.

Current treatment for acute pancreatitis is primarily supportive, consisting of bowel rest, intravenous fluids, and pain control. Because the majority of cases of acute pancreatitis resolve quickly, patients do not require parenteral nutritional support. Total caloric replacement should be 1.5–2.0 times the basal requirement. Protein replacement should be 1.5–2.5 gm/kg/day, depending on the extent of hypermetabolism. Fat can be given as 30–40% of total calories. There is evidence that intrajejunal enteral nutritional replacement can be given safely to patients without increasing pancreatic enzyme output or morbidity. Although immune-enhancing feeds containing glutamine, arginine, omega-3 fatty acids, and nucleotides have been shown to improve outcomes in critically ill and trauma patients, there are no controlled studies showing improved outcomes in acute pancreatitis. For patients whose GI tract is not functional and patients with severe multiorgan failure, parenteral nutrition should be given. Since significant malabsorption and chronic pain characterize chronic pancreatitis, treatment is primarily aimed at replacing pancreatic enzymes along with pain control. The use of enteral and parenteral nutrition has not been shown to have any positive effect on long-term outcome in chronic pancreatitis.

16. What are enterocutaneous fistulas?

Enterocutaneous fistulas are communications of the GI tract to the skin of the abdominal wall. Typically they occur after surgical intervention but may occur spontaneously as a complication of GI disease process such malignancy, pancreatitis, inflammatory bowel disease, or diverticulitis. They are classified by point of origin and whether they are high output (> 500 cc/day) or low output (< 500 cc/day). The more distal the fistula, the higher the likelihood that the fistula may heal with conservative measure. Complications of enterocutaneous fistulas include fluid and electrolyte disturbances, intra-abdominal abscess formation with sepsis, and malnutrition. Standard therapies for enterocutaneous fistulas include correcting fluid and electrolyte imbalances and localizing and treating potential septic foci in the abdominal wall or intra-abdominal cavity. Contrast studies need to be performed to identify the exact location of the fistula. If a complex cavity is identified, computed tomography should be performed to evaluate the abdominal cavity for an abscess or distal obstruction. Most patients with high-output fistulas need to be on either total bowel rest and parenteral nutrition or enteral feeding past the fistula site, if possible, while the fistula is healing. Patients with low-output fistulas may be placed on a low-residue diet. In all cases, careful evaluation of the nutritional status of the patient is important to ensure adequate substrates for optimal healing.

17. What are the nutritional consequences of enterocutaneous fistulas?
Malnutrition occurs in the majority of patients with enterocutaneous fistulas. Patients are typically hypermetabolic from the underlying disease process and persistent low-grade sepsis. They are unable to achieve adequate nutritional intake because of losses of significant amounts of protein and electrolyte-containing GI fluids. In all cases, careful evaluation of nutritional status is important to ensure adequate substrates for optimal healing. Patients who are unable to support caloric requirements orally should be started on nutritional support ideally by the enteral route. Although no studies prove that total parenteral nutrition is better than enteral nutrition, specific indications for total parenteral nutrition include the inability to achieve or tolerate enteral access or the presence of high-output fistulas. Novel treatments for treatment of fistulas include the use of somatostain and its long-acting synthetic analog octreotide. These polypeptides inhibit gastric, pancreatic, biliary, and enteric secretions dramatically as well as improve the absorption of fluids and electrolytes. To date, no studies have confirmed that the use of these agents accelerates the healing of enterocutaneous fistulas, but they decrease the amount of fistula output.

BIBLIOGRAPHY

1. Abou-Assi S, O'Keefe S: Nutrition in acute pancreatitis. J Clin Gastroenterol 32:203–209, 2001.
2. Jeejeebhoy KN: Management of nutritional problems in patients with Crohn's disease. J Can Med Assoc 166:913–918, 2002.
3. Latifi R, Killam RW, Dudrick SJ: Nutritional support in liver failure. Surg Clin North Am 71:567–578, 1991.
4. Latifi R, McIntosh JK, Dudrick SJ: Nutritional management of acute and chronic pancreatitis. Surg Clin North Am 71:579–595, 1991.
5. Lob DN, Memon MA, Allson SP, et al: Evolution of nutritional support in acute pancreatitis. Br J Surg 87:695–707, 2000.
6. Mahan K, Escott-Stump S (eds): Krause's Food, Nutrition and Diet Therapy, 10 ed. Philadelphia, W.B. Saunders, 2000.
7. Makhdoom ZA, Komar MJ, Still CD: Nutrition and enterocutaneous fistulas. J Clin Gastroenterol 31:195–204, 2000.
8. Matos C, Porayko MK, Francisco-Ziller N, et al: Nutrition and chronic liver disease. J Clin Gastroenterol 35:391–397, 2002.
9. Shils M, Olson J, Shike M (eds): Modern Nutrition in Health and Disease, 8th ed. Philadelphia, Lea & Febiger, 1994.
10. Swagerty DL Jr, Walling AD, Klein RM: Lactose intolerance. Am Fam Physician 65:1845–1850, 2002.
11. Verger JT, Schears G, Lord LM: Management of the patient with short bowel syndrome. AACN Clinical Issues: Advanced Practice in Acute & Critical Care 11:604–618, 2000.

28. NUTRITION IN THE MANAGEMENT OF CANCER

Angela M. Rialti, RD, and Alan B. Marr, MD

1. What is the incidence of malnutrition in cancer patients?
Fifty to eighty percent of cancer patients suffer from malnutrition. Malnutrition and inanition are the direct cause of death in 22% of all cancer patients. In the hospital, 45% of these patients will record a weight loss greater than 10%.

2. How does weight loss affect the prognosis of cancer patients?
Cancer patients who do not show weight loss have a significant improvement in survival rate, as compared to those who lose weight. Weight loss has been associated with a decrease in clinical status as defined by increases in cancer stage and in the number of tumor sites. The Eastern Cooperative Oncology Group Study analyzed the relationship between weight loss and diagnosis. They found that gastric and pancreatic cancer patients presented with the highest degree of weight loss. An intermediate weight loss was detected in unfavorable non-Hodgkin's lymphoma, and cancer of the colon, lung, and prostate. Those patients with favorable non-Hodgkin's lymphoma, acute non-lymphocytic leukemia, breast cancer, and sarcomas had the least association with weight loss. Weight loss negatively influences the prognosis of cancer patients undergoing surgery, chemotherapy, and radiotherapy. Patients who are in the malnourished group have increased complications and mortality from all three treatment modalities.

3. What impact does cachexia have in cancer patients?
Cancer cachexia is a syndrome characterized by progressive weight loss, inanition, anorexia, weakness, tissue wasting, and organ dysfunction. Its cause is multifactorial. Patients with cancer often have a loss of appetite as a result of their disease or treatment. Abnormalities in taste and smell contribute to decreased food intake and resulting weight loss. While tumors can prevent the passage of nutrition by direct compression, the metabolic pathways are altered by the tumor release of peptides and cytokines. Examples of these are tumor necrosis factor (TNF), interferon γ, interleukin-2, and interleukin-6. Intermediary metabolism is also altered, causing a high metabolic rate reflected in an increase in protein breakdown. This alteration occurs even in the face of starvation. The end result is an ineffective use of nutrients.

4. What happens to energy expenditure in the cancer patient?
Decreased energy expenditure is a normal response to starvation. But this response is not always seen in cancer patients. They can demonstrate a persistent increase in energy expenditure in the face of a decreased intake. This failure to conserve energy expenditure is one of the contributing factors to cancer cachexia. It is a maladaptation of cancer patients to a state of starvation. Little is known definitively in this area. Studies have produced conflicting results and the factors which determine energy expenditure in the cancer patient are not known with any degree of certainty.

5. How does cancer affect carbohydrate metabolism?
Tumor-bearing patients develop changes in carbohydrate metabolism. These patients have elements in common with both type II diabetes and stress. Cancer patients will develop a 25–40% increase in hepatic glucose production, similar to that seen in diabetic patients. But diabetic patients will decrease hepatic glucose production during starvation, while cancer patients will increase glucose production. This may be due to an increased availability of precursors of gluconeogenesis such as alanine, glycerol, and lactate. Increased circulating lactate, found in

cancer patients, is used by the liver to make glucose for both the tumor and the host. Early in their course, cancer patients demonstrate this as glucose intolerance. They have hyperglycemia and delayed clearance of both intravenous and oral glucose. Insulin resistance has been shown to be a major cause of this glucose intolerance. Cancer patients demonstrate an increased total body turnover of glucose, which according to Shaw and Wolfe, is proportional to the extent of disease. They show increased Cori cycle activity—increased recycling of carbon fragments derived from glucose.

6. What happens to fat metabolism in cancer patients?

Cancer patients have decreased fat reserves. A reduced food intake certainly contributes to this, but there are alterations in lipid metabolism secondary to the presence of tumor. Cancer patients have increased lipid mobilization with increased oxidation of free fatty acids. They also have a decreased clearance of serum lipids. This lipid mobilization is facilitated by lipolytic substances which induce the release of free fatty acids from adipose tissue. This mobilization is not suppressed by glucose infusion and appears to be a function of the type and amount of tumor burden.

7. Why is cancer referred to as a "nitrogen sink"?

Protein is the major source of nitrogen in the human body. Tumors derive protein at the expense of the host. Tumors act as "nitrogen sinks" by depleting the patient's protein mass and altering protein metabolism. Whole body turnover of protein is increased. Both hepatic synthesis of protein and protein catabolism are increased. Muscle protein synthesis is decreased and muscle protein breakdown increased. In simple starvation, by contrast, hepatic synthesis rates are decreased. The cancer patient shows a lack of the normal metabolic responses which conserve protein during both starvation and stress.

8. Does malnutrition affect tumor growth?

Protein calorie malnutrition may diminish tumor growth. Animal studies show significant reduction in tumor growth rates during protein calorie restriction. There have been no human studies to confirm this.

9. What relationship does malnutrition have to surgical therapy for cancer?

It is well established that cancer patients with severe malnutrition have worse surgical outcomes than patients who are adequately nourished. They have a higher rate of mortality, a higher rate of major complications, and more infectious complications. These complications include impaired wound healing, anastomotic leaks, abscess formations, infections, fistulas, and postoperative pneumonia. Malnourished cancer patients have impaired immunocompetence. Surgical therapy will further deplete the malnourished cancer patient. The stress response following surgery taxes depleted energy reserves. The patient is often unable to eat for several days after an operation, which further reduces energy reserves. A large cooperative study has demonstrated that in patients with severe malnutrition who must be operated on for cancer, use of perioperative total parenteral nutrition (TPN) can decrease complications and reduce mortality.

10. What relationship does malnutrition have to chemotherapy for cancer?

Severely malnourished patients have a diminished response to chemotherapy. These patients have difficulty completing the chemotherapy regime, being more likely to have hematopoietic side effects. Chemotherapy contributes to host malnutrition. Cancer drugs tend to be toxic and produce nausea, vomiting, mucositis, and gastrointestinal dysfunction. These side effects, in the already malnourished cancer patient, will actually influence the outcome of chemotherapy, by causing increased treatment morbidity and mortality.

There is little proof, however, that providing nutritional support to the patient undergoing chemotherapy will improve results, although it will increase the tolerance to chemotherapy and lower the impact of toxic side effects. A number of explanations have been offered for this, of which the most appealing is that the nutritional support feeds the tumor and helps the tumor survive the chemotherapy. But there is no clinical evidence that this is true.

11. What relationship does malnutrition have to radiation therapy for cancer?

Just as in other therapies for cancer, malnourished patients undergoing radiation therapy have increased morbidity and mortality. Radiation therapy can contribute directly to the malnutrition. The effect on the severity of malnutrition and amount of weight loss is dependent on the radiation dose, duration, volume of therapy, and body site being irradiated. Nutritional alterations may be site specific to local therapy. Example of this are nausea and vomiting caused by central nervous system irradiation, stomatitis caused by head and neck irradiation, dysphagia caused by thoracic irradiation, and enteritis and malabsorption caused by abdominal irradiation. These acute effects usually improve but may cause the dose of radiation to be limited which, in turn, leads to poorer response rates. As with chemotherapy, there is no evidence that provision of nutritional support to patients receiving radiotherapy can influence the end result.

12. How does nutritional repletion alter the response to surgery?

Several studies have demonstrated a marked reduction in complications and mortality of severely malnourished patients if given 7–10 days of preoperative nutritional support. These patients have improved serum proteins and immunocompetence. But still, the most common use of nutritional support is postoperative. Nutritional support should begin immediately postoperatively if the patient is either severely malnourished or not expected to have oral intake for 5–7 days. A number of studies support this. The question of whether to use TPN or total enteral nutrition (TEN) has yet to be answered conclusively. Enteral nutrition maintains the gut mucosa, promotes immunocompetence, and is associated with reduced septic mortality compared with TPN. However, most of the abdominal cancer operations interfere with the patient's tolerance for enteral nutrition. Early nutritional support can be carried out through surgical jejunostomy but this has not yet become common practice in surgical oncology.

13. How does nutritional repletion alter the response to chemotherapy?

Nutritional support may help to reduce the side effects of chemotherapy, and patients do exhibit weight gain. However, in large randomized trials, nutritional repletion has not resulted in increased lean body mass, increased response rate, or increased survival rates. Nutritional support does allow some patients to undergo chemotherapy who would not have be able to do so otherwise. An exception to this is the bone marrow transplant patient. Ten days of TPN prior to bone marrow transplant has resulted in an improvement in disease-free survival, relapse time, and overall survival.

14. How does nutritional repletion alter the response to radiation therapy?

The use of nutritional support in patients undergoing radiation therapy has not been studied as well as nutritional support in surgery or chemotherapy. Several retrospective and at least one prospective study have shown that patients on TPN have fewer toxicity-related interruptions and some weight gain, but no documented overall improvement in response or survival rates. Nutritional support should, therefore, be used to support the severely malnourished patient receiving radiation therapy and those patients with radiation enteritis.

15. What are the indications for TPN in the cancer patient?

Aggressive nutritional support should be used as an adjunct to the treatment of cancer patients. It is indicated if the patient is severely malnourished or if they are undergoing intervention with the intent of palliation or cure and enteral nutrition is otherwise contraindicated.

16. Can TPN induce cancer growth?

The results in humans are mixed but there is no definitive evidence that nutritional support actually stimulates growth or promotes metastasis in humans. Animal studies have been performed to demonstrate this by using enteral and parenteral nutrition. It is documented that malnourished tumor-bearing animals will gain weight and have an improvement in immunocompetence. Unfortunately these animals had a stimulation of tumor growth rate as well.

17. What is the difference between cancer-related weight loss and tumor-induced weight loss?
Patients with cancer often have specific problems that contribute to weight loss, such as physical obstruction of the GI tract, nausea, vomiting, constipation, depression, and pain as well as the side effects of treatment with radiation and chemotherapy. These causes are referred to as cancer-related weight loss. Tumor-induced weight loss (TIWL) is due to metabolic changes produced by the tumor or by the host in response to the tumor and is characterized by poor appetite, early satiety, change in taste, and classical anorexia. The fundamental difference is that TIWL is usually irreversible regardless of feeding.

18. Can fish oil and eicosapentanoic acid (EPA)-based formulas improve TIWL?
Studies have shown that fish oil and EPA (n-3 fatty acid) have an effect on the potential mediators of cachexia, including cytokine production, PIF, and APPR. Clinical studies providing 2.2 gm EPA to weight-losing pancreatic cancer patients suggest that these agents stabilize weight. They also have been shown to promote weight gain, prolong survival, cause a gain in lean body mass, reverse negative nitrogen balance, and improve appetite and functional ability. The evidence is promising, although much more research needs to be done to confirm its role in cancer treatment.

CONTROVERSIES

19. Can anabolic agents improve malnutrition in cancer patients?
The reason standard TPN fails to improve clinical outcomes is that standard TPN does not affect the changes in intermediary metabolism. The addition of metabolic agents or other biological response modifiers to TPN offers promise. Use of insulin improves protein balance in both cachectic animal and human studies. Growth hormone improves protein metabolism, wound healing, and immunologic status in surgical patients. Marrow stimulants can counteract toxic effects of chemotherapeutic agents. Further research is needed in these areas.

20. Can supplemental amino acids affect protein metabolism?
Branched-chain amino acid infusions can decrease protein catabolism in cancer patients. Whether this alters clinical outcomes is yet to be defined. Glutamine is a nonessential amino acid important for gastrointestinal mucosal growth that is often depleted in cancer patients. Because of its instability in simple amino acid form, it is not routinely added to TPN. Surgical patients have improved nitrogen balance, improved protein synthesis, and improved T-lymphocyte response when glutamine is repleted in addition to TPN therapy. Whether this will aid the cancer population requires further study.

BIBLIOGRAPHY

1. Askanazi J, Hensle TW, Starker PM, et al: Effect of immediate postoperative nutritional support on length of hospitalization. Ann Surg 203:236–239, 1986.
2. Barber MD, Rogers BB: Advances in the management of tumor-induced weight loss. Medscape CME, August 29, 2002. Available at <http://www.medscape.com/>.
3. Baron PL, Lawrence W Jr., Chan WM, White FK, Banks WL Jr.: Effects of parenteral nutrition on cell cycle kinetics of head and neck cancer. Arch Surg 121:1282–1286, 1986.
4. Bosaeus I, Daneryd P, Lundholm K: Dietary intake, resting energy expenditure, weight loss and survival in cancer patients. J Nutr 132(Suppl 11):3465S–3466S, 2002.
5. Bray GA: The underlying basis for obesity: Relationship to cancer. J Nutr 132(Suppl 11):3451S–3455S, 2002.
6. Brennan MF: Total parenteral nutrition in the cancer patient. N Engl J Med 305:375–382, 1981.

7. Brennan MF, Burt ME: Nitrogen metabolism in cancer patients. Cancer Treat Rep 65(Suppl 5):67–78, 1981.

8. Brennan MF, Pisters PW, Posner M, Quesada O, Shike M: A prospective randomized trial of total parenteral nutrition after major pancreatic resection for malignancy. Ann Surg 220:436–441; discussion 441–444, 1994.

9. Cameron IL: Effect of total parenteral nutrition on tumor-host responses in rats. Cancer Treat Rep 65(Suppl 5):93–99, 1981.

10. Chen MK, Souba WW, Copeland EMd, Copeland EM: Nutritional support of the surgical oncology patient. Hematol Oncol Clin North Am 5:125–145, 1991.

11. Copeland EM, Souchon EA, MacFadyen BV Jr., Rapp MA, Dudrick SJ: Intravenous hyperalimentation as an adjunct to radiation therapy. Cancer 39:609–616, 1977.

12. Copeland EMd, Copeland EM: Jonathan E. Rhoads lecture. Intravenous hyperalimentation and cancer. A historical perspective. JPEN J Parenter Enteral Nutr 10:337–342, 1986.

13. Daly JM, Reynolds HM, Rowlands BJ, Dudrick SJ, Copeland EMd: Tumor growth in experimental animals: Nutritional manipulation and chemotherapeutic response in the rat. Ann Surg 191:316–322, 1980.

14. Harrison LE, Brennan MF: The role of total parenteral nutrition in the patient with cancer. Curr Probl Surg 32:833–917, 1995.

15. Higdon JV, Frei B: Tea catechins and polyphenols: Health effects, metabolism, and antioxidant functions. Crit Rev Food Sci Nutr 43:89–143, 2003.

16. Holroyde CP, Reichard GA: Carbohydrate metabolism in cancer cachexia. Cancer Treat Rep 65 (Suppl 5): 55–59, 1981.

17. Kelly CJ, Daly JM: Perioperative care of the oncology patient. World J Surg 17:199–206, 1993.

18. Mullen JL, Buzby GP, Gertner MH, et al: Protein synthesis dynamics in human gastrointestinal malignancies. Surgery 87:331–338, 1980.

19. Pezner R, Archambeau JO: Critical evaluation of the role of nutritional support for radiation therapy patients. Cancer 55:263–267, 1985.

20. Popp MB, Wagner SC, Brito OJ: Host and tumor responses to increasing levels of intravenous nutritional support. Surgery 94:300–308, 1983.

21. Schein PS, Kisner D, Haller D, Blecher M, Hamosh M: Cachexia of malignancy: Potential role of insulin in nutritional management. Cancer 43:2070–2076, 1979.

22. Schwartz GF, Green HL, Bendon ML, Graham WPd, Blakemore WS: Combined parenteral hyperalimentation and chemotherapy in the treatment of disseminated solid tumors. Am J Surg 121:169–173, 1971.

23. Shaw JH, Wolfe RR: Glucose and urea kinetics in patients with early and advanced gastrointestinal cancer: The response to glucose infusion, parenteral feeding, and surgical resection. Surgery 101: 181–191, 1987.

24. Souchon EA, Copeland EM, Watson P, Dudrick SJ: Intravenous hyperalimentation as an adjunct to cancer chemotherapy with 5-fluorouracil. J Surg Res 18:451–454, 1975.

25. Strasser F, Bruera ED: Update on anorexia and cachexia. Hematol Oncol Clin North Am 16:589–617, 2002.

26. Tisdale MJ: Wasting in cancer. J Nutr 129(Suppl 1S):243S–246S, 1999.

27. Torosian MH, Daly JM: Nutritional support in the cancer-bearing host. Effects on host and tumor. Cancer 58:1915–1929, 1986.

28. Van Way, CW III: Handbook of Surgical Nutrition. Philadelphia, J. B. Lippincott, 1992.

29. Waterhouse C, Kemperman JH: Carbohydrate metabolism in subjects with cancer. Cancer Res 31:1273–1278, 1971.

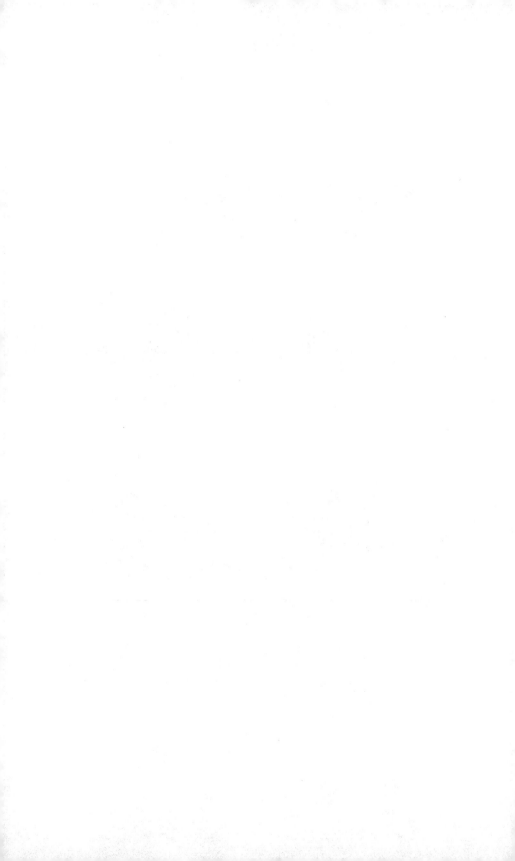

VII. Nutritional Science

29. NUTRITIONAL ASSESSMENT

Laura Clark, RD, LD, CNSD

1. What is nutritional assessment?

Nutritional assessment is a comprehensive approach to the definition of nutritional status. It includes information about medical history, social history, medications, physical examination, nutritional intake, diet history, laboratory data, and anthropometric measurements. It includes the measurement of somatic and visceral protein stores, nitrogen balance, and cell-mediated immunity. The assessment process usually includes two parts: screening and assessment. The purpose of screening is to identify patients at risk for nutritional problems. These include malnutrition and nutritionally related diseases such as diabetes and ulcerative colitis. Assessment is directed towards therapy. Assessment should identify the patient's deficits and needs, both for remedial nutrition therapy and for ongoing nutrition. The outcome of a nutritional assessment should be a care plan for the patient which identifies the appropriate medical nutrition therapies, both in patients requiring only modifications of a normal diet and in those who require aggressive nutritional repletion and support.

2. How is a nutritional assessment completed?

A formal assessment is completed by screening an individual and collecting information in the various areas described above. This information is obtained through interviewing, questionnaires, and reviewing the medical record. A nutrition screening/assessment form can be used in this process. Once the information is obtained it is analyzed. Sometimes the patient is given a score which reflects their nutritional status. A care plan is developed on the basis of the nutritional assessment.

3. What is meant by nutritional status?

Nutritional status is the expression of the degree to which physiologic needs for nutrients are being met. It is the balance of nutrient intake and nutrient requirements. It can be affected by many factors, including disease, cultural patterns, eating behavior or habits, psychological stress, economics, and nutrient absorption.

4. How is malnutrition classified?

Malnutrition is defined as a state of overnutrition or undernutrition. Overnutrition is usually called obesity, and malnutrition is usually taken to mean undernutrition. Classically, undernutrition falls into one of three categories. Marasmus is calorie malnutrition and is evidenced by physical wasting of energy stores, including somatic protein and fat. Serum proteins are typically preserved. Kwashiorkor is protein malnutrition and is produced by inadequate quantity and quality of protein, while calories remain adequate. Marasmic kwashiorkor is a combined protein and energy malnutrition. It is the most common form of undernutrition throughout the world. In clinical practice, it occurs when metabolic stress is placed on a chronically-starved individual. Malnutrition can be classified by loss of body weight, although one must consider the hydration status of the individual before doing so.

One calculates the percent of usual weight:

$$\text{actual weight} \div \text{usual weight} \times 100$$

The formula for percentage weight loss is calculated by the following formula:

$$\% \text{ Weight loss} = (\text{Usual weight} - \text{present weight}) \times 100 \div (\text{Usual weight})$$

The classification of malnutrition is as follows (based on percent of usual weight):

Mild   85–90%
Moderate   75–84%
Severe   < 74%

5. What is nutritional stress?

Many clinicians use this term to mean unintentional weight loss, especially in a context of increased demands. If the patient has lost 5 lb in a month or 10 lb in three months, he or she is at least mildly malnourished. Sometimes the term "nutritional stress" is used to indicate recent weight loss.

6. How does malnutrition affect functional status and disease outcomes?

The loss of 40% or more of the lean body mass (*not* the same as body weight) usually leads to the patient's death. Even lesser degrees of malnutrition may impair survival. Studies show that malnourished patients stay in the hospital longer, have higher hospital readmission rates, longer wound and fracture healing times, and have a higher death rate after surgery than well-nourished patients. Other studies show that immune function and muscle function are also affected. Malnutrition may contribute to heart failure and may even cause it in some circumstances.

7. What are the physical signs of malnutrition?

The hair is dry, dull, easily plucked, and discolored. Eyes are red, dry, or inflamed. The mouth, gums, and lips are red and swollen, often with sores. The sense of taste is diminished. Teeth show signs of gray or brown spots and can become loose. The skin is frail, pale, scaly, yellow colored, slow to heal, swollen, or flushed. Muscles lose strength, may appear wasted, and can exhibit twitching, cramping, and pain. The nervous system shows listlessness, loss of balance, hypoactive reflexes, memory impairment, neuropathy, and seizures.

8. What are anthropometric measurements and how are they used in nutritional assessment?

Anthropometric measurements include height, weight, skinfold thickness, and circumference measurements of various parts of the body. These measurements reflect present nutritional status and can be used to estimate the degree of obesity and even the percentage of body fat. They are most useful when taken accurately and compared over a period of time because they are not sensitive to acute changes in nutritional status. Height and weight are usually evaluated against reference norms such as the Metropolitan Life Insurance Tables. Body-frame size is also used in determining desired body weight.

Body composition may be measured by skinfold-thickness testing. This measurement can be useful but is valid only if the measurements are taken accurately. Skinfold sites typically measured are the triceps, biceps, below the scapula, above the iliac crest, and the upper thigh. Triceps skinfold estimates subcutaneous fat.

Circumference measurements can include the waist and hip circumference ratio (differentiates between gynoid and android obesity), mid-upper circumference (indicative of skeletal muscle mass), head circumference (typically used in children under the age of 3), and calf circumference. These numbers are then compared against norms. By measuring biceps, triceps, subscapular, and suprailiac skin folds, for example, one can consult an appropriate table and estimate the percentage of body fat.

9. What is the Body Mass Index (BMI)?

The BMI is commonly used to estimate the level of adiposity in individuals or in groups. It defines obesity as a relationship of weight to height. An index is usually a quantity divided by the body surface area, but the weight divided by the body surface area makes little sense either mathematically or clinically. So the BMI is defined as the ratio of the weight to the square of the height:

$$BMI = Weight\ in\ kg\ /\ (Height\ in\ meters)^2$$

The commonly used definition of normal BMI is 20 to 25 kg/m². A BMI of 20–25 shows the least risk for early death. A score above 25 is classified into three categories of obesity: mild,

25–29; moderate, 30–40; and severe, 40+. Generally, a BMI greater than 30 indicates clinical obesity and is associated with greater risk for the development of health problems and disease. This should be adjusted for age, as noted below.

The range of normal for the BMI increases with age.

Age group (yrs)	BMI (kg/m²)
19–24	19–24
25–34	20–25
35–44	21–26
45–54	22–27
55–64	23–28
65+	24–29

The BMI must be taken with a certain amount of skepticism. It is a convenient way of standardizing body size over the normal range of height and weight for adults but it does not eliminate the need to consider gender and frame size. An average man has a BMI about 2 kg/m^2 greater than an average woman of the same height. For a man 5' 10" in height, going from a small to a medium frame size increases the BMI by 1 kg/m^2; and going from a medium to a large frame size increases it by 2 kg/m^2.

10. What factors are used to carry out a nutritional assessment?
A medical history is the starting point. This should include diagnosis, metabolic needs, chronic or acute diseases, recent surgery, gastrointestinal problems, weight loss, alcohol use, and increased nutrient losses. Other factors important to assess are poor eyesight, physical disabilities, mental status changes, and drug side effects. A social history may include factors such as adequate income to purchase food, the ability to shop for and prepare food, and living conditions.

A nutrient intake history can be established by intake records such as a 24-hour recall, a 3–7-day diet history, observation of an individual at mealtime, and a food frequency record. These tools can help establish eating pattern histories and lead to a more comprehensive nutrient intake analysis to determine where deficiencies may be occurring.

11. How are visceral protein and somatic protein assessed?
Somatic protein (skeletal protein mass) measurements are assessed by height and weight measurements, creatinine-height index, and anthropometric measurements such as arm muscle circumference and triceps skinfold thickness. These are compared to normal value tables to assess the nutritional status.

Visceral protein status is assessed by using serum albumin, serum transferrin, and total lymphocyte count (TLC). Albumin should be over 3.5 gm/dl. A value lower than 3 is consistent with malnutrition and a value lower than 2 with severe malnutrition. These values will vary somewhat by laboratory. Transferrin should be greater than 200 mg/dL. A value of less than 160 is consistent with malnutrition. The TLC should be greater than 1800/ml. If it is less than 900/ml, there may be malnutrition. However, TLC is affected by many things, including infection and injury. None of the laboratory values are very dependable. If the laboratory values and the clinical picture are in conflict, the clinical findings should prevail.

12. What is nitrogen balance and how is it used in nutritional assessment?
Nitrogen balance is the difference between nitrogen intake and nitrogen output, as measured by excretion in the urine and the feces. Intake is determined by the dietary intake of protein (1 gram of nitrogen = 6.25 grams of protein). Output is determined by measuring total nitrogen output. For clinical purposes, fecal nitrogen is usually ignored, and total urinary nitrogen is estimated from the 24-hour urine urea nitrogen. Roughly 80% of the urine nitrogen is excreted as urea. To estimate total urinary nitrogen (TUN) from urine urea nitrogen (UUN), either of the following formulas can be used:

$$TUN = UUN + 4$$
$$TUN = UUN \times 1.25$$

The formula for nitrogen balance is:

N balance = (Protein intake (g) ÷ 6.25) − (UUN × 1.25)

A healthy person normally has a zero or slightly positive balance. A patient with a wasting disease will have a negative balance. Someone with high catabolism will have a large urea nitrogen excretion, often more than 20 gm/day. The goal for a patient recovering from an injury, an operation, or a major illness is a 2–4 gram positive nitrogen balance.

13. What is Subjective Global Assessment (SGA) and how is it used?

SGA is a method of assessing nutritional status as done by an experienced clinician. The clinician looks at the patient and decides if the patient is well-nourished, mildly malnourished, or severely malnourished. SGA relies on medical history, physical signs and symptoms, dietary changes or intolerances, physiologic stress, gastrointestinal symptoms, weight history, and functional capacity. The use of SGA gives a broad perspective of the nutritional status of a patient. Studies have shown that the SGA is as accurate as more elaborate techniques of nutritional assessment incorporating laboratory tests and anthropometric measurements. Putting it another way, the laboratory values and measurements add very little to the clinical evaluation. It is reassuring that an experienced clinician can assess nutritional status well enough for most purposes.

14. How is the immune system assessed?

Immunocompetence is difficult to assess. There is no such thing as an "immune function test." Immunocompetence may be estimated by using TLC and delayed hypersensitivity skin testing. TLC is an indicator of immune function and reflects T cells and B cells. A value of 1500–1800 cells/mm^3 shows mild depletion, 900–1500 is moderate depletion, and less than 900 shows severe depletion, which may be seen in the severely malnourished patient. Delayed hypersensitivity skin testing measures cell-mediated immunity, and is clinically significant because it can be used as an indicator of postoperative sepsis and mortality. But no measurement of immune function can be relied upon to predict the patient's susceptibility to infection.

15. How are nutritional requirements determined?

Requirements for vitamins and minerals are defined by the Recommended Dietary Allowances as published by the Food and Nutrition Board of the National Research Council-National Academy of Sciences. These are established for the general, healthy population. In critically ill people, these needs may change according to their disease or condition. Nutrient requirements change according to particular disease states. Calorie requirements can be established using the Harris Benedict Equations or other formulas to calculate the basal energy expenditure and multiplying this by the appropriate stress and activity factors to determine the patient's caloric needs. A resting energy expenditure (REE) may also be measured using indirect calorimetry with a metabolic cart to determine calorie needs. The subject is considered in detail in Chapter 30.

BIBLIOGRAPHY

1. American Dietetic Association: Pocket Resource for Nutrition Assessment. Chicago, ADA, 1996.
2. ASPEN: Nutrition Support Dietetics, Core Curriculum. Silver Spring, MD, ASPEN Publications, 1993.
3. Detsky A, McGlaughlin J, Baker J, et al: What is subjective global assessment of nutritional status? JPEN J Parenter Enteral Nutr 11:8–13, 1987.
4. Hill G: Body composition research: Implications for the practice of clinical nutrition. JPEN J Parenter Enteral Nutr 16:197–218, 1992.
5. Mahan LK, Escott-Stump S (eds): Krause's Food, Nutrition, and Diet Therapy, 9th ed. Philadelphia, W.B. Saunders, 1996.
6. Zeman FJ, Neiy DM: Clinical Nutrition and Dietetics. New York, MacMillan, 1991.

30. DETERMINING ENERGY REQUIREMENTS

Carol Ireton-Jones, PhD, RD, LD, CNSD, FACN

1. What are the components of a normal person's daily energy expenditure?
- Basal metabolic rate (BMR), or the amount of energy expended in voluntary and involuntary bodily functions, accounts for the majority of energy expended daily.
- Energy expended for the digestion and absorption of food (the thermic effect of food) ranges from 8% to 10% above BMR.
- Energy expended in daily activities and exercise accounts for the balance of daily energy expenditure.

Gender and stature affect BMR. The variance in individual daily energy expenditures usually is based on the amount of energy expended in activities, including exercise. Energy expenditure is related to body weight, especially lean body mass and to a lesser degree body fat.

2. What are the components of an ill or injured patient's daily energy expenditure?
Energy expenditure is increased above BMR due to the degree of stress of the illness or injury. Although malnutrition alone may cause a decrease in BMR, a patient with increased stress due to an operation or illness is most likely to have an increase in BMR, even in the presence of malnutrition. The stress caused by the catabolic state results in increased daily energy expenditure. Activity level is usually not included in the daily energy expenditure, because moderately to severely stress patients do not participate in normal daily activities.

Previous and ongoing studies have shown that metabolic rate and therefore daily energy expenditures are increased in moderately to severely stressed patients, such as those with traumatic injuries, burns, or head injuries. Treatment regimens, age, and body composition also affect individual energy expenditure in response to injury and illness.

3. How can daily energy expenditure be determined for normal persons and patients?
Energy expenditure can be measured using indirect calorimetry or estimated using predictive equations for both normal persons and ill or injured patients. For normal persons, the accuracy of the estimation or prediction of energy needs (i.e., kcal/day) can be assessed by the maintenance of body weight. Persons who lose weight need more kcal/day, and persons who gain need to decrease kcal intake per day. There are individual differences in daily activities and energy expenditure that cannot be accounted for exactly in energy equations. For patients who are ill or injured, even more variations exist in relation to individual response to disease or injury. Energy equations can be used to predict daily energy expenditure; however, improved accuracy can be achieved by measuring energy expenditure using indirect calorimetry.

4. What equations are used to estimate energy expenditure?
The most commonly used equations for estimating energy expenditure in both normal adults and ill or injured patients are the Harris Benedict Energy Equations (HBEEs). These equations were developed from indirect calorimetric measurements of energy expenditures of normal persons at rest. HBEEs, which are different for males and females, estimate basal energy expenditure (BEE) or BMR. However, the BMR is more likely to be considered resting metabolic rate (RMR) because true BMR can be estimated only under highly rigorous research conditions. Additional kcal must be factored in and added to the RMR to account for the thermic effect of food and activity to estimate daily energy expenditure.

Male

HBEE = 66.47 + 13.75 × wt (kg) + 5.0 × ht (cm) – 6.76 × age (years)

Female

HBEE = 655.1 + 9.56 × wt (kg) + 1.85 × ht (cm) – 4.68 × age (years) where HBEE = kcal/day; wt = actual body weight in kg; ht = height in cm; and age = current age in years

Factors to account for daily energy expenditure in normal persons include the following:
• Light activity: HBEE × 1.1
• Moderate activity: HBEE × 1.2–1.3
• Heavy activity: HBEE × 1.4–1.5

These equations have also been applied to ill or injured patients, extrapolating the effect of the stress of the disease or injury in place of the activity factor. Factors to account for daily energy expenditure in ill or injured patients include the following:
• Mild stress (e.g., after surgery): HBEE × 1.1
• Moderate stress (e.g., moderate injury or infection): HBEE × 1.2–1.3
• Severe stress (e.g., multiple system organ failure): HBEE × 1.4–1.5

5. Are there better equations to estimate the energy expenditure of ill or injured adults?

Energy expenditures vary widely but can be estimated for ill or injured patients using readily available data such as weight, height, age, sex, disease state, and ventilatory status as described by the Ireton-Jones energy equations (IJEEs). The factors related to energy expenditure in the IJEE are the same factors described above. Obesity is a negative factor in the equation for spontaneously breathing patients but is not included in the equation for ventilator-dependent patients. However, the factors related to body weight are lower in the equation for ventilator-dependent patients than in the equation for spontaneously breathing patients, effectively accounting for the variation in body weight.

Spontaneously breathing patients
IJEE (s) = 629 – 11(A) + 25(W) – 609(O)

Ventilator-dependent patients
IJEE (v) = 1784 – 11(A) + 5(W) + 244(S) + 239(T) + 804(B)

where IJEE = kcal/day, s = spontaneously breathing, v = ventilator-dependent, A = age (years), W = actual body weight (kg), S = sex (male = 1, female = 0); T = diagnosis of trauma (present = 1, absent = 0), B = diagnosis of burn (present = 1, absent = 0), O = obesity > 30% above IBW from 1959 Metropolitan Life Insurance tables or BMI > 27 (present = 1, absent = 0)

The IJEEs have been validated and found to correlate significantly with energy expenditure measured by indirect calorimetry; therefore, they are useful for application to the clinical setting.

6. What other equations are used to estimate the energy expenditure of normal adults?

Other equations used to estimate the energy expenditures of normal individual range from simple to complex. The RDA tables suggest a range of calorie requirements based on age for both adults and children. A simple equation is to estimate daily energy expenditure from current body weight:
• Weight loss = weight in pounds × 10
• Weight maintenance = weight in pounds × 15
• Weight gain = weight in pounds × 20

7. What is indirect calorimetry?

Indirect calorimetry is the determination of energy expenditure through measurement of oxygen consumption and carbon dioxide production during respiratory gas exchange. Indirect calorimetry is based on the premise that the energy released by oxidative processes and by anaerobic glycolysis is ultimately transformed into heat or external work. Energy expenditures of both ventilator-dependent and spontaneously breathing patients can be measured by indirect calorimetry. Most measurements are now done with the use of a portable indirect calorimeter. Some of the larger indirect calorimeters are also capable of providing respiratory function analyses and may be used in other venues. A recently developed, small, handheld device measures oxygen consumption only but has been validated for accurate measurement of energy expenditure in spontaneously breathing patients.

When patients are measured using indirect calorimetry, the effect of the disease or injury is assessed as metabolic rate is measured; therefore, it is not necessary to add an additional factor to account for the illness or injury. Some clinicians add an additional factor of 10% to account for slight increases in energy expenditure that may occur during the day as a result of movement; however, the need for this adjustment has not been validated. Gottschlich has shown that patients can be measured any time during the day because there is no difference in energy expenditures in critically ill patients throughout the day and night.

8. What is respiratory quotient?

Respiratory quotient (RQ) is calculated from the ratio of carbon dioxide produced (VCO_2) to oxygen consumed (VO_2):

$$RQ = VCO_2/VO_2$$

During measurement of energy expenditure, this ratio reflects net substrate utilization. Oxidation of each major nutrient class occurs at a known RQ (ranging from 0.7 for fat oxidation to 1.0 for glucose oxidation) because the amounts of oxygen consumed and carbon dioxide produced are characteristic and constant for protein, carbohydrate, and fat. When the RQ is greater than 1.0, net fat synthesis occurs; however, RQs greater than 1.0 can also occur when carbohydrate (glucose) intake or total caloric intake is excessive. An RQ of 0.85 is said to reflect a mixture of substrate utilization. Use of the RQ alone as a tool for assessing nutrient intake adequacy has been suggested; however, evaluation of RQ alone cannot adequately depict the entire clinical process of the patient and therefore must be assessed along with clinical factors and energy expenditure determinations. An RQ that is out of physiologic range (less than 0.65 or greater than 1.2) usually indicates that the indirect calorimetric measurement of energy expenditure was faulty and that both RQ and energy expenditure data are false.

9. How do you estimate energy requirements of overweight patients?

It is more difficult to estimate the energy expenditures of overweight and obese patients because their variation in body composition affects overall energy expenditure. Body weight is a factor in most energy expenditure equations. In addition, energy expenditure is related to body weight. Therefore, actual body weight rather than ideal body weight or any other variation of body weight should be used in any predictive equation. The Ireton-Jones equations for ill or injured patients account for obesity in relation to the factor multiplied by the body weight; a specific factor related to obesity is also used in the equation for spontaneously breathing patients.

It is best to measure the energy expenditures of overweight or obese patients using indirect calorimetry to obtain a more accurate assessment of energy expenditure. Energy requirements may not equal energy expenditure. Nutritional support should be based on measured or predicted energy expenditure, the clinical status of the patient, and the goal of therapy. Energy needs may be greater or less than that predicted or measured. Weight loss is usually not a goal of therapy in a patient who is moderately or severely ill because the catabolic effect is exacerbated by malnutrition.

10. Is there a simple way of estimating daily energy needs in adults of normal weight and obese patients?

The American College of Chest Physicians consensus statement, published in 1997, suggests that providing 25 kcal/kg of usual body weight is adequate to promote anabolic functions for patients in the intensive care unit. McCowen and colleagues found 25 kcal/kg to be the optimal nutritional support regimen for normal-weight and obese patients requiring parenteral nutrition. It should be noted that usual or current body weight is referenced by these authors, regardless of the presence of obesity. As with any equation for ill or injured patients, the body weight used in an equation should be the best estimate of dry weight or preresuscitation body weight. The excessive weight added from fluid administration should not be included in the body weight used in an energy expenditure equation.

11. How do I determine how many calories a patient really needs?

The goal of nutritional support—that is, maintenance or repletion of nutritional status—is the final determinant of the amount of energy (number of calories) to be provided to the patient. Energy expenditure equations and measurement of energy expenditure provide the basis or starting point for provision of nutritional support. Clinical judgment may lead to the addition of calories to allow for repletion or anabolism or subtraction of calories to avoid glucose intolerance or substrate or fluid tolerances or to meet weight loss goals. Energy requirements should be individualized using the predicted or measured energy expenditure as a guide. In addition, because energy needs may change over time, reassessment is important.

12. How do I know how many calories my patient is receiving?

Estimating the caloric and protein intake of patients receiving an oral diet is accomplished by monitoring daily intake and calculating the nutrient composition of the intake. This task may be tedious because all intake must be recorded, including exact amounts. Most hospitals have the ability to provide a "calorie count" for patients whose energy intake is in question by working with the nutrition services (dietary) department. The nutrient composition of each menu item is available; however, accuracy can be questionable when data are obtained from a busy hospital ward unit where patient meal trays may be inadvertently removed or discarded. These are usually mere estimations of intake. For patients receiving continuous nutritional support either enterally or parenterally, more complete intake records are usually kept. The following table lists the caloric content of protein, carbohydrate, dextrose, and fat:

PROTEIN	CARBOHYDRATE	DEXTROSE	FAT
4 kcal/gm	4 kcal/gm	3.4 kcal/gm (dextrose is in the hydrous form with one molecule of water per molecule of glucose, yielding less energy)	9 kcal/gm

Enteral tube feeding product labels provide nutrient composition by milliliter, which simplifies calculation of actual caloric intake. Most enteral formulas contain either 1.0. 1.2, 1.5, or 2.0 kcal per ml. Parenteral nutrition formulas usually have the individual nutrient listed in grams provided per total volume of the container (bag). It is often easiest to calculate the total kcals of the nutrients per liter and then multiple by the actual number of milliliters that the patient received.

13. How important is it for the patient to be in calorie balance?

Calorie balance simply means that the number of calories calculated for the patient to consume is equivalent to the number that the patient received. Calorie balance can be a significant problem in hospitals. Patients may be on nothing-by-mouth (NPO) status for tests; upon returning from the test, their meal may be delayed. Enteral feedings may be turned off due to tests or perceived intolerance; they also may be turned off to change the feeding and not readily restarted. It has been estimated that patients on enteral feedings in the hospital receive 80% of their recommended energy intake. This estimation affects the other nutrients as well. The detriment can be best defined by examining cumulative caloric balance. If a patient requires 2000 kcal/day and each day receives only 1600 kcal, in a 54-day period the patient has lost over one full day of nutrient intake. This calorie deficit can occur with any nutritional support regimen. In addition, delay in initiating nutritional support should be included when cumulative caloric balance is calculated. Ill and injured patients who do not receive adequate nutritional support experience a loss in lean body mass, which leads to increased incidence of infection, longer hospital stays, and poorer outcomes.

BIBLIOGRAPHY

1. Cerra FB, Benitez MR, Blackburn GL, et al: Applied nutrition in ICU patients: A consensus statement of the American College of Chest Physicians. Chest 111:769–778, 1997.

2. Gottschlich MM, Jenkins M, Mayes T, et al: Lack of effect of sleep on energy expenditure and physiologic measures in critically ill burn patients. J Am Diet Assoc 1997;97(2):131–139.

3. Ireton-Jones CS: Estimating energy requirements in nutritional considerations in the intensive care unit. In Shikora S, Martindale R, Schwaitzberg S (eds): TITLE OF BOOK? CITY? Kendall Hunt Publishing, pp 31–38, 2002.

4. Ireton-Jones CS, Turner WW, Liepa GU, et al: Equations for estimation of energy expenditures in patients with burns with special reference to ventilatory status. J Burn Care Rehabil 13:330–333, 1992.

5. Ireton-Jones CS, Turner WW: The use of respiratory quotient to determine the efficacy of nutritional support regimens. J Am Diet Assoc 87:180–183, 1987.

6. Ireton-Jones C, Jones J: Improved equations for predicting energy expenditure in patients: The Ireton-Jones equations. Nutr Clin Pract 17(4):236–239, 2002.

7. Jequier E: Measurement of energy expenditure in clinical nutritional assessment. J Parent Ent Nutr 11(5):86S–89S, 1987.

8. McClave SA, Snider HL: Use of indirect calorimetry in clinical nutrition. Nutr Clin Prac 7(5):208–221, 1992.

9. McClave SA, Lowen CC, Kleber MJ, et al: Clinical use of respiratory quotient obtained from indirect calorimetry. J Parent Ent Nutr 27(11):21–26, 2003.

10. McClave SA, Spain DA, Skolnick JL, et al: Achievement of steady state optimizes results when performing indirect calorimetry. J Parent Ent Nutr 27(1):16–20, 2003.

11. McCowen KC, Friel C, Sternberg J, et al: Hypocaloric total parenteral nutrition: Effectiveness in prevention of hyperglycemia and infectious complications—a randomized clinical trial. Crit Care Med 28:3606–3611, 2000.

12. Nieman DC, Trone GA, Austin MD: A new hand held device for measuring resting metabolic rate and oxygen consumption. J Am Diet Assoc 103:588–592, 2003.

13. Porter C, Cohen N: Indirect calorimetry in critically ill patients: Role of the clinical dietitian in interpreting results. J Am Diet Assoc 96(1):49–57, 1996.

14. Spain DA, McClave SA, Sexton LK, et al: Infusion protocol improves delivery of enteral tube feeding in the critical care unit. J Parent Ent Nutr 23(5):288–292, 1999.

15. Turner WW: Nutritional considerations in the patient with disabling brain disease. Neurosurgery 16(5):707–713, 1985.

31. BODY COMPOSITION

Stanley M. Augustin, MD, and Charles W. Van Way III, MD

1. What are the major compartments of the body?

Chemically, the human body is composed primarily of water, followed by proteins, fats, minerals, and carbohydrates. These components are located in several different tissue compartments. Total body water includes extracellular water and intracellular water, and total body mass is composed of lean body mass and body fat.

By studying the composition of the various body components, we can better understand how change in any one can affect an individual. Alterations in lean body mass can influence muscle function and the risk for disability. For example, athletes use body composition information to maximize nutrition and training programs. The measurement of body fat has become important in research, educational, and clinical settings to determine the risk for disease. Since the prevalence of obesity has increased in the U.S., there has been an additional increase in obesity-related disease, such as type 2 diabetes and hypertension.

Average Values for Body Weight Compartments (in kilograms)

COMPARTMENT	MEN	WOMEN
Weight	76 (100%)	61 (100%)
Fat	20 (26%)	19 (31%)
Lean body mass	56 (74%)	42 (69%)
Extracellular mass	29 (38%)	22 (36%)
Body cell mass	27 (36%)	20 (33%)

2. What is the water content of the human body?

In adult males approximately 60% of total body weight is water. This percentage decreases with age. All of the body water is contained in the lean body mass. Since fat essentially contains no water and females have a larger percentage of body fat, water accounts for less of their weight.

Total body water can be estimated by having a person ingest a known quantity of water labeled with tritium (^3H) or deuterium (D_2O), then measuring the plasma water enrichment or the corresponding stable isotope after equilibration. Total body water also can be estimated through bioelectrical impedance, in which the conductance of a small alternating electrical current is measured. These measurements are related to known prediction equations, and total body water is then calculated.

3. What comprises total body water?

Total body water is composed of intracellular water (ICW) and extracellular water (ECW). Since the water content of cells remains fairly constant, intracellular water is found only within the lean body mass. Extracellular water includes plasma volume, interstitial water, cerebrospinal fluid, and joint fluid. Extracellular fluid can be measured by using radio-labeled $^{82}Br^-$. Although technically difficult to measure, intracellular water can be estimated by using radio-labeled $^{42}K^+$. The more common method is to subtract extracellular water from total body water to derive intracellular water.

Average Values for Body Fluid Compartments (in liters)

COMPARTMENT	MEN	WOMEN
Total body water (TBW)	41	31
Extracellular water (ECW)	17	14
ECW/TBW	0.41	0.44
Intracellular water (ICW)	24	17
ICW/TBW	0.59	0.56

4. What is total body mass?

Total body mass is composed of lean body mass and body fat. Lean body mass is composed of the extracellular mass (extracellular fluid, plasma, bone minerals, bones, tendons, teeth, and other substances) and body cell mass (metabolically active tissue such as skeletal muscles, viscera, and the cells of the blood and immune system).

5. How is lean body mass determined?

Lean (fat-free) body mass is the largest body compartment. The most straightforward method to calculate lean body mass is by percentage of normal weight (74% of the body mass of a healthy man and 69% of a healthy woman).

But since the amount of fat varies with individuals, other methods exist. Lean body mass can be measured by densitometry. This method takes advantage of the fact that the specific gravity of lean body mass is heavier than that of body fat. By weighing a person underwater, one can determine overall specific gravity and calculate lean body mass and fat.

Another research method takes advantage of the fact that all of the intracellular water is located in the body cell mass. To determine body cell mass, divide intracellular water by 0.70.

6. How do you measure human body fat?

Methods for determination of human body composition range from indirect measures that depend on mathematical models to direct measurement. Indirect models include descriptive methods such as anthropometry, volume displacement, and bioelectric impedance. Direct measurement includes computed tomography (CT), magnetic resonance imaging (MRI), and dual-energy x-ray absorptiometry (DEXA).

7. What are the benefits of the various techniques?

Anthropometry, the most basic and least expensive method, involves measurement of skinfold thickness in various parts of the body. These results are subsequently placed into known equations to determine fat-free mass or fat mass based on body density. The reliability of anthropometry depends on sex, age, race, and the skill of the examiner.

Volume displacement, a more cumbersome method, can be used to estimate body density and fat by measuring the volume of water displaced when a person is submerged. Air displacement also can be used to determine volume. Body density is obtained by dividing weight by the volume measured. Body fat is then estimated from the above equation.

Radiologic methods of direct measurement, such as MRI and DEXA, are becoming more widespread because of their speed, ease of use, and low operation cost. DEXA measures body fat based on a three-compartment model in which adipose tissue, bone, and other lean muscle tissue attenuate energy from x-rays in a tissue-specific manner. Most whole-body MRI scanners can be used to quantify whole-body adipose tissue using T1-weighted images when the proper software is used.

8. How is body composition affected by malnutrition?

Body cell mass decreases and extracellular fluid usually increases in malnourished or stressed patients. Since severe malnutrition hinders metabolism, these patients have less protein and fat. Because there is little fat in the total body mass, the percentage of protein relative to body weight may be higher than normal.

BIBLIOGRAPHY

1. Desai BB: Handbook of Nutrition and Diet. New York, Marcel Dekker, 2000.
2. Goodpaster BH: Measuring body fat distribution and content in humans. Curr Opin Clin Nutr Metabol Care 5:481–487, 2002.
3. Kim J, Wang Z, Heymsfield SB, et al: Total-body skeletal muscle mass: Estimation by a new dual-energy x-ray absorptiometry method. Am J Clin Nutr 76:378–383, 2002.

4. Mazess RB, Barden HS, Bisek JP, Hanson J: Dual-energy x-ray absorptiometry for total-body and regional bone-mineral and soft tissue composition. Am J Clin Nutr 51:1106–1112, 1990.
5. Pietrobelli A, Formica C, Wang Z, Heymsfield L: Dual-energy x-ray absorptiometry body composition model: Review of physical concepts. J Physiol E941–E951, 1996.
6. Van Der Ploeg, Withers R, Laforfia J: Percent body fat via DEXA: Comparison with a four-compartment model. J Appl Physiol 94:499–506, 2003.

32. HORMONAL CONTROL OF METABOLISM

Thomas S. Helling, MD, and Thomas S. Helling, Jr., MD

1. What is Cuthbertson's ebb and flow theory of metabolism?

Dr. David Cuthbertson first derived his theory of ebb and flow for a lecture at the Royal College of Surgeons of England in 1942. He divided the metabolism after injury into two phases: the ebb phase, a period of depressed metabolism immediately following injury, and the flow phase, a subsequent rise in metabolism which supports the healing process. The ebb phase begins with the initial injury and is characterized by a period of "anti-anabolism." This includes hyperglycemia, restoration of circulating volume, raised sympathetic nervous activity, and restoration of tissue perfusion. Once the circulating volume and tissue perfusion is restored, the flow phase begins. The flow phase is characterized by increased metabolism of protein reserves, including negative nitrogen balance, hyperglycemia, heat production, and increased metabolic rate. While the ebb phase only lasts for a few hours, the flow phase can last from days to weeks, depending on the severity of injury.

2. What is metabolism?

Most simply, metabolism can be thought of as the sum of catabolic and anabolic reactions. Catabolism is the breakdown of energy-rich compounds such as glucose and triglycerides to a form of energy more usable by the cell, such as adenosine triphosphate (ATP). Catabolism occurs via two pathways, aerobic and anaerobic. Aerobic catabolism is the primary pathway for production of ATP using O_2 as the final electron acceptor during non-stressed states. The anaerobic pathway produces ATP using pyruvate as the final electron acceptor. Catabolism occurs during stressed and non-stressed states but is accentuated during stressed states with increased oxygen consumption and nitrogen wasting. Anabolism is the formation of energy rich compounds and tissues from simpler compounds. Anabolism uses the energy provided by the catabolic reactions to "drive" the energetically unfavorable anabolic reactions. Anabolism occurs primarily during non-stressed states and is associated with growth and development and with system maintenance.

3. What are hormones?

The word "hormone" is derived from the Greek root "hormaein" which means to excite, arouse, or set in motion. This word was proposed by Starling to describe chemical agents that are released by one group of cells, travel through the blood stream, and affect other cell populations. It was once believed that hormones only acted over great distances but over the past decades three classes of hormones have been determined, based on their radius of effect. *Endocrine* hormones are synthesized in a tissue or gland and travel long distances to reach target cells. *Paracrine* hormones are synthesized by a cell and travel shorter distances to target cells. *Autocrine* hormones are synthesized by the same cell that they affect.

There are at least three chemical types of hormones, as well, depending on the structure of the molecules from which they are derived. The first type, *peptide* hormones, are synthesized from amino acids under the control of genes, just like proteins. Hormones released from the hypothalamus and pituitary are peptides. Some examples are corticotropin releasing factor (CRF), adrenocorticotropic hormone (ACTH), insulin, glucagon, growth hormone, and β-endorphin. The second type of hormones are *catecholamines* and are synthesized from tyrosine. The third type of hormones are *steroid* hormones. All steroid hormones are synthesized from the cholesterol ring. Steroid hormones are divided into two groups: the androgen hormones and the adrenal hormones. Cortisol and aldosterone are steroid hormones released from the adrenal cortex during stress.

Hormones act through a cascade system which amplifies the original signal. For humans, many hormonal signals initiate in the brain, particularly in the hypothalamus-pituitary-adrenal axis (HPA). The hormonal response to stress is initiated in the hypothalamus, which sends hormonal signals to the pituitary via a closed portal circulation. Hormones released from the pituitary travel through the blood and act on target organs, most notably the adrenal cortex, pancreas, and liver. The response to stress is produced by the sympathetic nervous system and the endocrine system.

4. What is the hormonal response to stress?

A number of hormones are released in response to stress. ACTH is released from the anterior pituitary and is under the control of CRF which is produced by the hypothalamus. When stress occurs, signals from the autonomic nervous system are processed by the brain and a signal is sent to the hypothalamus. CRF is then released to the anterior pituitary where it causes the release of ACTH. The glucocorticoid cortisol is released (under the influence of ACTH) to establish the metabolic availability of glucose from the liver, amino acids from skeletal muscle, and fatty acids from adipose tissue. Cortisol inhibits the action of insulin in the liver and inhibits the pentose phosphate pathway (producing nicotinamide adenine dinucleotide phosphate (NADPH) and ribose sugars). Cortisol, glucagon, and epinephrine all keep the blood sugar elevated. ACTH also causes the release of aldosterone, a mineralocorticoid released from the adrenal cortex. Aldosterone is responsible for the reabsorption of sodium and chloride ions in the early distal convoluted tubule which increases fluid reabsorption during periods of stress.[3]

Glucagon is normally secreted by the alpha cells of the pancreatic islets in response to a state of hypoglycemia. However, during stress, glucagon maintains a state of hyperglycemia by inhibiting the action of insulin, promoting the breakdown of glycogen and adipose tissue, and by stimulating the glycogenolytic and gluconeogenic pathway. Epinephrine, the endogenous opioid β-endorphin, and cortisol all cause the release of glucagon.

Growth hormone is synthesized by the acidophilic cell of the anterior pituitary. Growth hormone increases amino acid uptake and protein synthesis in hepatocyte and skeletal muscle cells and inhibits the action of insulin. Growth hormone also supplies substrate for gluconeogenesis by breaking down adipose tissue into glycerol and fatty acids and stimulates the secretion of catecholamines.

Catecholamines are neurotransmitters (indicating very close association with the sympathetic nervous system) that can also act as hormones. Epinephrine is secreted from the adrenal medulla and, aside from its vasoactive properties, is primarily a hormone that acts on the pancreas, liver, muscle, and heart. In the pancreas, epinephrine stimulates the release of glucagon while inhibiting insulin. During stress it is thought that epinephrine "adjusts the set points" of the hormonal response of the endocrine pancreas and these hormones (glucagon and insulin) in turn control the disposition of key substrates. In the liver, epinephrine stimulates the breakdown of glycogen and stimulates gluconeogenesis. In muscle, epinephrine stimulates the breakdown of muscle glycogen to lactic acid which is then transported to the liver for gluconeogenesis (Cori cycle).

5. What changes in response to insulin occur in stress?

Insulin is the primary storage signal for metabolic fuels such as glucose, fatty acids, and protein. During non-stressed states, insulin facilitates the transport of glucose across cellular membranes. In the liver and muscle, insulin promotes the synthesis of glycogen, the storage form of glucose. Insulin also promotes the storage of energy-rich triglycerides in adipose tissue. In insulin's absence, adipose tissue is broken down. Insulin does not promote storage during the hyperglycemia of stress because it is opposed by other hormones. Cortisol, epinephrine, glucagon, β-endorphins, and the catecholamines are known as the *counter-regulatory* hormones.

6. What substances other than hormones are involved in stress?

Hormones are not the only mediators of stress responses in tissue. Another class of peptide molecules, the *cytokines*, are also involved in the stress response. *Interleukin-1* (IL-1) is synthesized by blood monocytes and tissue macrophages and is produced in almost all inflammatory responses. IL-1 elicits a variety of effects. IL-1 acts on the central nervous system, most notably the hypothalamus. This in turn stimulates the release of local prostaglandins causing a raised body temperature, an increased metabolic rate and O_2 consumption, and affects the satiety center. IL-1 also increases the transcription of IL-2 and its receptors which in turn increases T-cell proliferation. IL-1 is also a potent stimulator of hepatic acute phase proteins synthesis as well as connective tissue and bone remodeling.

Another cytokine is *tumor necrosis factor* (TNF). TNF-$_\alpha$ or cachectin is produced by blood monocytes, pulmonary macrophages, hepatic Kupffer cells, and peritoneal macrophages. A number of inflammatory and infectious stimuli such as lipopolysaccharide, viral particles, exotoxins, hypoxia, ischemia, and fungi are responsible for the release of TNF$_\alpha$. TNF orchestrates the synthesis and proliferation of the immune response by promoting the release of neutrophils, transendothelial passage, production of superoxides, release of lysozymes, and production of macrophages. While TNF release facilitates the immune response, high levels are detrimental. In experimental animal studies, elevated TNF levels have induced anemia due to decreased red blood cell mass. TNF affects metabolism by increasing the transport of glucose across cellular membranes and increasing cellular loss of lactate, breaking down adipose tissue, and releasing amino acids from tissue. TNF is responsible for increasing transcription of hepatic acute phase proteins and increased hepatic uptake of amino acids resulting in precursors for gluconeogenesis. This increased release of amino acids results in whole body tissue wasting that over a prolonged period of time induces a cachexic state.

Eicosanoids are a separate class of biological mediators which are, chemically, lipids. Formed from arachidonic acid, they are intimately associated with the inflammatory response. There are four major groups of eicosanoids: *prostaglandins* (PGE, PGF), *prostacyclins* (PGI$_2$), *thromboxanes* (TXA$_2$, TXB$_2$), and the *leukotrienes*. The eicosanoids are primarily autocoids, having their greatest effect on the cells from which they are released. The endothelium converts arachidonic acid to prostacyclin, while platelets convert arachidonic acid to thromboxane. Prostaglandins are not stored by cells but rather synthesized *de novo* when stimulation occurs. Their actions are the most varied of any natural occurring compound. There are many types of stimuli such as hypoxia, ischemia, tissue injury, pyrogen, endotoxin, thrombin. Prostacyclin has the ability to inhibit platelet aggregation, while thromboxane has the ability to stimulate platelet aggregation. It is believed that a decrease of PGI$_2$ and an increase of TXA$_2$ play a role in coagulation during shock. Prostacyclins and prostaglandins are endogenous vasodilators whereas thromboxanes are potent vasoconstrictors. Leukotrienes have the ability to stimulate leukocyte adherence and vascular permeability. Leukotrienes are also potent vasoconstrictors and bronchoconstrictors modulating changes found in acute lung injury and the adult respiratory distress syndrome (ARDS). For every action elicited by one eicosanoid there is an opposite action elicited by another eicosanoid.

Platelet activating factor (PAF) is yet another lipid hormone which aggregates platelets and affects the breakdown and synthesis of glucose. PAF is secreted by a number of cells: platelets, leukocytes, and endothelium. Increased levels of PAF correlate with an increase in glucose turnover and synthesis, increased levels of glucagon, and increased levels of catecholamines in experimental models.

7. What hormones are involved in anabolism following stress?

Growth hormone and insulin are thought to be primarily anabolic in nature. Growth hormone is a potent stimulator of cell division and protein synthesis. Growth hormone reduces the deamination of amino acids, increases insulin secretion, increases protein synthesis in the liver, and may aid in retaining the essential elements nitrogen, potassium, and phosphorus. Growth hormone may exert its mitogenic effects through the somatomedins, or insulin-like growth factors; however, its mitogenic ability has yet to be fully elucidated. Insulin is the main effector of glucose homeostasis. Insulin is responsible for the transport of glucose across cellular membranes and promoting the synthesis of glycogen. Insulin is also responsible for the maintenance of fatty acids in adipose tissue. Insulin plays a role in the transport of certain amino acids from the liver to muscle tissue, ensuring that muscles have an adequate supply of amino acids for tissue maintenance. It must be kept in mind that the anabolic actions of these hormones are suppressed initially after stress and their effects occur hours or days after the initial injury.

8. What are the metabolic differences between starvation and stress?

During starvation, the body does not receive adequate nutrients to supply day-to-day metabolic demands. A state of hypoglycemia results and the body uses alternate fuels for energy, primarily fatty acids for muscles and ketone bodies for the brain. During starvation, levels of glucagon and insulin do not change. Rather, the availability of glucose determines the rate of glycogen, fatty acid, and protein breakdown, controlling the substrate for the resulting gluconeogenesis. The availability of substrate determines the rate of metabolic processes. Liver mass is depleted due to glycogen breakdown and the kidney's role in gluconeogenesis becomes more important. During prolonged periods of starvation, substrate availability is reduced and the role of gluconeogenesis becomes less important for energy. The body depends more on fatty acid and ketone body oxidation for energy. Cardiac output and oxygen consumption are both decreased during starvation. With conservation of protein, ureagenesis is diminished.

In stress, metabolism is raised to meet the demands of inflammation, tissue injury, and wound repair. Initially an increase in sympathetic nerve activity results in increased cardiac output and a increased vascular resistance in order to maintain blood pressure and tissue perfusion. An increase in counter-regulatory hormones such as glucagon, cortisol, epinephrine, and catecholamines synergistically act to suppress the release and action of insulin, establishing a state of hyperglycemia. Energy can be derived from carbohydrates, protein, and fat but glucose is the primary energy source for nearly all tissues. In order to maintain hypermetabolism and the resulting hyperglycemia, an increased demand for gluconeogenic precursors are derived from amino acids, glycerol, and protein. A state of hypermetabolism will quickly deplete nutritional stores if caloric demands are not met and sustained. As a result of hypermetabolism, protein oxidation, ureagenesis, glycogenolysis, and lipolysis are elevated.

9. What substrates are used to make glucose during stress?

Gluconeogenesis is the primary glucose source during periods of stress. Many stress-related hormones help provide precursors for this pathway in order to maintain the hyperglycemic state. All amino acids except leucine and lysine can provide the carbon skeleton necessary for gluconeogenesis; however, the primary amino acids used are alanine, glutamine, and glycine. A number of other amino acids are metabolized to form the intermediates pyruvate (from glycine, serine, cysteine) and α-ketoglutarate (arginine, proline), which then can give rise to alanine or glutamine. Adipose tissue is broken down giving fatty acids and glycerol. The glycerol can be used in gluconeogenesis while the fatty acids cannot. The fatty acids are broken down by β-oxidation and used by many tissues such as muscle for energy.

There are two cycles which are important for providing glucogenic substrates in the liver. Both of these cycles operate between muscle and the liver via the vascular system. The *Cori cycle* provides lactate from muscle which is transported in the blood to the liver for gluconeogenesis. Similarly, the *alanine cycle* provides alanine from muscle which is then used to produce glucose in the liver.

10. What is the hormonal response to hemorrhagic shock?

Hemorrhagic shock is due to a large volume of blood loss resulting in hypotension, loss of vascular tone, and cardiovascular dysfunction. The neuroendocrine response to hypovolemic shock is to maximize cardiac function, to conserve salt and water, and to provide oxygen and nutrients to vital organs such as the heart and the brain. The human body has many types of receptors that are able to detect changes due to hemorrhagic shock. Changes in pressure, tonicity, osmolarity, pH, oxygen, carbon dioxide, and glucose are all monitored by receptors in the central nervous system. Loss of blood volume is detected by baroreceptors in the heart, aorta, and other arteries. These afferent nervous signals are processed primarily by the hypothalamic-pituitary-adrenal axis. The loss of blood volume elicits the response of many of the hormones that are released in the stress response. The most common hormones are ACTH (anterior pituitary), cortisol (adrenal gland), glucagon (pancreas), and vasopressin (posterior pituitary). The effects of these hormones cause a state of hyperglycemia by suppressing the action of insulin and promoting the breakdown of adipose tissue, muscle, and glycogen. The hyperglycemic state has two results. First, glucose raises the blood osmolarity and causes a shift of fluid from the cells into the intravascular space. This helps to restore and maintain circulating volume and, at the same time, lowers the blood osmolarity to or below normal levels. This decrease in blood osmolarity is sensed by osmoreceptors in the hypothalamus and vasopressin is released from the posterior pituitary. Vasopressin conserves sodium and water. It also increases splanchnic vasoconstriction, helping to maintain blood flow to vital organs such as the heart and the brain. Second, glucose provides the energy needed for vital tissue maintenance and repair.

11. What are some common clinical syndromes of altered metabolism?
Hypoglycemia, diabetes, diabetic ketoacidosis, obesity, and syndrome X.

12. What is diabetic ketoacidosis?
Diabetic ketoacidosis (DKA) is an example of an altered ratio of insulin to glucagons, epinephrine, norepinephrine, and cortisol. DKA is usually seen in type I diabetics, although it may be seen in type II diabetics. DKA occurs because insulin levels are low, whereas levels of glucagons, epinephrine, and cortisol are increased. This altered ratio causes a catabolic state in which fatty acids and protein are broken down, leading to increased gluconeogenesis and hepatic ketone formation. A hyperglycemic state ensues, leading to profound dehydration, acidosis, and electrolyte abnormalities. Treatment entails correction of any underlying illness, rehydration, insulin administration, and electrolyte repletion.

13. How important is glucose control in the critically ill patient?
Insulin resistance is common in critically ill patients, even patients with no prior history of diabetes. A recent randomized controlled study demonstrated that keeping blood sugar tightly regulated between 80 and 110 mg/dl reduces morbidity and mortality in the surgical ICU compared with conventional insulin therapy. The investigators found a decrease in the use of antibiotics and blood transfusions, a decreased risk of polyneuropathy, and prevention of acute renal failure.[9]

BIBLIOGRAPHY

1. Amaral JF, Shearer JP, Mastrograncesco B, et al.: The temporal characteristics of the metabolic and endocrine response to injury. J Trauma 28:1335–1352, 1988.
2. Cuthbertson D: The metabolic response to injury and its nutritional implications: Retrospect and prospect. JPEN J Parenter Enteral Nutr 3:108–129, 1979.
3. Davis JH, Sheldon GF: The biologic response to injury. In Schwartz SI (ed): Surgery: A Problem Solving Approach. New York, Mosby, 1995.
4. Feldman M, Kieser RS, Unger RH, Li CH: Beta endorphin and the endocrine pancreas. Studies in healthy and diabetic human beings. N Engl J Med 308:349–353, 1983.
5. Fong Y, Moldawer LL, Shires GT, Lowry SF: The biologic characteristics of cytokines and their implications in surgical injury. Surg Gynecol Obstet 170:363–378, 1990.
6. Harris RA, Crabb DW: Mechanisms involved in switching the metabolism of the liver between the well-fed state and the starved state. In Devlin TM (ed): Textbook of Biochemistry with Clinical Applications. New York, Wiley-Liss, 1992.
7. Lang CH, Dobrescu C, Hargrove DM, et al: Platelet-activating factor-induced increases in glucose kinetics. Am J Physiol 254:E193–E200, 1988.
8. Maier RV, Bulger EM: Endothelial changes after shock and injury. In Waxman K (ed): New Horizons: What mediates tissue injury after shock? 4:211–223, 1996.
9. Van Den Berghe G, Wouters P, Weekers F, et al: Intensive insulin therapy in critically ill patients. N Engl J Med 345:1360–1366, 2001.
10. Wilmore D: Hormonal responses and their effects on metabolism. Surg Clin North Am 56:999–1018, 1976.

33. AMINO ACIDS: GLUTAMINE AND ARGININE

Chau N. Nguyen, MD, Scott W. Kujath, MD, and Animesh Dhar, PhD

1. What is the role of glutamine in human physiology?
Glutamine is the most abundant free amino acid in the human body. It is formed from glutamate and ammonia by glutamine synthetase. Skeletal muscle is the primary site of glutamine synthesis. It acts, among other things, as a nitrogen donor during protein and nucleic acid synthesis. Circulating concentrations of glutamine decrease during catabolic stress, such as major surgery, trauma, sepsis, and burn, despite peripheral release. This decrease in glutamine concentration is related to susceptibility to infections. It has been shown that the intestinal mucosa uses glutamine as a primary source of fuel during stress, sparing glucose for other tissues. The kidney also takes up glutamine, using the amide nitrogen to form urinary ammonium and leaving the carbon skeleton for gluconeogenesis. During sepsis, glutamine is used extensively in the liver for gluconeogenesis, ureagenesis, and the synthesis of proteins, nucleic acid, and glutathione. Glutamate, the γ-amide of glutamine, can be decarboxylated to produce γ-aminobutyrate (GABA), an inhibitory CNS neurotransmitter.

2. Is glutamine an essential or nonessential amino acid?
In general, glutamine is considered a nonessential amino acid because it can be synthesized by the human body from other amino acids. As noted above, glutamine concentrations decrease during stress—sepsis, trauma, major surgery, and burns—with concomitant increased release of glutamine from skeletal muscle. Increased uptake of glutamine by other organs, such as intestine, liver and kidney, contributes to the decreased levels of glutamine. This increased requirement for glutamine has prompted many researchers to label it as a "conditionally essential" amino acid. Multiple studies have shown that supplementing glutamine intake helps to avoid depletion of muscular protein stores and decreases the morbidity associated with major illness.

3. How is glutamine metabolized by the body?
The small intestine mucosa apparently uses glutamine as a primary fuel during stress. The amide nitrogen is released as ammonia and citrulline; the latter plays a key role in continuing the urea cycle. From there, approximately 50% of glutamine is converted to alanine, which is then taken up by the liver for gluconeogenesis. The rest of glutamine in the small intestine is further deaminated to its carbon skeleton and oxidized, generating 30 moles of adenosine triphosphate (ATP) per mole of glutamine. This makes glutamine almost as good an energy source as glucose. Glutamine supplementation has been shown to preserve the health of gut mucosal cells and decrease bacterial translocation with gut-associated lymphoid tissue (GALT), while leaving glucose available for obligate glycolytic organs. The intestinal mucosa is a rapidly growing tissue, using significant amounts of glutamine for protein and nucleic acid synthesis.

4. What effect does glutamine have on the immune system?
Glutamine is an important fuel for some cells of the immune system, especially the macrophages, polymorphonuclear leukocytes (PMN), and lymphocytes. In fact, glutamine is required for lymphocyte cell culture. Indirectly, it also has a significant effect on gut integrity by maintaining gut lymphocytes. It decreases the risk of bacterial translocation through the maintenance of tight junctions between enterocytes and GALT. GALT, as part of the host defense, secretes IgA as well as assists in phagocytosis of bacteria, preventing bacteria from entering the blood stream. Glutamine also causes significant increase in PMN free glutamine, alanine, asparagines, aspartate, glutamate, ornithine, arginine, serine, and glycine concentrations and subsequently increases PMN functions. In the presence of lipopolysaccharide (LPS), an important

component of bacterial cell wall, glutamine has been found to reduce the level of tumor necrosis factor (TNF). During periods of reduced glutamine concentration, stress response of human lymphocytes is impaired. Therefore, glutamine is directly and indirectly essential to minimize the cytotoxic inflammatory effects during stress.

5. Should glutamine be added to parenteral nutritional formulas?
Glutamine is not stable in solution with other amino acids because it spontaneously decomposes to glutamic acid and ammonia. This decomposition is negligible over a few days and appears only after a month or more in solution. But commercial production of amino acids requires them to be stable in solution for 6 months or longer. Stability may also be poor when glutamine is mixed with acidic total parenteral nutrition (TPN) solutions. Glutamine must be added to the TPN mixture at the time of its preparation, shortly before administration. This addition, while possible, adds to the cost of the TPN and has not been considered important in the past. However, the benefits of glutamine outweigh the cost. More and more studies have shown that glutamine supplementation decreases the incidence of sepsis, shortens the length of hospital stay, and hence reduces hospital costs. The effects are greatest in patients with severe trauma, patients undergoing major surgery, bone marrow transplant patients, patients who are critically ill (including patients with existing infection), and low-birth-weight infants. Glutamine use in TPN is still experimental.

Glutamine is a component of most enteral preparations. It has been speculated that one of the major reasons for the superiority of enteral nutrition over parenteral nutrition is that the former usually contains glutamine.

6. How is arginine utilized in the human body?
Arginine is important in the urea cycle for detoxifying ammonia. It is cleared by arginase, almost exclusively in the liver, to form urea and ornithine. Ornithine then re-enters the cycle. Arginine is considered a nonessential amino acid because the human body can synthesize it. But similar to glutamine, it has also been classified as a conditionally essential amino acid because of its rapid depletion during stress periods.

Arginine is a starting point for the synthesis of creatine and creatine phosphate. Creatine phosphate is especially critical to the energy metabolism of the body. In muscle, it is the energy reservoir for the adenosine nucleotide system. While ATP provides the chemical energy that allows the actin and myosin fibrils to move along one another, it is creatine phosphate that reforms ATP from adenosine diphosphate (ADP) and adenosine monophosphate (AMP). During ischemia, ATP remains at normal levels for a considerable period, while creatine phosphate is progressively depleted in order to maintain ATP levels. Only when the creatine phosphate is completely depleted does ATP begin to fall to levels too low to permit continued muscular activity.

7. How does the body's use of arginine change with stress?
With stress, there is an increase in protein breakdown and production of urea. More arginine is used in the urea cycle. As noted above, arginine is a starting point for the synthesis of creatine and creatine phosphate. Both are upregulated during stress.

8. Does arginine have any pharmacologic effect?
Arginine stimulates the production of several anabolic hormones, including pituitary growth hormone, prolactin, and insulin. Arginine supplementation has been shown to increase wound healing by enhancing collagen synthesis. Arginine given in amounts exceeding requirements appears to enhance the immune system. These effects are seen only when arginine is given as a supplement to an otherwise adequate nutritional regimen.

9. What effect does arginine have on the immune system?
As indicated earlier, arginine enhances the immune system. Similarly to glutamine, it upregulates the function of T lymphocytes, macrophages, and PMNs. Arginine acts through nitric

oxide and polyamine synthesis. Nitric oxide, an important internal chemical messenger, vasodilates and may provide a constant vasodilatory tone throughout the cardiovascular system. For this reason, several studies have been done to determine the effect of arginine on the myocardium. Nitric oxide also participates in immunologic reactions, including the killing activity of macrophages. In PMNs, arginine causes significant increases in the concentration of arginine, ornithine, citrulline, aspartate, glutamate, and alanine and also stimulates hydrogen peroxide formation and myeloperoxidase activity while superoxide anion formation is reduced. A recent prospective, randomized, double-blind, controlled study shows that immunonutrition, containing arginine, n-3-fatty acids, and nucleotides, significantly reduces the number of systemic inflammatory response syndrome (SIRS) days per patient and also lowers the multiple organ failure score. Last but not least, arginine produces an increase in lymphocyte interleukin-2 release and receptor activity.

BIBLIOGRAPHY

1. Alexander JW: Nutritional pharmacology in surgical patients. Am J Surg 183(4):349–352, 2002.
2. Andrews FJ, Griffiths RD: Glutamine: Essential for immune nutrition in the critically ill. Br J Nutr 87 Suppl 1:S3–8, 2002.
3. Bastian L, Weimann A: Immunonutrition in patients with multiple trauma. Br J Nutr 87 Suppl 1:S133–134, 2002.
4. Cynober LA: Do we have unrealistic expectations of the potential of immuno-nutrition? Can J Appl Physiol:S36–44, 2001.
5. Mates JM, Perez-Gomez C, et al: Glutamine and its relationship with intracellular redox status, oxidative stress and cell proliferation/death. Int J Biochem Cell Biol 34(5):439–458, 2002.
6. Muhling J, Fuchs M, et al: Effects of arginine, L-alanyl-L-glutamine or taurine on neutrophil (PMN) free amino acid profiles and immune functions in vitro. Amino Acids 22(1):39–53, 2002.
7. Pithon-Curi TC, Trezena AG, et al: Evidence that glutamine is involved in neutrophil function. Cell Biochem Funct 20(2):81–86, 2002.
8. Takeuchi K, Simplaceanu E, et al: L-Arginine potentiates negative inotropic and metabolic effects to myocardium partly through the amiloride sensitive mechanism. Jpn J Physiol 52(2):207–215, 2002.
9. Van Way CW: Amino acids. In Van Way CW (ed): Handbook of Surgical Nutrition. Philadelphia, J.B. Lippincott, 1992.
10. Wischenmeyer PE, Kahara M, et al: Glutamine reduces cytokine release, organ damage and mortality in a rat model of endotoxemia. Shock 16(5):398–402, 2001.

34. NUTRITION AND THE IMMUNE SYSTEM

Bill K.W. Chang, MD, Craig G. Chang, MD, and Animesh Dhar, PhD

1. Why is good nutrition important to the immune system?

The immune system, like all organ systems, is constantly turning over its cells and protein components. It undergoes even more rapid turnover than most systems. The immune system regenerates much of itself each day. It must be able to recognize antigens and synthesize many proteins, such as immunoglobulins, complement, and enzymes. It must produce various cells, such as lymphocytes, plasma cells, macrophages, and neutrophils. Like all of the body's systems, the immune system depends on adequate daily nutrition: amino acids for protein synthesis, fat and carbohydrates for energy production, and vitamins and minerals for their specific roles in cellular growth and protein synthesis.

2. What happens to the immune system in protein malnutrition?

Protein malnutrition deprives the immune system of amino acids that are used for cellular replication. The immune system response requires that certain cell lines dramatically increase in number. This "feed-forward" mechanism is called clonal expansion. Neutrophils and macrophages, both of which phagocytize bacteria and particulate debris, have half-lives of less than 12 hours. The body completely replaces these cells twice daily.

Amino acids are also used for the synthesis of various immune substances. Immunoglobulins (antibodies) are proteins that attach to foreign substances (antigens) and enhance the ability of the neutrophils and macrophages to phagocytize the immunoglobulin-antigen complex. These processes cause killing of bacteria and viruses. To support protein synthesis, the body depends on dietary protein to keep amino acid pools at high enough levels because there is constant loss of protein in the urine and stool as urea and ammonia. If the intake is inadequate, the only alternative is the breakdown of muscle protein.

In reality, pure protein deprivation is not especially common, but it clearly causes a diminished immune response, mostly involving the humoral arm of the immune system. In general, plasma protein levels are depressed, but resting immunoglobulin levels may be normal. Diminished lymphoid tissue as well as depression of polymorphonuclear leukocyte and macrophage activity is also evident. The number of T-helper cells is also decreased. The overall effect is a combination of diminished activity of the antigen-presenting cells, diminished stimulation of B cells by T cells, and impaired protein synthesis. These deficits result in the clinical findings of increased numbers of infections and susceptibility to infection.

3. What is the effect of calorie or protein-calorie malnutrition (PCM) on the immune system?

PCM is the most prevalent disease in the world. Pure calorie malnutrition by itself is relatively rare and is usually combined with one or more specific nutrient deficiencies. This full-spectrum malnutrition is usually referred to as protein-calorie malnutrition. The effect of protein-calorie malnutrition is extensive, affecting all organ systems. The host immunity is affected broadly, with particular detrimental effects on the cell-mediated immunity. The thymus and spleen may be atrophic, and the lymphoid tissue is poorly developed. The number and functions of T cells, phagocytic cells, and secretory immunoglobulin A antibody response are reduced. Delayed hypersensitivity reactions, which are mediated by T cells, are often suppressed. In addition, levels of many complement components are reduced. Together these deficiencies result in increased opportunistic infection and increased morbidity and mortality in hospitalized patients.

Despite these specific defects, the immune system is fairly resistant to malnutrition. Both adults and children suffering from PCM are still capable of antibody responses and can mount both lymphocyte response and leukocytosis. In animal studies the gut immune system is preserved despite significant PCM. Putting it another way, immunity is maintained at the expense of other tissues. Muscle serves as a reservoir of energy and amino acids that can be drawn upon in illness or malnourishment. Malnourished people show muscle wasting long before the immune system fails.

PCM has effects somewhat similar to those of AIDS. The specific defect produced by AIDS is depletion of T helper cells (CD4 cells) and depression of the T cell-mediated immune response. Infections that are thereby facilitated include Pneumocystis carinii pneumonia, herpes, and tuberculosis. The similarity between PCM and AIDS suggests a synergy between the two conditions. Indeed, this scenario can be seen in Africa, where AIDS is known as the "slim disease" because of its link with malnutrition. Thus, prevention and treatment of PCM is an important part of the management of the patient with AIDS.

4. Why is glutamine important in the immune system?

Glutamine is a unique amino acid. It has at least two distinct functions in the body, both of which are important for the immune system.

First, it is a preferred energy source for rapidly proliferating cells. It supplies nearly as much adenosine triphosphate (ATP) as glucose when metabolized completely and is preferred to glucose in such tissues as the gut mucosa. It helps to maintain bowel mucosal integrity and prevent atrophy. The functional result is that translocation of bacteria from the bowel to the tissues and vessels is lessened or prevented. The gut mucosal barrier is one of the body's "outer wall" defenses against infection. If glutamine is not provided to the gut mucosa, the barrier begins to fail and the internal components of the immune system must deal with bacteria invasion of the portal circulation. The normal route of glutamine into the mucosal cells is through the intestinal lumen, but glutamine is also taken up by the mucosa if given intravenously. It appears likely that intravenous glutamine is sufficient to maintain the gut mucosal barrier.

Second, glutamine is a nitrogen donor in protein, purine, and pyrimidine synthesis. It seems to be essential for cellular replication. It acts as a "nitrogen carrier" between cells. It is a precursor to the synthesis of DNA and RNA. The need for glutamine is particularly acute when metabolism is increased, as in surgical stress, sepsis, injury, and burns. This is especially true in the immune system, with its high level of protein synthesis and rapid cellular turnover.

Increasing evidence suggests that glutamine is a critical substrate for cells of the immune system. Glutamine depletion in lymphocytes prevents late activation. Glutamine deprivation in monocytes lowers surface antigens responsible for phagocytosis. Clinical studies have demonstrated lower nitrogen losses, fewer infections, and shorter hospital stays in bone marrow transplantation patients who were supplemented with glutamine. The use of glutamine appeared to lower the mortality rate as well (see Chapter 33).

5. What minerals are important to immunity?

Selenium has gained much attention. Its role in the immune system appears to be intertwined with that of vitamin E. Together, they can increase antibody titers and maintain biologic membranes. They protect unsaturated membrane phospholipids and protein sulfhydryl groups from oxidants that may impair cellular function. Selenium is a component of glutathione peroxidase, which reduces hydrogen peroxide and other peroxides in the cytosol to prevent the formulation of free radicals. Animal studies have shown that selenium deficiency suppresses lymphocyte response to mitogens, reduces phagocytic activity, and lowers intracellular killing of polymorphonuclear (PMN) cells. Selenium excess does not suppress immune function. Selenium can spare vitamin E and vice versa. When both are deficient, immune function is impaired more severely than when only one is inadequate.

Other electrolytes and trace elements are important as well. Excessive calcium interferes with leukocyte function by displacing magnesium and thereby reducing cell adhesion. Copper is a cofactor for enzymes that are vital for lymphocyte and macrophage function. A functional copper deficiency resulting in impaired neutrophil phagocytosis has been documented in animal studies. Zinc has an important role in immune function also (see below).

6. Why is zinc important to the immune system?

Zinc deficiency results in impaired wound healing as well as an increased susceptibility to infection. Adequate zinc status is essential for T-cell division, maturation, and differentiation; lymphocyte response to mitogens; apoptosis of lymphoid and myeloid cells; gene transcription; and membrane stability. Zinc is also the structural component of a wide variety of proteins, neuropeptides, hormone receptors, and nucleotides. Among the zinc-dependent enzymes is thymulin, which is essential for the formation of T lymphocytes. Zinc deficiency rapidly diminishes cell-mediated responses, results in marked atrophy of the thymus, and causes lymphopenia. Primary and secondary antibody responses are also reduced in zinc deficiency. Zinc also inhibits the production of tumor necrosis factor, which causes cachexia and wasting in patients with AIDS and cancer.

7. What particular vitamins are important to immune response?

Vitamin A has been studied most extensively. Experiments have shown that dietary vitamin A increases the expression of the major histocompactibility complex class I molecule HLA-DR and the adhesion molecules of monocytes and macrophages. These molecules enhance cell-mediated immune responses. Vitamin A deficiency causes declines in cellular immunity, as measured by delayed hypersensitivity skin tests. As the deficiency progresses, humoral immunity, as measured by serum immunoglobulin M (IgM) responses to a protein antigen, also declines. Vitamin A also antagonizes some of the deleterious effects of steroids on immunity and wound healing.

Vitamin E also has gained much attention. Vitamin E is widely recognized as a major lipid-soluble antioxidant in the body, where it scavenges free radicals and protects cellular structures against oxidative stress. Experiments have shown that antioxidants may modulate signal transduction and gene expression in immune cells. Evidence also indicates that vitamin E plays a role in protecting the immune system of elderly people.

The water-soluble vitamins are important to the immune system as well. Folic acid, pyridoxine (vitamin B_6), and vitamin B_{12} deficiencies produce depression of both antibody and cell-medicated responses. Biotin and pantothenic acid deficiencies also impair antibody response and cellular immunity. Finally, vitamin C deficiency produces scurvy, which is characterized by a diminished resistance to infection due to inhibition of both leukocyte and monocyte chemotaxis.

8. What is the effect of fatty acid malnutrition on the immune system?

Essential fatty acid deficiency (EFAD) is associated with depressed inflammatory responses. For example, depressed neutrophil chemotaxis may be related to reduced generation of the arachidonate metabolite leukotriene B4 (LTB4). In animal studies, neutrophils from EFAD rats and monkeys showed decreased membrane depolarization and superoxide anion formation and depressed bactericidal capacity. EFAD also impairs the capacity of macrophages to spread and adhere. Early in life, it appears that EFAs are necessary for normal development of the T-cell lines and splenic lymphocytes.

9. What effect does omega-3 fatty acid have on immunity?

Omega-3 polyunsaturated fatty acid, also known as linolenic acid, is an essential fatty acid found in fish oil. Omega-3 fatty acid metabolizes to form eicosapentanoic acid, which is the precursor of prostaglandins (PGE_3, PGI_3, TXA_3). In one study, linolenic acid deficiency in three humans caused a reduced mitogenic response in isolated lymphocytes. Another study involving burn-injured rats found that cellular immunity was better maintained in rats fed with diets mixed with eicosapentanoic acid. Omega-3 fatty acids also seem to prolong the survival of malnourished patients with malignancies.

10. What is the immune response to obesity and weight loss?

Obesity appears to be associated with impaired immunity. Overweight patients are at greater risk for infection and bacteremia. Obesity is a risk factor for poor wound healing after surgery.

Impaired T- and B-cell function has been noted in comparison with nonobese patients. Obese children and adolescents have impaired delayed-type hypersensitivity, mitogen-stimulated lymphocyte proliferation, and bactericidal capacity of neutrophils. However, this general view may not be completely true. One study showed that phagocytosis was not affected by obesity and that the activated monocyte oxidative burst was actually higher among the obese. Although there appears to be a predisposition to certain infections in obese people, the exact effect on the immune system has not been well defined.

Rapid weight loss and fasting negatively affect immunity and are associated with decreased mitogen-stimulated lymphocyte proliferation. Significant decreases in neutrophil, monocyte, and natural killer cell counts, but not T- or B-cell counts, have also been reported following rapid weight loss. However, studies of acute fasting in volunteers revealed no increase in the incidence of infection. It is believed that acute fasting in the presence of adequate protein stores is well tolerated by the immune system.

11. Can the immune system be stimulated or augmented with certain types of nutrition?

Yes. A balanced nutrition supports the immune system, and provision of certain nutrients to stressed trauma or burn patients has been shown to lower septic complications. A study in 1994 found a significantly decreased incidence of abdominal abscess and multiorgan failure after the use of feeding formula enriched with glutamine, arginine, omega-3, polyunsaturated fatty acid (PUFA), nucleotides, and branched-chain amino acids. Decreased ventilator use, shorter stays in the intensive care unit (ICU), and fewer total hospital days were also noted in the study. Other work with arginine and omega-3 PUFA in burns showed fewer wound infections and improved lymphocyte blastogenesis. Recently, more studies involving glutamine have shown that infectious morbidity was decreased in the critically ill patients and bone marrow transplantation patients when feedings were supplemented with glutamine. Multiple other studies also demonstrated beneficial effects of diets enriched with glutamine in immune system.

12. What are the effects of enteral feedings on the immune system?

Enteral feeding is the body's preferred route of nutrition when the gastrointestinal tract is functional. Compared with total parenteral nutrition (TPN), enterally fed patients have a lower number of septic complications, including bacteremia, abdominal abscess, and pneumonia. It is speculated that the beneficial effects result from prevention of mucosal atrophy and decreased bacterial translocation as well as maintenance of the gut-associated lymphoid tissue (GALT) in mucosal immunity. It has been shown that overgrowth of bacteria results when the gut is not used for feeding. Subsequently, these bacteria have an increased tendency to be cultured from the respiratory tract of patients in the ICU. Experimental work has shown that upper respiratory immunity is compromised if the gut is not used.

The beneficial effects of enteral feedings occur even with small volumes of "trophic" feeds. In head-injured patients, the effect has been noted to occur only if the feedings were started early in the course. The current concept is one of a "common mucosal immune system." Once initial activation of precursor IgA-producing cells occurs within the Peyer's patches, the antigen-sensitized cells undergo mitotic changes and the resulting B lymphoblasts migrate to regional lymph nodes and eventually to the systemic circulation via the thoracic duct. This process, in turn, enhances the systemic response to infection.

However, some studies have failed to show a clear clinical benefit for the enteral route compared with TPN. The jury may be still out. Nevertheless, the consensus favors enteral feeding whenever possible.

BIBLIOGRAPHY

1. Bjerve K, Fischer S, Wammer F, Egeland T: alpha-Linolenic acid and long-chain omega-3 fatty acid supplementation in three patients with omega-3 fatty acid deficiency: Effect on lymphocyte function, plasma and red cell lipids, and prostanoid formation. Am J Clin Nutr 49(2):290–300, 1989.

2. Cerra FB, Lehman S, Konstantinides N, et al: Improvement in immune function in ICU patients by enteral nutrition supplemented with arginine, RNA, and menhaden oil independent of nitrogen balance. Nutrition 7:193–199, 1991.

3. Daly JM, Goldfine J, et al: Enteral nutrition with supplemental arginine, RNA and omega-3 fatty acids in patients after operation: Immunologic, metabolic and clinical outcome. Surgery 56:112, 1992.

4. Daly JM, Reynolds J, Sigal RK, Shou J, Liberman MD: Effect of dietary protein and amino acids on immune function. Crit Care Med 18(2 Suppl):S86–S93, 1990.

5. Fraker PJ, King LE, Garry BA, Medina CA: The immunopathology of zinc deficiency in humans and rodents. In Klurfeld DM (ed): Human Nutrition—A Comprehensive Treatise, vol. 8: Nutrition and Immunology. New York, Plenum Press, 1993.

6. Gottschlich MM, Jenkins M, Warden GD, et al: Differential effects of three enteral dietary regimens on selected outcome variables in burn patients. JPEN J Parenter Enteral Nutr 14:225–226, 1990.

7. Holm P, Palmblad J: Acute energy deprivation in man: Effect on cell-mediated immunological reactions. Clin Exp Immunol 25:207–211, 1976.

8. Kramer TR, et al: Lymphocyte responsiveness of children supplemented with vitamin A and zinc. Am J Clin Nutr 58:566–570, 1993.

9. Kubena KS, McMurray DN: Nutrition and immune system: A review of nutrient-nutrient interactions. J Am Diet Assoc 96(11):1156–1164, 1996.

10. Kudsk KA, Li J, Renegar KB: Loss of upper respiratory tract immunity with parenteral feeding. Ann Surg 223:629–635, 1996.

11. Kudsk KA, Minard G: Enteral versus parenteral nutrition in the critically ill and injured. Curr Opinion Crit Care 1:255–260, 1995.

12. Moore FA, Moore EE, Kudsk KA, Brown RO, Bower RH, Koruda MJ, Baker CC, Barbul A: Clinical benefits of an immune-enhancing diet for early postinjury enteral feeding. J Trauma, 37(4):607–615, 1994.

13. O'Leary MJ, Coakley JH: Nutrition and immunonutrition. Br J Anaesth 77:118–127, 1996.

14. Plusa SM, Webster N, Primrose JN: Neutrophil adhesion molecule expression and response to stimulation with bacterial wall products in humans is unaffected by parenteral nutrition. Clin Sci 91:371–374, 1996.

15. Roth E, Spittler A, Oehler R: Glutamine: Effects on the immune system, protein balance and intestinal functions. Wien Klin Wochensch 108(21):669–676, 1996.

16. Sirisinha S, Suskind R, Edelman R, Asvapaka C, Olson RE: Secretory and serum IgA in children with protein-calorie malnutrition. Pediatrics 55(2):166–170, 1975.

35. OMEGA-3 FATTY ACIDS AND HEART DISEASE

William S. Harris, PhD

1. Why the interest in fish oil?

Medical reports in the 1970s linked a high-fish diet with reduced heart disease rates in Greenland Eskimos. There has since been a rising interest in the potential health benefits of fish oil. Recent studies have largely confirmed that a component of fish oil called omega-3 fatty acids has cardioprotective effects. The two omega-3 (n-3) fatty acids found in fish oils are eicosapentaenoic acid (EPA) and docosahexaenoic acid (DHA). These fatty acids are unique to fish oils and are not found in plant-derived oils such as corn or soybean oil.

2. How do omega-3 (n-3) fatty acids affect coronary heart disease (CHD) risk factors?

The beneficial properties of omega-3 fatty acids can be attributed to their effects upon four of the body's components: blood lipoproteins, blood platelets, inflammation process, and heart muscle. Briefly, n-3 fatty acids lower lipoproteins, inhibit platelets, decrease the inflammatory reaction, and protect the myocardium.

3. How do omega-3 fatty acids affect blood lipoproteins?

At intakes of 3–4 gm/day, omega-3 fatty acids have their greatest impact on blood triglyceride levels, not on cholesterol. Since they don't change cholesterol levels, some people have questioned whether they can be helpful. But it appears that lowering triglyceride levels may be good for the heart. EPA and DHA have a small but often significant effect on HDL-cholesterol levels in some patients. However, one "down side" of omega-3 fatty acids is their tendency to raise LDL levels in patients with high triglyceride levels. This effect is also shared by triglyceride-lowering drugs such as fibrates, and we don't yet know if it is an adverse effect. Fish oil supplementation can also lower levels of chylomicron triglycerides which enter the blood after eating. These particles may be contribute to coronary artery disease as well, but this is a relatively new area of research and definitive answers are still not in hand.

4. What effect do omega-3 fatty acids have on platelets?

One of the first recognized effects of omega-3 fatty acids is their ability to "thin the blood." They make the blood less likely to clot (somewhat like aspirin). This is believed to be a good effect and may contribute to the observed reduction in heart disease seen in some studies. Early concerns about excessive bleeding from fish oil use have proved to be unfounded.

5. What are the effects of omega-3 fatty acids on the inflammatory reaction?

Part of the process of atherosclerosis is an inflammatory reaction in damaged blood vessels. High blood cholesterol levels, high blood pressure, diabetes, cigarette smoke, and possibly homocysteine can damage arterial linings and initiate repetitive cycles of injury, inflammation, and repair. These inflammatory cycles, continuing over decades, are thought to contribute to the growth of obstructive plaques. Omega-3 fatty acids have a significant generalized anti-inflammatory effect which is mediated through the formation of inhibitory prostaglandins. Particular prostaglandins can inhibit the immune system in general and the inflammatory reaction in particular. Administration of omega-3 fatty acids may inhibit the inflammatory component of atherosclerosis and help slow the rate of progression of the disease.

6. Does the administration of omega-3 fatty acids protect the myocardium?

All of the preceding effects of omega-3 fatty acids are seen on the blood or the vessel wall, including the coronary vessels which feed the heart. But n-3 fatty acids, incorporated into the heart itself, may help keep the muscle from dying when its blood supply is cut off during a heart attack. This is an active field of research and some current examples may serve to demonstrate the point.

In one study, oily fish (such as sardines, mackerel, and salmon) was taken for two years by men who had already survived one heart attack. The researchers found that the number of fatal heart attacks was reduced, although the total number of heart attacks was not significantly lowered. The most convincing study, however, was the GISSI-prevention study, in which over 11,000 post-MI patients were treated with 850 mg of EPA and DHA, 300 mg of vitamin E, both, or neither. After 3.5 years, there was no benefit in the vitamin E group, but the total death rate was reduced by 20% in the omega-3 group. Interestingly, the greatest impact (a 45% reduction) was seen in sudden cardiac death (SCD), a pathology usually caused by malignant arrhythmias. This effect became statistically significant within 4 months of beginning supplementation. The antiarrhythmic theory of omega-3 action is also supported by a report from the Physicians Health Study, in which high blood levels of omega 3 fatty oils were associated with up to a 90% reduction in risk for SCD. Exactly how omega-3 fatty acids reduce risk for SCD is under investigation.

7. How much should a patient take?

One must first determine whether omega-3 fatty acids are being taken in order to lower triglycerides or simply to help prevent heart disease. If the intent is to lower triglycerides, 3–4 grams per day of n-3 fatty acids are required. This would require the patient to eat over 4 pounds of a low-fat fish like sole every day, or a half pound of oily fish such as mackerel, herring, or salmon. Supplementation is the only practical option. But to obtain 3–4 grams from capsules is not easy. The typical fish oil capsule at the health food store contains 30% n-3 fatty acids, which means that 10–12 capsules per day are required. More concentrated products (50%) are available via mail-order, reducing the dose to "only" 6–8 capsules per day. In the future, highly concentrated products containing 85% n-3 fatty acids will become available, bringing the dose down to 4 capsules per day. The current cost for obtaining 3–4 grams of n-3 fatty acids from supplements is currently $0.75–$1.00 per day.

If n-3 fatty acids are being taken (like aspirin) for cardioprotection, much lower intakes may suffice. Intakes of 2–3 servings of oily fish per week or about 1 gm of EPA and DHA/day are recommended. This level of fish oil is equivalent to 2–3 capsules of fish oil concentrates per day. Since the safety of fish oils, especially in these low doses, is beyond question, their widespread use, especially in secondary prevention, is anticipated. As with any treatment for the prevention of heart disease, a decision to take n-3 fatty acids should be made in consultation with the physician managing the patient's overall care.

BIBLIOGRAPHY

1. Albert CM, Campos H, Stampfer MJ, et al: Blood levels of long-chain n-3 fatty acids and the risk of sudden death. N Engl J Med 346:1113–1118, 2002.
2. Burr ML, Fehily AM, Gilbert JF, et al: Effects of changes in fat, fish, and fibre intakes on death and myocardial reinfarction: diet and Reinfarction Trial (DART). Lancet 2:757–761, 1989.
3. Daviglus ML, Stamler J, Orencia AJ, Dyer AE, et al: Fish consumption and the 30 year risk of fatal myocardial infarction. N Engl J Med 336:1046–1053, 1997.
4. Endres S, von Schacky C: N-3 polyunsaturated fatty acids and human cytokine synthesis. Curr Opin Lipidol 7:48–52, 1996.
5. Harris WS: N-3 fatty acids and lipoproteins: Comparison of results from human and animal studies. Lipids 31:243–252, 1996.
6. Kris-Etherton PM, Harris WS, Appel LJ: Fish consumption, fish oil, omega-3 fatty acids, and cardiovascular disease. Circulation 106:2747–2757, 2002.
7. Leaf A, Kang JX, Xiao YF, Billman GE: Clinical prevention of sudden cardiac death by n-3 polyunsaturated fatty acids and mechanism of prevention of arrhythmias by n-3 fish oils. Circulation 107:2646–2652, 2003.
8. Leaf A: Cardiovascular effects of fish oils: Beyond the platelet. Circulation 82:624–628, 1990.
9. Marchioli R, Barzi F, Bomba E, et al: Early protection against sudden death by n-3 polyunsaturated fatty acids after myocardial infarction: Time-course analysis of the results of the Gruppo Italiano per lo Studio della Sopravvivenza nell-Infarto Miocardico (GISSI)-Prevenzione. Circulation 105:1897–1903, 2002.
10. Thies F, Garry JM, Yaqoob P, et al: Association of n-3 polyunsaturated fatty acids with stability of atherosclerotic plaques: A randomised controlled trial. Lancet 361:477–485, 2003.

36. NUCLEIC ACIDS AND NUCLEOTIDES IN NUTRITIONAL SUPPORT

Rifat Latifi, MD, and Gerard A. Burns, MD

1. What are nucleotides and nucleic acids?

Nucleotides are low–molecular-weight biological compounds involved in virtually all biochemical processes. They consist of a nitrogenous base, a 5-carbon sugar, and at least one phosphate group. Nucleic acids, ribonucleic acid (RNA), and deoxyribonucleic acid (DNA) are high–molecular-weight compounds that are made up of long chains of nucleotides. They form the genetic code and are essential for protein synthesis. They function as an energy source in cellular metabolism and as intermediates in biosynthetic and oxidative pathways.

The synthesis of nucleotides is a major activity of the cell. Next to protein synthesis, nucleotide synthesis consumes more amino acids than any other biologic activity. Nucleotides contain either purine or pyrimidine bases. Adenine, inosine, and guanine are purine bases, while thymidine, cytosine, and uracil are pyrimidine bases. Purine nucleotides are synthesized de novo from glutamine, glycine, aspartate, CO_2, and phosphoribosylpyrophosphate (PRPP), while pyrimidines are synthesized from aspartate or glutamine, NH_3, and CO_2.

Purine nucleotides, with their high-energy phosphate side chains, are fundamental to cellular energy metabolism and are intermediaries in biosynthetic and oxidative pathways. Purine nucleotide biosynthesis produces inosine monophosphate (IMP), adenosine monophosphate (AMP), and guanosine monophosphate (GMP). IMP is synthesized by the de novo pathway of purine biosynthesis from glycine and is then converted to AMP and GMP.

2. What are the main sources of nucleotides?

The three main sources of nucleotides are:
1. Dietary nucleotides
2. Salvage of nucleotides released by intracellular metabolism
3. De novo synthesis from amino acids and sugars

3. What are nucleosides?

The addition of a pentose sugar to a nitrogen base produces a nucleoside. Depending on which sugar is added to the nitrogen base, a nucleoside can be ribonucleoside or a deoxyribonucleoside. Nucleosides, unlike nucleotides, contain no phosphate group. Many nucleosides are biologically active. Adenosine, a vasodilator, is used as a pharmacologic agent. Nucleosides are produced by intracellular metabolism and are used for purine biosynthesis via the salvage pathway. The most common pathway is the resynthesis of IMP from inosine, which is a product of adenosine nucleotide metabolism.

4. What is the function of nucleotides?

Nucleotides, as building blocks of DNA and RNA, are essential to the genetic mechanism, protein synthesis, regulation, and structure. Adenosine triphosphate (ATP) and adenosine diphosphate (ADP) are energy sources for many intracellular reactions and synthetic processes. Nucleotides are required in all cells, but they are especially important in tissues with rapid cell proliferation such as intestine, liver, and lymphoid tissue. T lymphocytes require nucleotides to maintain a normal cellular immune response. Various tissues in the body, such as liver, are capable of synthesizing nucleotides de novo. When tissues are unable to synthesize purine nucleotides, purines are transported from another tissue. For example, adenosine is released from the liver and taken up by the lung in large amounts.

173

5. What is the rationale for using diets supplemented with nucleotides?
The small intestinal mucosa requires a constant supply of nucleotides to produce DNA and RNA. In these rapidly proliferating cells, the content of DNA and RNA must double for cell division to occur. However, in these cells, the enterocyte has a limited capacity for de novo biosynthesis. The small intestine must rely on the salvage pathway to synthesize nucleotides from nucleosides. The nucleosides—inosine, adenosine, and so on—come either from the blood or from luminal nucleosides. The latter may come from the diet, from the sloughing of enterocytes, or from bacterial breakdown. In addition, nucleotides themselves can be absorbed from the intestinal lumen.

It is clear that the small intestinal mucosa relies partially on intestinal nucleotides and nucleosides to meet its synthetic demands. There are at least two significant implications. The first is that diets that contain no nucleotides or nucleosides may not offer sufficient support to the intestinal mucosa in some circumstances. This includes many enteral diets, especially elemental diets, and includes all varieties of total parenteral nutrition (TPN). The second implication is that nucleotide or nucleoside supplementation could be beneficial to critically ill patients. This type of supplementation has been implemented clinically in certain enteral products.

6. What is the role of nucleotides on intestinal mucosa?
Nucleotides exert multiple protective actions on the intestinal mucosa and facilitate repair of injured mucosa. Experimental rats receiving TPN supplemented with nucleotides showed higher protein and DNA content in intestinal mucosa, increased maltase activity, higher villous height, and more proliferative activity in crypt cells compared with rats receiving nucleotide-free TPN. In mice, intraperitoneal and oral administration of a mixture of nucleotides and nucleosides reduced bacterial translocation and improved repair of mucosal injuries.

Clinically, the frequency of diarrhea in children was reduced from 68% to 52% when milk formulas were supplemented with nucleotides.

7. What is the mechanism by which nucleotides protect intestinal mucosa?
The basis for this protective action is unclear, although it is known that dietary nucleotides enhance intestinal epithelial cell proliferation and differentiation.

8. How are dietary nucleotides typically processed?
The metabolic fate of any exogenously administered nucleotide depends on its entry position in the overall pathway of purine metabolism.

Nucleic acids undergo partial hydrolysis in the stomach, after which they are subjected to pancreatic nuclease to yield nucleotides. Phosphodiesterases and alkaline phosphatases cleave phosphate groups to form nucleosides. Nucleosidases release the sugar moiety leaving free nitrogen bases. The presence of charged phosphates in nucleotides impedes their transport across cell membranes. Phosphates remove the charged phosphates and together with nucleotidase facilitate transport across the cell membrane. Dietary nucleotides converge in the cell cytoplasm in the form of nucleosides, which are then used in the salvage pathway to reform nucleotides.

9. Does it matter how nucleotides are supplied in order to exert their beneficial actions?
Nucleotides may be supplied either enterally or parenterally. Parenterally administered purine and pyrimidine derivatives are effectively used via salvage pathways. TPN formulas supplemented with a mixture of nucleotides and nucleosides can promote intestinal ulcer healing in rats by restoring villose architecture and accelerating cell proliferation. TPN supplemented with a mixture of nucleotides and nucleosides in animals undergoing massive intestinal resection resulted in significantly higher residual jejunal total mucosal weight, protein, DNA, RNA, and the ratio of proliferating cells per crypt as compared with a standard TPN formula.

10. What is the role of nucleotides in liver injury or resection?
The clinical use of nucleotides in liver disease has been suggested in order to improve healing of the liver. Experimental studies have suggested beneficial effects. A mixture of nucleotides

and nucleosides given subcutaneously prevented ethionine-induced liver injury by suppressing the accumulation of triglycerides in the liver, reducing the increase of liver enzymes, and preventing the decrease of hepatic ATP concentration. In rats undergoing a 70% hepatectomy, supplementation of TPN regimens with nucleotides and nucleosides improved both nitrogen balance and whole body protein turnover. Nucleotide supplementation was beneficial in galactosamine-induced liver injury by reducing the extent of injury histologically and by improving clinical biochemical liver indices.

11. Are nucleotides standard components of TPN solutions?
No. Currently nucleotides are not included in standard TPN solutions. Some patient populations have been shown to benefit from nucleotide-enriched TPN, however. There are now enteral formulas fortified with nucleotide (in addition to arginine, omega-3 fatty acids, and glutamine) that are intended to enhance the immune system in patients receiving them. Since enteral immunonutrition has been proved to be clinically beneficial, no doubt TPN solutions will be fortified with nucleotides, nucleosides, and other immune-enhancing substrates in the near future.

12. What are the immunologic functions of nucleotides?
The immunologic role of nucleotides has been studied mainly in experiments with nucleotide-free diets. In the early 1980s, it was observed that renal transplant patients receiving standard nucleotide-free TPN had better graft function with few rejection episodes and required lower doses of immunosuppressants. Once on a regular diet, these patients required increased doses of immunosuppressants to maintain graft function and prevent rejection.

Animal studies have demonstrated the consequences of nucleotide-free diets. Such diets diminish T-cell mediated immune responses such a delayed-type cutaneous hypersensitivity to various antigens, decreased mitogenic response, and reduced interleukin-2 production. There is also evidence of decreased survival from systemic infections caused by *Staphylococcus aureus* and *Candida albicans* in animals fed a nucleotide-free diet. The increased susceptibility to systemic infections has been shown to reverse with RNA supplementation.

Administration of nucleotides to animals previously fed nucleotide-free diets restores concanavalin A and phytohemagglutinin-stimulated T-cell mitogenesis. Enhanced levels of mitogenesis are associated with RNA- and uracil-supplemented diet in mice.

Nucleotide deficiency reduces splenic stem cell proliferation. This can be reversed with RNA supplementation. Dietary nucleotides modulate T helper cell–mediated antibody production and have a preferential effect on antigen-driven T helper cell–mediated immune response.

13. Are nucleotides essential nutrients in critically ill patients?
Nucleotides and nucleosides are major and essential components of all cells. The metabolic rate of nucleotides is accelerated in hypermetabolic conditions such as sepsis, trauma, or surgical stress. Substantial evidence suggests that these nutrients are conditionally essential for normal stress responses. The conditions that increase nucletoide requirements are rapid cellular proliferation and include hepatic injury or resection, intestinal development and adaptation following massive intestinal resection, and other nonspecific challenges to the host immune system.

14. What is the role of immune-enhancing diets in trauma patients and critically ill patients?
Nucleotides are a component of several immune-enhancing formulas that also contain glutamine, arginine, and omega-3 fatty acids. These formulas have been shown to be beneficial in multiple clinical trials.

Glutamine, arginine, nucleic acids, and omega 3 fatty acids supplemental enteral feeding in severe trauma patients reduced major infection rate, decreased the use of antibiotics, and shortened hospital stays. In a prospective, randomized, placebo-controlled, double-blinded, multicenter trial of patients in the surgical intensive care unit, early enteral feeding supplemented with arginine, nucleotides, and omega-3 fatty acids was shown to reduce postoperative and wound complications. Septic patients fed early enterally with the same supplemented diet (in another double-blinded multicenter study) had a substantial reduction in the hospital stay.

No clinical study has examined the beneficial effect of isolated nucleotide supplementation in enteral feeding formulas in critically ill or trauma patients. However, as a component of an immune-enhancing formula, nucleotides appear to have a role in nutritional support of the critically ill.

15. Should nucleotides be given as a calorie source?

No. Nucleotides should not be administered as a calorie source, only as a promoter of protein synthesis and cellular immunity. It seems likely that nucleotides will one day become an essential component of nutri-pharmacologic intervention in critically ill and trauma patients.

16. Is there standardized nomenclature to use when discussing nucleotides?

Published studies have used different terms to describe various nucleotide supplementation regimens including nucleotides, polynucleotides, nucleotide-nucleoside mixtures, RNA, and purines and pyrimidines.

BIBLIOGRAPHY

1. Adjei A, Yamamoto S, Kulkarni A. Nucleic acids and/or their components: A possible role in immune function. J Nutr Sci Vitaminol 41:1–16, 1995.
2. ASPEN Guidelines for the use of parenteral and enteral nutrition in adult and pediatric patients. J Parent Ent Nutr 26(Suppl), 2001. (See pages 885A–895A [burns] and 909A–925A [critical illness].)
3. Bower RH, Cerra FB, Bershadsky B, et al: Early enteral administration of a formula (impact) supplemented with arginine, nucleotides, and fish oil in intensive care unit patients: Results of a multicenter, prospective, randomized, clinical trial. Crit Care Med 23:436–449, 1995.
4. Grimble G: Why are dietary nucleotides essential nutrients? Br J Nutr 76:475–478, 1996.
5. Grimble GK: Dietary nucleotides and gut mucosal defence. Gut Suppl 1:S46–S51, 1994.
6. Heyland DK, Cook DJ, Guyatt GH: Does the formulation of enteral feeding products influence infectious morbidity and mortality rates in the critically ill patient? A critical review of the evidence. Crit Care Med 22:1192–1202, 1994.
7. Iijima S, Tsujinaka T, Kishibuchi M, et al: Total parenteral nutrition solution supplemented with nucleoside and nucleotide mixture sustains intestinal integrity, but does not stimulate intestinal function after massive bowel resection in rats. Am Inst Nutr 589–595, 1995.
8. Jyonouchi H, Sun S, Goodman D, et al: Dietary fatty acid modulates actions of nucleotides of humoral immune responses. Nutrition 11:437–443, 1995.
9. Jyonouchi H, Sun S, Sato S. Nucleotide-free diet suppresses antigen-driven cytokine production by primed T cells: Effects of supplemental nucleotides and dietary fatty acids. Nutrition 12:608–615, 1996.
10. Kishibuchi M, Tsujinaka T, Yano M, et al: Effects of nucleosides and a nucleotide mixture of gut mucosal barrier function on parenteral nutrition in rats. J Parenteral Enteral Nutr 21:104–111, 1997.
11. Kudsk KA, Minard G, Croce MA, et al: A randomized trial of isonitrogenous enteral diets after severe trauma. Ann Surg 224:531–543, 1996.
12. Kulkarni AD, Rudolph FB, Van Buren CT: The role of dietary sources of nucleotides in immune function: A review. Am Inst Nutr 1442S–1446S, 1994.
13. LeLeiko NS, Walsh MJ: The role of glutamine, short-chain fatty acids, and nucleotides in intestinal adaptation to gastrointestinal disease. Pediatr Gastroenterol 43:451–469, 1996.
14. LeLeiko NS, Walsh MJ, Abraham S: Gene expression in the intestine. The effect of dietary nucleotides." Adv Pediatr 42:145–166, 1995.
15. Martinez-Augustin O, Boza JJ, Navarro J, et al: Dietary nucleotides may influence the humoral immunity in immunocompromised children. Nutrition 13:465–469, 1997.
16. Matsumoto Y, Adjei AA, Yamauchi K, et al: A mixture of nucleosides and nucleotides increases bone marrow cell and peripheral neutrophil number in mice infected with methicillin-resistant Staphylococcus aureus. Am Inst Nutr 817–822, 1994.
17. Matsumoto Y, Adjei AA, Yamauchi K, et al: Nucleoside-nucleotide mixture increases peripheral neutrophils in cyclophosphamide-induced neutropenic mice. Nutrition 11:296–299, 1995.
18. Schloneb PR: Immune-enhancing diets: Products, components, and their rationale. J Parent Ent Nutr 25(Suppl):S3–S7, 2001.
19. Senkal M, Mumme A, Eickhoff U, et al: Early postoperative enteral immunonutrition: Clinical outcome and cost-comparison analysis in surgical patients. Crit Care Med 25:1489–1496, 1997.
20. Sukumar P, Loo A, Magur E, et al: Dietary supplementation of nucleotides and arginine promotes healing of small bowel ulcers in experimental ulcerative ileitis. Dig Dis Sci 42:1530–1536, 1997.

21. Tsujinaka T, Iijima S, Kido Y, et al: Role of nucleosides and nucleotide mixture in intestinal mucosal growth under total parenteral nutrition. Nutrition 10:203–204, 1994.

22. Uauy R, Quan R, Gil A: Role of nucleotides in intestinal development and repair: Implications for infant nutrition. Am Inst Nutr 1436S–1441S, 1994.

23. Van Buren CT, Rudolph F: Dietary nucleotides: A conditional requirement. Nutrition 13:470–472, 1997.

24. Walker WA: Exogenous nucleotides and gastrointestinal immunity. Transplant Proc 28:2438–2441, 1996.

25. Yamamoto S, Wang MF, Adjei AA, Ameho CK: Role of nucleosides and nucleotides in the immune system, gut reparation after injury, and brain function. Nutrition 13:372–374, 1997.

VIII. *Total Parenteral Nutrition*

37. INDICATIONS FOR TOTAL PARENTERAL NUTRITION

David S. Seres, MD

1. What is total parenteral nutrition?
Total parenteral nutrition (TPN) is a means of providing patients who are unable to tolerate enteral nutrition, either orally or by tube, with all of their nutritional requirements. It is administered through a central venous catheter and contains protein, calories, vitamins, and minerals. Crystalline amino acid solutions are the source for protein; nonprotein calories are provided by dextrose solutions and lipid emulsions. Lipid emulsions may be mixed with the other components of TPN in what is called a "3-in-1" admixture or infused as a separate "piggy back." Peripheral veins will not tolerate the high osmotic load required when administering TPN. Therefore, TPN must be administered into a central vein. Peripheral parenteral nutrition (PPN) is similar to TPN but must be far more dilute and therefore in a much larger volume.

2. What is hyperalimentation?
Hyperalimentation, which means over-feeding, was used in the past to refer to parenteral nutrition. Hyperalimentation delivered excess calories and protein to overcome the increase in metabolic rate in acutely ill patients. It has now been clearly shown that doing so significantly increases the risk of metabolic and infectious complications.

3. What are the indications for TPN?
TPN is indicated for patients who cannot be fed adequately via the bowel (e.g., patients with intestinal blockage, malabsorption, or a gut that is inaccessible to nourishment). Because of the risks associated with TPN and the lack of clear evidence that early initiation of TPN improves outcomes, patients who will be without nourishment for a short time should not receive TPN. The amount of time patients may be without nourishment is the subject of debate amongst experts in the field. Previously well-nourished patients who are unable to receive enteral nutrition should receive TPN only when at least 5–7 days have passed and an additional 5–7 days without adequate enteral nutrition is expected. Malnourished patients should receive TPN immediately when a total of 5–7 days without enteral nutrition is expected.

4. What are the contraindications for TPN?
The contraindications for TPN are the converse of the indications. Patients who are able to receive adequate nourishment via enteral means should not receive TPN. Well-nourished patients generally tolerate 5–7 days with no nourishment without adverse effect. Some authors advocate allowing 14 days or more without nourishment before initiating TPN in patients without preexistent malnutrition. This discrepancy is due to the lack of clear data from randomized controlled trials indicating that TPN is beneficial in such patients. Malnourished patients should not receive TPN if it is expected that their nutritional needs will be met with enteral nutrition within 5–7 days. In addition, TPN is contraindicated if the expected benefit is outweighed by the risks of metabolic and infectious complications, by psychological or financial burdens, or by a reduction in quality of life. Competent patients may refuse all forms of nutrition support. Advance directives must be respected when patients lose the capacity for medical decision-making.

5. Is the absence of bowel sounds an indication for TPN?

Bowel sounds are, for the most part, the result of colonic peristalsis. When an ileus occurs, peristalsis is lost in the colon and stomach (more precisely foregut and hindgut) but persists in the small intestine despite a lack of bowel sounds. On the other hand, bowel sounds may be heard in the presence of complete obstruction. Therefore, patients may be fed with tubes placed into the small intestine whether or not bowel sounds are heard. Tube feeding is usually contraindicated in patients with obstruction, because dangerous distention is likely to occur. Finally, patients who are hemodynamically unstable risk bowel infarction when fed enterally prior to fluid resuscitation and should not receive enteral feeds, whether or not bowel sounds are present, until resuscitated.

6. Is TPN indicated for patients who can receive but refuse enteral feeding?

A great deal of attention has been paid by the lay press to the use of feeding tubes to prolong vegetative states "unnecessarily." As a result, patients may feel that they are doomed to such a state if they accept a feeding tube. Patients may also believe that the placement of a feeding tube precludes eating by mouth and other normal activities. Because of these and other misconceptions, the process of deciding whether to allow the insertion of a feeding tube may be one of the most emotionally challenging experiences facing patients, and tube feeding may be one of the most difficult therapies for us to convince patients to accept.

The risks from malnutrition, which increase while waiting for acceptance of a feeding tube, may exceed the risks from parenteral nutrition. Therefore, it may be appropriate to start TPN while the issues surrounding the patient's refusal of a feeding tube are addressed.

7. Is TPN indicated for patients in whom esophageal obstruction is the only known gut dysfunction?

Many, if not most, patients with esophageal obstruction are malnourished on presentation. Malnutrition increases the risk of surgical morbidity and mortality. Surgery is often required to obtain enteral access in such patients when the obstruction prevents the placement of a nasogastric tube or the passing of an endoscope for a percutaneous endoscopic gastrostomy (PEG). TPN may be required to improve the nutritional state of the patient until the obstruction can be relieved or enteral access gained. The benefit of improved nutritional state may outweigh the risk of TPN prior to any intervention in severely malnourished patients such as these. Rapid conversion to enteral feeding, however, is always the goal.

8. Is preoperative TPN beneficial?

Preoperative TPN may improve surgical outcome in *severely* malnourished patients with cancer. In minimally and moderately malnourished patients, preoperative TPN has not been shown to have any beneficial effect and may increase morbidity and mortality. Preoperative TPN should be used only if the patient is severely malnourished and unable to receive enteral feeding.

9. Is postoperative TPN beneficial?

The risk of complications due to TPN outweighs any potential benefit in the well-nourished surgical patient, unless the patient is unable to tolerate enteral feeds for an extended period. Five to seven days without nourishment is safer for these patients than TPN for the same period.

In malnourished patients, TPN should be started immediately after surgery when it is expected that enteral nutrition will not be possible within 5–7 days. However, with the increased use of jejunal feeding in patients with ileus, the use of TPN in this population has greatly diminished.

10. Is TPN indicated for patients with inflammatory bowel disease?

Adequate nourishment is critical for the patient with inflammatory bowel disease and may actually help reduce disease activity. However, the route of administration makes no difference in this regard.

11. Do all patients with gastrointestinal fistulas require TPN?

Patients with high-output fistulas often require TPN to keep up with the large quantities of nutrients lost through the fistulas. However, putting the bowel at rest has not proved to be an effective means for speeding the healing of fistulas. Therefore, enteral feedings may be used for most of these patients. Patients with upper intestinal fistulas may have feeding tubes placed below or, occasionally, through the fistula. Patients with colonic fistulas may be fed with a low residue diet either by mouth or via tube.

12. Will a patient requiring TPN for short-bowel syndrome require TPN for a lifetime?

Patients with short-bowel syndrome often require long-term TPN for all or part of their nutritional requirements. The gut does have the ability to adapt to the loss of length. This adaptation depends on a number of factors, in particular the presence or absence of the ileocecal valve and/or colon. Absorption of nutrients improves during the first 2 years after bowel excision. The amount of function regained is individual, as is the length of residual bowel required for a patient to become independent of TPN. Specific nutrients and growth factors are under investigation and show some promise in improving bowel adaptation. However, at this time these agents are investigational and should not be considered standard treatment.

13. Is TPN indicated for patients with pancreatitis?

Pancreatitis is by itself not an indication for parenteral nutrition. Most patients with acute pancreatitis are well nourished or able to tolerate oral or tube feeding within 5–7 days. In more protracted cases, enteral feeding through a long nasoenteric or jejunal tube has been shown to be safe and effective, even when pancreatitis is severe. Patients with necrotizing pancreatitis, pancreatic abscesses, and pancreatic pseudocysts may require TPN.

14. Is intravenous fat contraindicated for patients with pancreatitis?

Intravenous fat is safe for patients with pancreatitis as long as serum triglyceride levels are monitored. Hypertriglyceridemia may be a cause of acute pancreatitis when serum levels exceed approximately 1000 mg/dl. In patients with pancreatitis in whom a triglyceride level of 400–450 mg/dL is noted, intravenous lipid may be withheld. Fat-free TPN for an extended period results in essential fatty acid deficiency and therefore should be avoided. However, unless the patient has an underlying lipid disorder, it is unusual for triglyceride levels to be increased to this degree by TPN when current standards for formulation and infusion of TPN are followed.

15. Should patients on TPN receive intravenous fat at all?

Intravenous lipid emulsions are made of phospholipids, which must be taken up in the reticuloendothelial system before being utilized. Large amounts may overwhelm this system and lead to immune dysfunction. Additionally, the only intravenous lipids available in the United States are made entirely of omega-6 long-chain fatty acids, which are the precursors to proinflammatory eicosanoids. Theoretically, when omega-6 fatty acids are the predominant fatty acids administered to a patient, immunosuppression and the stimulation of the inflammatory cascade may result, which may be deleterious to septic patients.

The benefit from the inclusion of fat in TPN is a reduction in the incidence of hyperglycemia by providing the same calories using less dextrose. This benefit may be nullified in the current era of tight glycemic control and requires more study.

It is commonly accepted that intravenous fat may be included in the TPN of patients without severe infections and that the discontinuation of intravenous fat may be considered in patients with severe sepsis. Furthermore, it is advised that the practice of increasing the ratio of fat to dextrose in TPN to improve glycemic control be discontinued until the impact of intravenous fat on patient outcome is better understood.

16. Is intravenous fat contraindicated in patients with thoracic duct leak?

Only enteral fat restriction is required in patients with thoracic duct leak. Intravenous fat has no impact on flow in the thoracic duct because it does not directly enter the intestinal lymphatics.

Therefore, there is no contraindication to the use of intravenous fat in patients with thoracic duct leak.

17. Is TPN indicated for patients with cancer?

Operative outcome may be improved in severely malnourished patients with cancer when given TPN for 1–2 weeks prior to surgery. However, when compared calorie for calorie to enteral nutrition, TPN does not provide superior nourishment to patients with cancer or any other systemic illness. As with any clinical situation, TPN should be considered in patients with cancer only when full enteral nutrition is not possible and the patient's prognosis is sufficiently favorable.

18. Is TPN required for patients with hypoalbuminemia?

Even severely hypoalbuminemic patients may be fed enterally. Most hypoalbuminemic patients tolerate and absorb enteral nutrition well enough to meet their needs. Specialized oligopeptide formulas may be necessary if standard feeds are not tolerated. Patients with intractable diarrhea may need supplementation with parenteral nutrition if weight maintenance cannot be achieved with enteral nutrition alone.

It should be noted that a persistently low albumin or prealbumin (transthyretin) in a patient on nutritional support is an indicator of continued catabolism—not of inadequate nourishment. Metabolism is significantly altered in any condition associated with an elevation of inflammatory mediators, such as cancer, HIV/AIDS, and sepsis. Lean mass is lost due to the breakdown of muscle and organs into their component amino acids. Amino acids are then utilized less as a substrate for protein synthesis and more as a fuel for energy. In this situation, it is not possible to regain lean mass without the use of anabolic agents (which have not been shown to impact outcome), and any weight gain that is achieved will be in the form of fat. Therefore, unless the underlying condition is resolved, no nutritional support of any kind will overcome the effect of catabolism.

19. Does TPN provide better nourishment to patients with HIV/AIDS?

TPN has not been shown to provide nourishment more efficiently or more safely than enteral nutrition in patients with HIV/AIDS. Enteral nutrition has salutary effects on immunity and may be associated with fewer risks. As with any chronic disease, prognosis must be weighed before starting any form of nutritional support.

20. Is TPN indicated for patients with hyperemesis gravidarum or gastroparesis?

Patients with hyperemesis and gastroparesis can be successfully fed orally or enterally with nasogastric tubes. Long nasoenteric tubes placed past the pylorus may be used to feed vomiting patients, although there is the risk of dislodgement of the tube up into the stomach. TPN may be used when enteral feeds and medical therapies have failed.

BIBLIOGRAPHY

1. ASPEN Board of Directors and the Clinical Guidelines Task Force: Guidelines for the use of parenteral and enteral nutrition in adult and pediatric patients. J Parenter Enter Nutr 26(1 Suppl):1SA–138SA, 2002.
2. Koretz RL, Lipman TO, Klein S: American Gastroenterological Association technical review on parenteral nutrition. Gastroenterology 121(4):970–1001, 2001.

38. CENTRAL TOTAL PARENTERAL NUTRITION

Kimberly Alexander, RD, LD, CNSD, and Charles W. Van Way III, MD

1. Who should receive central total parenteral nutrition (TPN)?

Central TPN is a nutritional strategy of last resort. Simply, it is given to patients who must have nutritional support but who cannot be fed orally or enterally. Sometimes such patients are given peripheral TPN (see Chapter 39). The decision to give central TPN is based upon:

- *Diagnosis.* Early initiation of parenteral nutrition is indicated for such hyper-metabolic states as burns, trauma, and sepsis. If the gastrointestinal tract is nonfunctional (see below), then TPN may be the only available means of support. Perioperative use should be initiated only if there is severe malnutrition. Most postoperative patients do not need TPN, nor would they benefit from it.

- *Nutritional Status.* Patients with inadequate nutrition or malnutrition, defined as greater than 10% weight loss, must receive nutritional support. If a patient has been without adequate oral intake for more than 5–7 days, nutritional support must be started. Patients with hypermetabolic conditions, such as burn or head injury, should be started on support after 3–4 days.

- *Gastrointestinal function.* The major causes of gastrointestinal malfunction are paralytic ileus, gastric atony, and mechanical obstruction. Any of these can be seen with injury or sepsis, postoperatively, or with diseases such as peritonitis, perforated bowel, abdominal abscess, or bowel ischemia. A number of these diseases require surgical treatment with nutritional support indicated as a perioperative adjunct to surgery. Still other causes for gastrointestinal dysfunction include fistula, short bowel syndrome, and acute pancreatitis.

- *Intravenous access.* From a practical standpoint, the decision to use central versus peripheral parenteral nutrition often depends on whether there is a central venous catheter already in place. If a central line has been placed for other reasons, then it makes good sense to use it for nutritional support. Similarly, the simple nonavailability of peripheral sites may mandate central TPN. On the other hand, any reluctance to use a central line would push the decision to peripheral parenteral nutrition.

2. How is central TPN put together?

The traditional TPN formula was made up by mixing 50% glucose with 8.5% amino acids and then adding electrolytes, vitamins, and trace elements. This produced a formula with 250 grams of glucose and 42.5 grams of amino acid per liter. But over the past few years it has become more usual to substitute fat calories for some of the glucose calories. For example, at St. Luke's Hospital, the "standard" central TPN solution contains 150 grams of glucose and 34 grams of fat (170 ml of 20% fat emulsion), in addition to 42.5 grams of amino acids, per liter. The formula contains about 1 calorie per milliliter. Automated mixing devices have made it feasible to make up custom formulas for many patients. For example, a diabetic patient might be given a 10% glucose formula while a patient with higher protein needs might be given 60–65 grams of amino acids.

The other components are vitamins, trace elements, and electrolytes (see Chapters 4, 5, and 6). Vitamins are added in the form of a multivitamin solution, which is made up according to the recommendations of the AMA Council on Food and Nutrition. For patients in renal failure, the standard vitamin package is modified to contain only the water-soluble vitamins. Trace elements are also given in a standard package, containing zinc, copper, chromium, manganese, and, sometimes, selenium. Electrolytes are given in two ways. In the TPN solution are maintenance amounts of sodium, potassium, chloride, calcium, magnesium, and phosphate. Electrolyte deficiencies are usually made up by giving separate intravenous electrolytes.

3. What is a "3 in 1" system?

Most hospitals have adopted the 3 in 1 approach to central TPN. The formula for each patient is mixed in a single 3-liter bag and administered over 24 hours. The more traditional formulations were dispensed in one-liter units; three of the old units can be placed in a 3-liter bag, hence the 3 in 1 name. The intravenous solution is changed only once a day, mixing costs are reduced, and the whole process is simplified, reducing the chance for error. Disadvantages are longer time to initiate changes in TPN and less ability to adjust electrolytes. Glucose control in particular is affected, because if one puts too much insulin in a 3-liter bag, the TPN for the day must be discontinued. As discussed below, glucose control should be done more often with a separate intravenous solution containing insulin (an "insulin drip").

4. How is central TPN ordered?

If a standard TPN formula is used in the hospital, then simply assess the calorie requirements and give that amount of standard TPN. Determine if there are any further fluid and electrolyte requirements and give supplemental intravenous fluid to meet them.

To determine an individualized formula, the process is much more complex:

• Assess calorie, protein, and fluid requirements.
• Fat: Calculate fat calories as 30% of estimated caloric needs
  (Fat calories) = (Total calories) × (0.3)
  Convert fat calories to amount of lipid emulsion (1.1 cal/ml for 10% emulsion, 2 cal/ml for 20%)
  (Lipid emulsion in ml) = (Fat calories) ÷ 1.1 (2 for 20% emulsion)
• Protein: Determine calories to be provided from protein.
  A good general rule is 17% of total calorie needs. With high protein needs, this can be raised to 20% or even to 25%. Estimate the amount of amino acids (protein) by dividing the protein calories by 4 kcal/gm protein.
  (Protein calories) = (Total calories) × (0.17) (Or 0.2 to 0.25)
  (Grams protein) = (Protein calories) ÷ 4
  Calculate the amount of standard amino acid solution (8.5% amino acids): (Amino acid solution in ml) = (Grams protein) ÷ 0.085 or ÷ 0.1 for 10% amino acids or ÷ 1.5 for 15% amino acids
• Dextrose: Determine calories to be provided from carbohydrates by subtracting fat and protein calories from total calories. Convert to grams of dextrose.
  (Dextrose calories) = (Total calories) − (Fat calories) − (Protein calories)
  Then calculate the amount of 50% dextrose solution which must be added to the TPN mixture:
  (Dextrose 50% in ml) = (Dextrose calories) ÷ 1.7 cals/ml for 50% or 2.38 cals/ml for 70% dextrose or 1.36 cals/ml for 40% dextrose
• Determine the free water requirements by subtracting the fat emulsion, protein solution, and dextrose solution from the total fluid requirements.
• Finally, combine all of the above into a prescription:
  _____ ml 50% dextrose
  _____ ml 8.5% amino acids
  _____ ml 10% (or 20%) fat emulsion
  _____ ml water
• Add electrolytes, and trace elements.

In the above calculations, amino acid calories are counted as part of total calories. While it is possible to calculate "non-protein calories" and to do the entire set of calculations on that basis, this is probably unnecessary. Amino acids are given primarily to replace body protein stores, which metabolize and produce energy. A particular molecule of amino acids given to the patient may wind up as a component of body protein but it is replacing another molecule from the body which was broken down for energy. The energy balance calculations should therefore include the amino acids given to the patient.

5. What laboratory studies should be monitored and how often should they be obtained?

LAB STUDY	BASELINE	DAILY	EVERY 2–3 DAYS	WEEKLY
Electrolytes	X		X	
Blood urea nitrogen, creatinine	X		X	
Blood glucose	X	X First 3 days	X	
Magnesium and phosphorus	X			X
Calcium	X			X
Liver function tests	X			X
Albumin and prealbumin	X			X
Cholesterol and triglycerides	X	X First 2 days		X
Hemoglobin, WBC	X		X	
Prothrombin time	X			X
Urine glucose*	X	4–6/day, First 3 days	X	
Urine urea nitrogen (24 hr)				X

* The adjustment of blood glucose during the first 3 days on central TPN is critical. Monitoring should be as often as necessary (see below).

6. How should blood glucose be regulated?

The greatest danger from TPN during the first 24 hours is that the patient will become hyperglycemic. This may lead to osmotic diuresis as glycosuria leads to excessive excretion of free water by the kidney, and thence to hyperosmolar dehydration. Hyperosmolar dehydration, otherwise known as non-ketotic hyperosmolar coma, is a potentially lethal disorder and is capable of killing within 24–48 hours unless it is treated by lowering the blood sugar and giving free water. It is best treated by prevention, so it is important to keep the blood glucose below the renal threshold. This is usually cited as 250 mg/dl but can be as high as 400 or as low as 150 in some patients. So it is important to measure the urine glucose, especially for the first two or three days, in order to be absolutely sure that the patient is not having glycosuria and osmotic diuresis. Measuring the blood sugar alone may not be completely reliable.

Recent studies have shown that the glucose is best maintained between 120 and 180 mg/dl. This is a relatively low target range and is much lower than has been traditional. But higher levels of blood glucose appear to interfere with white cell function and impair the immune system.

Managing glucose is usually done by putting up to 20 units of insulin per liter in the TPN solution. If this does not control the glucose, then an insulin drip should be started. The insulin drip typically begins at 2–5 units of insulin per hour but, in an insulin-resistent patient, may need to be considerably higher. Many patients, especially those who are diabetic, will exhibit insulin resistence. The normal pancreas secretes the equivalent of 40–60 units of insulin per day. But diabetic patients may require as much as several hundred units to control their blood sugar. Insulin resistance is seen in patients on TPN in such conditions as sepsis, pancreatitis, and trauma. As the patient recovers, however, the insulin resistence may diminish and the insulin requirements may change greatly over a few days. Close glucose monitoring several times a day is mandatory in patients receiving supplemental insulin.

7. How are electrolytes managed?

Electrolyte management of patients on TPN is no different from that for anyone else receiving intravenous fluids. It is generally best to give maintenance amounts in the TPN and give any other requirements separately (see Chapter 6).

Potassium is often a particular problem in patients on TPN. When hypertonic glucose and insulin are given together, potassium is driven into the cells and the serum potassium is lowered. Indeed, this is the standard emergency treatment for hyperkalemia. So, when TPN is started, the serum potassium often drops. This is best prevented by giving a generous replacement amount of potassium. Patients should receive at least one mEq of potassium per kilogram of body weight.

8. What is "refeeding syndrome"?

During a period of starvation, the body adapts to use less carbohydrate and more fat metabolism for energy. Tolerance for carbohydrates in general and dextrose in particular may be greatly impaired. Tolerance for fluid loads is impaired. When such a patient is abruptly given TPN, the sudden influx of carbohydrates may cause intracellular passage of potassium, magnesium, and phosphorus and result in low serum levels that can be resistant to treatment. Fluid overload may be produced by standard amounts of TPN. Respiratory failure is the greater danger from refeeding syndrome.

9. How should refeeding syndrome be prevented?

Patients at risk are those in whom there has been inadequate intake for one to two months, as well as severe weight loss (> 5% over one month or > 10% over six months). Such patients should be started on TPN or other forms of nutritional support quite slowly. Only one-third of estimated basal energy needs should be given during the first 24 hours and the amount should be gradually increased over three to four days to estimated needs. Fluid overload should be avoided by monitoring intake and output and measuring daily weights. A weight gain of more than 1 kg per week is fluid retention and should be avoided.

It is best to begin with one-third of caloric needs per day and increase by one-third over 3–4 days while monitoring potassium, phosphorus, and magnesium levels for the first 3–4 days to avoid complications in the starved or malnourished patient. Specifically, at the start of therapy, glucose intake should be less than 150 gm/day and sodium to less than 20 mEq/day. Total fluids should be less than 800 ml/day. Potassium, calcium, magnesium, and phosphorus should be carefully monitored and replaced as necessary.

After the first week of therapy, the patient's metabolism will have shifted back to normal and the nutritional regimen adjusted to provide more than estimated needs in order to promote weight gain.

10. How much calcium and phosphorus can be given together?

Calcium phosphate is only minimally soluble. Combining calcium and phosphate ions in solution may result in precipitation of calcium phosphate. The amounts usually given in TPN are calculated by the pharmacy to produce no difficulty. But if it is necessary to increase either calcium or phosphate, attention should be paid to the solubility product, which is the maximum amount of the two ions which can be given together. The rule of thumb is that the sum of the calcium concentration in mEq/l and the phosphate concentration in mMol/l should not exceed 30. This provides a safety factor to allow for variations in pH, volume of solution, and mixing procedures.

11. How can TPN be monitored for adequacy and repletion?

Prealbumin (thyroxin-binding prealbumin) is a serum transport protein with a half-life of only 2 days. It will show a response to an adequate nutritional regimen in less than one week. In the absence of inflammatory response or liver failure, prealbumin will increase approximately 0.1 mg/dl/day if adequate protein is provided. However, during the catabolic phase of injury response, which lasts for a few days following minor trauma and three weeks following a major injury or burn, the liver does not make transport proteins or albumin. The prealbumin may stay depressed even though adequate calories and protein are provided.

Albumin can be monitored but is usually slow to respond because of its longer half-life. Albumin levels also respond to fluid shifts, making changes difficult to interpret.

The urinary nitrogen balance in patients without renal failure can be very helpful. If the corrected urine urea nitrogen (UUN) is subtracted from the nitrogen intake as calculated from the nutritional regimen, the nitrogen balance is obtained. This can indicate if a patient is anabolic (values +3 to +5), in balance (values –2 to +2), or catabolic (values less than –2). If the patient is catabolic, then one should make sure that the caloric intake is adequate, increase the protein intake, and then re-measure the UUU in two or three days.

12. How can one evaluate and prevent overfeeding?
A metabolic cart study provides more than an estimate of energy balance. It also measures the respiratory quotient (RQ), which is the ratio of the carbon dioxide production to the oxygen production. An RQ level > 1 indicates overfeeding by total calories or total carbohydrate. A level 0.7 or less represents underfeeding, while an RQ of 0.8 to 0.9 is normal on a mixed nutrient regimen. Overfeeding is best avoided by giving no more than the estimated needs and by measuring metabolic the needs with a metabolic cart. Limiting the amount of carbohydrate helps to avoid overfeeding.

13. What are the maximum units of substrate per kg in TPN for maximum utilization and absorption with minimal complications?
Carbohydrates. The liver can use 4–6 mg/min/kg of carbohydrates, or 6–9 gm/kg/day. This corresponds to 500–600 grams of dextrose for an average man. This is a relatively generous allowance.
Fat. The recommendations of the manufacturer of fat emulsions is to use a limit of 2.5 gm/kg/day. However, a smaller limit helps to avoid the complications of excessive fat, including elevation of triglycerides, interference with clotting, and possible inhibition of the immune system. We recommend that 1.5 gm/kg/day not be exceeded. This corresponds to more than half of the normal caloric requirements. Most patients need about 1 gm/kg/day to obtain 30% of their estimated calories from fat.
Protein. Protein is simply used for energy if given in excess. However, too much protein may cause a rise in the blood urea nitrogen. A practical rule is to give no more than 25% of the caloric requirements as protein, which corresponds to 1.5–2 gm/kg/day of protein or amino acids.

14. How do I identify TPN-induced liver disease?
Elevation of liver enzymes within 1 to 3 weeks after starting parenteral nutrition (PN) is not uncommon. These usually return to within normal limits within 1 to 2 weeks after cessation of PN. However, liver enzymes should be monitored weekly since fatty liver infiltration is a known complication of overfeeding. Other etiologies should be ruled out, including sepsis, essential fatty acid deficiency, and carnitine deficiency.
Cholestasis is a common complication of extended PN with NPO status, possibly related to lack of intraluminal nutrient stimulation of hepatic bile secretion. Total serum bilirubin and serum alkaline phosphatase should be monitored weekly. If elevation of bilirubin is seen, other causes should be ruled out, such as impaired bile flow, toxic tryptophan metabolites, overfeeding, and biliary tract obstruction.

15. Can other medications or blood be run through the PN catheter?
To prevent contamination, no blood or other meds should be run through the same lumen. Likewise, no specimens or CVP should be obtained from TPN. If multiple solutions need to be infused, a triple-lumen catheter is necessary.

16. Are lipids harmful or beneficial?
It has been documented that fat emulsions have a vascular protective effect and lengthen patency of vascular endothelium. It is well known that triglyceride levels increase rapidly in sepsis and it has been documented that lipoproteins combine and inactivate endotoxins. This becomes a risk of overfeeding with too many fat calories (greater than 45% of total calories) or overfeeding total calories (which can lead to hyperglycemia).

BIBLIOGRAPHY

1. American Society for Parenteral and Enteral Nutrition: Guidelines for the use of parenteral and enteral nutrition in adult and pediatric patients. Section VI: Normal requirements—Adults. J Parent Ent Nutr 26(1 Suppl):235A–255A, 2002.

2. Kelly DG: Guidelines and available products for parenteral vitamin and trace elements. J Parent Ent Nutr 26(5 Suppl):534–536, 2002.
3. Latifi R, Dudrick SJ (eds): Current Surgical Nutrition. Austin, R.G. Landes, 1996.
4. Parenteral Nutrition Products: Drugs for human use. Drug Efficacy Study Implementation. Fed Reg 65:21200–21201, 2000.
5. Parenteral nutrition. Chapter 13 in Heimburger DC, Weinsier RL (eds): Handbook of Clinical Nutrition. 3rd ed. St. Louis, Mosby-Year Book, 1997.
6. Parenteral nutrition. Chapter 22 in Williams SR (ed): Nutrition and Diet Therapy. 7th ed. St. Louis, Mosby-Year Book, 1993.
7. Rombeau JL, Caldwell MD (eds): Clinical Nutrition: Parenteral Feeding. 2nd ed. Boston, Little, Brown, 1991.
8. Souba WW: Nutritional support. N Engl J Med 336:41–48, 1997.
9. Van Way CW (ed): Handbook of Surgical Nutrition. Philadelphia, J.B. Lippincott, 1992.
10. Veterans Affairs Total Parenteral Nutrition Cooperative Study Group: Perioperative total parenteral nutrition in surgical patients. N Engl J Med 325:525–532, 1991.

39. PERIPHERAL PARENTERAL NUTRITION

Paul G. Cuddy, PharmD, Ellen P. Dooling-McGurk, RPh, BCNSP,
Pamela A. Orr, MSN, RN, FNP, and L. Beaty Pemberton, MD

1. What is peripheral parenteral nutrition (PPN)?

PPN refers to the complete delivery of all required protein and calories through a peripheral venous catheter. This therapy started in the 1970s and continues to be a widely used means of delivering nutritional support to patients unable or unwilling to take nutrition via the gastrointestinal tract. The goal of PPN is the same as total parenteral nutrition (TPN)—complete provision of required calories and nitrogen. Advantages of PPN include avoidance of central venous catheters and the resulting potential complications, such as line sepsis, and lower start-up costs. Disadvantages of PPN include difficulty with meeting predicted energy and protein needs using tolerable volumes of fluid and fat and difficulty with maintaining adequate peripheral venous access sites due to the hypertonic nature of the nutritional fluids.

2. How is PPN different from TPN?

The route of administration dictates the differing composition of the two fluids. TPN involves administration of highly concentrated dextrose that typically ranges from 25% to 30%. Such highly concentrated dextrose solutions are hyperosmolar at 1200–1500 mOsm/L. The glucose concentration in PPN is 5–10%, which is only 250–500 mOsm/L. This osmolality difference underlies the need to administer TPN through a central vein while allowing PPN to be administered through a peripheral vein.

Another difference is the need to use fat as a primary calorie source with PPN. If desired, fat can be virtually eliminated in central TPN. Finally, because PPN is more dilute, it requires administration of larger fluid volumes. TPN can be more highly concentrated, allowing delivery of total nutrition support with lower fluid volumes.

Nonetheless, the differences between PPN and TPN are diminishing. Current practice is to use larger amounts of fat in TPN to lower glucose concentrations. It is common to provide 30% of calories as fat, which lowers the glucose requirements considerably. Glucose in TPN is often 15% or even less.

3. How is PPN similar to TPN?

Regardless of the route of administration, both PPN and TPN involve administration of glucose, fat, protein, electrolytes, vitamins, and trace elements. The therapeutic objectives are similar: preservation of body protein stores to promote positive nitrogen balance and delivery of adequate calories, vitamins, and minerals. Generally, similar metabolic monitoring is involved—visceral proteins, electrolytes, and assessment of nitrogen balance.

4. What are the prerequisites for successful PPN?

Successful PPN requires the complete delivery of all required calories and protein without undue complications. To accomplish this goal, patients must have good peripheral venous access to accommodate delivery of hypertonic feeding solutions. Similarly, large fluid loads are inevitable with PPN, and good candidates should not have any fluid intolerance (e.g., oliguric renal failure, congestive heart failure, ascites). Since intravenous fat is the main caloric source, patients receiving PPN must tolerate significant fat loads (e.g., 40–60% of total calories).

5. Why is intravenous fat essential for successful PPN?

Glucose at 3.4 calories per gram cannot supply adequate nonprotein calories to meet the anticipated metabolic needs of patients requiring PPN. For example, a patient requiring 1500 calories needs roughly 440 grams of dextrose to meet estimated needs, which equates to roughly 4.5 L of 10% dextrose per day. This estimate ignores the additional obligatory fluid load that results from protein and electrolyte delivery. For this reason, an isotonic, calorie-dense nutrient is needed, and intravenous fat at 9 calories per gram fulfills this criterion perfectly. Using 750 ml of 20% intravenous fat delivers those same 1500 calories of energy in an isotonic emulsion.

6. Which patients are good candidates for PPN?
Good candidates for PPN need partial or total parenteral nutrition support that is anticipated to last a few days to less than 2 weeks. It is especially attractive in patients whose caloric needs are not particularly great and who have good peripheral venous access. A representative candidate might be a patient with coagulopathy or other condition in which central vein catheterization is inadvisable or a surgical candidate with only mild nutritional deficits, or a patient with damaged central veins. Good candidates should be able to tolerate large volumes of fluid, lipid, and electrolyte solutions.

7. Which patients are poor candidates for PPN?
Conditions that identify poor PPN candidates include tenuous cardiac status, renal impairment, hepatic failure, moderate-to-severe nutritional deficits, and poor peripheral venous access. Any of these conditions prevents delivery of the amounts of fluids, electrolytes, or lipids needed to provide adequate calories and protein.

8. What special nursing care is required for patients receiving PPN?
Good nursing care is essential for the safe delivery of PPN. Routine care for the PPN patient should include:
- Weighing the patient at least 3 times weekly
- Checking vital signs (frequently dictated by the condition of the patient)
- Mouth care if the patient cannot receive anything by mouth
- Recording intake and output fluid daily
- Attending to the local catheter (dressing should be occlusive and dry at all times)
- Changing tubes daily
- Maintaining a dedicated intravenous line for PPN (no secondary tubing or blood draws)
- Observing line insertion site for signs of inflammation or infiltration

9. What procedures should be followed if the PPN is interrupted?
Because the final dextrose concentration in PPN is typically between 5% and 10%, concerns over hypoglycernia resulting from solution interruption are much less worrisome than with TPN, in which dextrose concentrations are 15–25%. It is not necessary to hang a replacement solution if PPN is unexpectedly interrupted. Glucose monitoring should be performed if indicated by the patient's clinical status.

10. How does monitoring for PPN differ from monitoring for central venous TPN?
Because the goal of both methods is to provide nutrition and avoid complications, monitoring is, for the most part, very similar. For PPN in particular, extra attention should be directed to identifying signs and symptoms of fluid overload, such as weight gain, elevated heart rate, respiratory distress, edema, unmatched fluid intake and output, or hyponatremia. Triglyceride levels should be monitored with the understanding that continuous infusion of lipids may produce moderately elevated levels. Caution is warranted if levels exceed 350 mg/dl. The peripheral IV site should be observed frequently and changed at the first sign of erythema, swelling, or pain. Finally, it is wise to review the medication profile daily. The triple IV antibiotic therapy initiated for a new fever may significantly add to the daily fluid load while decreasing the number of peripheral IV sites available.

11. What are the differences between PPN and peripheral protein-sparing therapy?
Peripheral protein-sparing therapy uses 3–5% amino acid solutions alone or in conjunction with hypocaloric amounts of dextrose or glycerol to provide 1–2 gm of protein per kg per day in

an attempt to minimize nitrogen losses. The rationale and indications for peripheral protein sparing therapy are different from those for PPN, and unlike PPN, no effort is made to deliver the anticipated caloric need with protein-sparing therapy. Although PPN solutions are designed to provide equivalent levels of protein, they also provide dextrose and lipids to deliver estimated daily energy requirements.

12. What is a 3-in-1 formulation?

A 3-in-1 formulation is a parenteral nutrition product that contains amino acids, dextrose, and lipid emulsions in the same container. Advantages of this type of solution include convenience, slower infusion rates of lipid emulsions, and cost savings related to use of fewer tubes and pumps. The 3-in-1 product is especially useful for PPN because the isotonic lipid emulsion significantly decreases the osmolality of the nutritional solution.

Disadvantages of 3-in-1 solutions include coloring that inhibits visual inspection of the parenteral nutrition solution for particulate matter or precipitates, more complicated admixture compatibility and stability issues, and the large molecule size of the lipids that precludes use of a 0.22 micron ("sterilizing") filter. Although 3-in-1 solutions are more likely to promote bacterial growth than traditional amino acid-dextrose combinations, they are less likely to support bacterial growth than lipid emulsions alone.

13. What treatment modalities have been used to prevent thrombophlebitis?

The development of thrombophlebitis is multifactorial. Precipitating factors include endothelial injury, inflammatory response, venoconstriction, and thrombus formation. Buffers such as sodium bicarbonate and sodium hydroxide have been added to PPN solutions to raise the pH to 7.2–7.4, in hope of preventing chemical injury to the vein. These have been successful. Other PPN additives that have been used successfully are heparin, which may minimize the formation of the fibrin clot at the tip of the catheter that leads to thrombus formation, and hydrocortisone, which may affect both the inflammatory response and the clotting cascade. Unfortunately, compatibility and stability issues of nutrition solutions are complex, and empirical dosing guidelines are not available. Consult a nutrition support team or IV pharmacist before initiating these therapies.

Some topical preventive therapies have been tried as well. Transdermal nitroglycerin patches applied near the IV site produce a local vasodilation. Topical nonsteroidal anti-inflammatory creams and gels not only may inhibit the local inflammatory response but also may help prevent platelet aggregation.

Medical practices that may be useful in preventing or reducing thrombophlebitis associated with PPN include follow-up by nutrition support teams, placement of fine-gauge catheters into large veins, use of in-line filters, and use of lipids and glycerol as calorie sources instead of glucose.

14. What is ProcalAmine?

ProcalAmine is a commercially prepared solution of 3% amino acids and 3% glycerol with electrolytes. It can be administered alone as a protein-sparing regimen, or lipid emulsions can be added to increase calorie delivery. One liter provides 30 gm of protein, 30 gm of glycerol, and 240 total calories. The solution has an osmolality of 735 mOsm/L, and the pH ranges from 6.5 to 7.0.

Nutrition Product Reference Table

COMPONENT	CALORIES PER LITER	MOSM PER LITER	GRAMS PER LITER
10% dextrose	340	504	100
20% dextrose	680	1008	200
5.5% amino acids	220	575	55
8.5% amino acids	340	890	85
10% lipids	1100	260	100
20% lipids	2000	260	200
Electrolytes	NA	235	NA

NA = not applicable.

15. Based on the information in the reference table, what is the osmolality of the final solution if a PPN solution is prepared using 1 liter each of 10% dextrose, 5.5% amino acids, and 10% lipids, with electrolytes (assume negligible volume)? How many calories does it provide? How much protein?

To calculate the osmolality, first add the osmolalities together (504 + 575 + 260 + 235 = 1574 mOsm). However, because osmolality is an expression of concentration, the total mOsm is divided by the total volume (1574/3 = 525 mOsm/L). **Total** calories delivered would be 1660 (340 + 220 + 1100), although 66% would be from fat (1100/1660 × 100). This formula delivers only 55 gm of protein.

16. You decide to begin peripheral parenteral nutrition in a 55-kg patient who is under mild stress. Your nutritional goals are 1 gm/kg (55) of protein, 30 calories/kg (1650) of total energy, and 2500 ml of water. Using the reference table in question 14, what orders should be written to meet these goals?

A reasonable prescription calls for 1 L of 10% dextrose (provides 340 calories, 504 mOsm/L), 1 L of 5.5% amino acids (provides 55 gm of protein, 220 calories, 575 mOsm/L), 500 ml of 20% fat emulsion (1000 calories, 130 mOsm/L), plus standard electrolytes, vitamins, and trace elements (235 mOsm/L). This prescription provides roughly 1560 calories of total energy, 55 gm of protein, and 2.5 L of water; the final osmolality is 579 mOsm/L.

BIBLIOGRAPHY

1. ASPEN Board of Directors: Guidelines for the use of parenteral and enteral nutrition in adult and pediatric patients. J Parenter Enter Nutr 17:1SA–52SA, 1993.
2. Evans NJ, Bamba M, Rombeau JL: Care of central venous catheters. In Rombeau JL, Caldwell MD (eds): Parenteral Nutrition, 2nd ed. Philadelphia, W. B. Saunders, 1993, pp 353–356.
3. Fairfull-Smith RJ, Freeman JB: Nutrition in Clinical Surgery, 2nd ed. Baltimore, Williams & Wilkins, 1985, pp 200–205.
4. McEvoy GK (ed): American Hospital Formulary Service Drug Information. Bethesda, MD, American Society of Health-System Pharmacists, 1997.
5. Payne-James JJ, Khawaja HT: First choice for total parenenal nutrition: The peripheral route. J Parenter Enter Nutr 17:468–478, 1993,
6. Van Way CW (ed): Handbook of Surgical Nutrition. Philadelphia, J.B. Lippincott, 1992.
7. Waxman K, Day AT, Stellin GP, et al: Safety and efficacy of glycerol and amino acids in combination with lipid emulsion for peripheral parental nutrition support. J Parenter Enter Nutr 16:374–378, 1992.

40. VENOUS ACCESS FOR NUTRITION

Ezra Steiger, MD, FACS, CNSP, and Susan Curtas, RN, MSN

1. What is the most appropriate vascular access for a fluid-restricted patient who is severely malnourished and requires parenteral nutrition support?

Fluid-restricted patients require markedly hypertonic solutions to meet their caloric requirements in as small a volume as possible. This requirement precludes the use of peripheral veins for the administration of a peripheral lipid system. Central venous access is required in such circumstances. Any technique that allows positioning of the catheter tip near the junction of the vena cava and right atrium, including a peripherally inserted central venous catheter (PICC), is appropriate.

2. How often should a central venous catheter used for parenteral nutrition be changed in the intensive care unit?

The routine changing of central lines to prevent infections has not been found to be of value. This includes both removal and reinsertion of another catheter and guidewire exchanges. The catheter should be changed only if there is a suspicion of possible catheter-related sepsis or if there is mechanical catheter malfunction. If there is strong suspicion of catheter sepsis, the old catheter should be removed and cultured and a new catheter placed on the other side. If catheter removal is planned to rule out catheter sepsis or for mechanical dysfunction, the catheter can be changed over a guidewire and the tip cultured. If the tip culture is positive, a new catheter should be placed on the opposite side

3. What preparation techniques should be used to place a central venous line at the bedside?

Maximum barrier techniques should be used, including hand washing, sterile gown, gloves, mask, and hair covering. The area being cannulated should be prepared with a 2% tincture of chlorhexidine, and sterile drapes should be used to isolate the area in a sterile fashion. Although not as well studied, these recommendations are probably applicable to the insertion of PICCs, especially when the catheter is to be used for parenteral nutrition.

4. What are the symptoms and signs of a central venous catheter-related axillary or subclavian vein thrombosis?

The patient notices pain and swelling in the arm, shoulder, or chest wall area on the ipsilateral catheter side. Other symptoms may include dilated, visible chest wall veins, axillary area tenderness, and a slight bluish discoloration of the same arm. A mild temperature elevation may also occur even in the absence of infection. There may be difficulty in infusing or withdrawing from the catheter if the thrombus extends beyond the tip of the catheter. The diagnosis is confirmed by axillary and subclavian venous ultrasound or by contrast venography.

5. What are the symptoms and signs of an infected central venous catheter?

Central venous catheters may become infected at the exit site or the hub, or the intravascular catheter segment may be the source. Fever is usually present and may be low grade or present as markedly elevated temperature spikes. In the patient who may already have an ongoing infection elsewhere, a change in the fever pattern may be indicative of a possible central line infection. The development of glucose intolerance may precede the onset of fever. Leukocytosis may be present in bacterial infections, whereas leukopenia may be indicative of a fungal infection. If the catheter exit site is infected, erythema, tenderness, and exudate may be present. This condition may also occur along the tract of a subcutaneously tunneled catheter, with or without purulent drainage. In PICC lines the erythema, swelling and tenderness can be along the peripheral vein through which the catheter was placed, with or without exit site drainage. A history of shaking chills and elevated temperature commensurate with or beginning shortly after the initiation of the infusion in the home parenteral nutrition patient is almost always indicative of a catheter infection.

6. How do you diagnose a central venous catheter infection?

A history is taken and physical exam is performed to rule out other obvious potential sources of infection. Blood, urine, and, if appropriate, exit site cultures are sent for analysis. Quantitative blood cultures are obtained through the central venous catheter and a peripheral vein. A greater colony count of the blood withdrawn via the catheter compared with the colony count of blood drawn through the peripheral vein is presumptive evidence of catheter infection. Endoluminal brush techniques to diagnose catheter infections are used with increasing frequency. Culturing the removed catheter tip has the disadvantage of requiring catheter removal to obtain a diagnosis. If there is doubt that a central line is the cause of the fever, it can be managed most safely by changing it over a guidewire and culturing its tip. If the tip is positive, the catheter should be removed and a new catheter inserted in another location.

7. How do you treat central venous access line infection?

Removal of the catheter and administration of appropriate antibiotics usually treat purulent exit site infections of noncuffed catheters. Exit site infections in cuffed-tunneled catheters can usually be treated with antibiotics and frequent dressing changes. Tunnel or cuff infections in tunneled catheters must be treated by removing the catheter and giving antibiotics. Intravascular catheter infections may be treated with antibiotics if it is due to *Staphylococcus epidermidis* or other susceptible non–slime-forming organisms. Removing the venous access device best treats fungal and other bacterial infections.

8. How can the incidence of catheter-related infections be minimized?

Quality assurance and continuing education are essential to reducing the rate of catheter infections. Review and evaluation of new materials and methods should take place routinely. Catheter insertion and care protocols should be evidence-based and incorporate the latest technology and recommendations. Educational programs for new employees and personnel in training should be available. Teams who specialize in the use and care of access devices have been shown to be both cost-effective and efficacious at reducing the incidence of catheter infections and complications. These principles may be difficult in the setting of a nursing shortage. However, infection risk increases when the nursing staff levels falls below a critical mass.

9. What is the most likely cause of chest pain associated with infusion of TPN solutions?

The pain is usually due to the catheter tip pushing up against the side wall of the superior vena cava. This problem most often occurs with left-sided catheters when the tip has not been directed inferiorly enough to be at the junction of the superior vena cava and right atrium. The catheter can become malpositioned over time due to positional changes that may be related to Valsalva efforts such as coughing, sneezing, or straining. A chest x-ray shows the catheter tip directed against the side wall of the superior vena cava instead of going directly downward toward the right atrium. If the catheter is not changed or repositioned, the tip may erode through the superior vena cava.

10. What is withdrawal occlusion? How do you treat it?

Withdrawal occlusion is the inability to aspirate fluid or blood from the catheter while still being able to infuse through it. It is thought to be due to a thrombus near the tip of the catheter that acts in a ball valve fashion to occlude the tip of the catheter when it is being aspirated. It is usually treated with tPA (Tissue Plasminogen Activator) placed in the catheter for 30–90 minutes and then aspirated. Longer dwell times might be needed to clear the thrombus from the catheter tip.

11. How do you restore flow through an occluded catheter?
The first attempt to restore catheter flow is made by trying to instill a dilute heparin-saline solution through the catheter with a moderate amount of pressure using a 1- to 3-ml syringe. If this strategy is unsuccessful, tissue plasmingen activator can be instilled and left to dwell for 30–90 minutes if the obstruction is thought to be due to clotted blood. A similar procedure can be done with 70% alcohol if the blockage is thought to be due to lipid material and with 0.1 N hydrogen chloride if the occlusion is thought to be due to crystalline material.

BIBLIOGRAPHY

1. Cobb DK, High KP, Sawyer RG, et al: A controlled trial of scheduled replacement of central venous and pulmonary-artery catheters. N Engl J Med 327:1062–1069, 1992.
2. Cook D, Randolph A, Kernerman P, et al: Central venous catheter replacement strategies: A systematic review of the literature. Crit Care Med 25:1417–1424, 1997.
3. Eyer S, Brummitt C, Crossley K, et al: Catheter-related sepsis: Prospective, randomized study of three methods of long-term catheter maintenance. Crit Care Med 18:1073–1079, 1990.
4. Fridkin SK, Pear SM, Williamson TH , et al: The role of understaffing in central venous catheter-associated bloodstream infections. Infect Control Hosp Epidemiol 17:150–158, 1996.
5. Grady NP, Alexander M, Dellinger EP, et al: Guidelines for the prevention of intravascular catheter-related infections. MMWR, August 9, 2002.
6. Kite P, Dobbins BM, Wilcox MH, et al: Evaluation of a novel endoluminal brush method for in situ diagnosis of catheter-related sepsis. J Clin Pathol 50:278–282, 1997.
7. Loughran SC, Borzatta M: Peripherally inserted central catheters: A report of 2506 catheter days. J Parent Enter Nutr 19:133–136, 1995.
8. Lowell JA, Bothe A: Venous access. Surg Clin North Am 71:1231–1246, 1991.
9. Mosca R, Curtas S, Forbes B, et al: The benefits of isolator cultures in the management of suspected catheter sepsis. Sugery 102:718–723, 1987.
10. Passaro M, Steiger E, Curtas S: Long term silastic catheters and chest pain. J Parent Enter Nutr 18:340–343, 1994.
11. Sheretz RJ, Ely EW, Westbrook DM, et al: Education of physicians-in-training can decrease the risk for vascular catheter infection. Ann Intern Med 132:641–648, 2000.

41. COMPLICATIONS OF TOTAL PARENTERAL NUTRITION

Pamela A. Orr, MSN, RN, FNP, Douglas M. Geehan, MD, and
L. Beaty Pemberton, MD

1. What are the types of complications of total parental nutrition (TPN)?
Complications can arise from four main categories, all of which should be monitored: adequacy of delivery, mechanical, metabolic, and infectious complications. Adequate delivery of nutrition includes complications due to excess or under feeding.

2. What is meant by mechanical complications?
Mechanical complications can occur during insertion and maintenance. The most common complication during insertion is a pneumothorax or hemothorax. Another is puncture of the subclavian artery or other major vessel. Injury to the brachial plexus, thoracic duct, and mediastinum can occur but is uncommon. An air embolism, clotted catheter, or venous thrombosis are commonly seen complications. Misplacement of the catheter can occur with the catheter tip in the heart or crossing the mediastinum into the opposite subclavian vein. Catheter breakage, with catheter embolus, is well known.

3. What are some of the ways to avoid mechanical complications of the central venous catheter?
One way to avoid complications of line misplacement and diagnose a pneumothorax or a hemo-thorax is to read a chest x-ray prior to running fluids through the line. Also, suturing the central venous catheter in place will stabilize the line to prevent slippage in or out of the superior vena cava. Utrasound guidance may minimize catheter placement time and allow fewer attempts to locate an appropriate vein.

4. Is one vein better than the others for infusing TPN?
The most commonly used central vein to cannulate for TPN infusion is the subclavian vein, because it can be stabilized on the chest wall and is the most comfortable for the patient. The internal jugular vein approach allows the use of ultrasound imaging for localization and has a lower incidence of pneumothorax or hemothorax than the subclavian approach, but catheter dressings and stability are more difficult to maintain with an internal jugular approach than the subclavian. Internal jugular placement may be more uncomfortable for the patient and can interfere with tracheotomy dressings. The femoral vein for long-term TPN is discouraged as well because of the increased risk of infection from not being able to maintain cleanliness of the area and increased danger of thromboembolism from pelvic vein thrombosis.

5. Should the central line be removed if the patient has a fever?
The central line is suspected as a source when a fever of unknown origin develops after the line has been placed. Line sepsis should be suspected if any fever occurs in the presence of a central line. Even worse, a line can become infected even if the infection starts elsewhere. An infected line may show no erythema or purulent drainage at the catheter site. A patient with an infected central venous catheter may show fever or increased white blood cell count.
If infection is confirmed, the line should be removed. The patient should be treated with antibiotics long enough to clear any bacteremia, and the line should be replaced in a different site. If an infection is only suspected, it is sometimes undesirable to remove the line. In this case, the

line should be changed over a wire and a catheter tip culture obtained. If the tip culture is positive, the new line should be completely removed.

6. How is central venous catheter bacteremia determined?

A central venous catheter that is infected can cause a bacteremia. To confirm a central venous catheter bactermia, a tip culture from the line is done at the same time blood cultures from a peripheral vein are obtained. If the infection is caused by the same organism on the tip and in the blood, then the central venous catheter is the probable cause.

7. What type of catheters are best for long-term TPN?

Nontunneled catheters can be used safely in the acute care setting, but for home TPN, tunneled catheters are better. Tunneled catheters provide better catheter stability and decrease the risk of infection. A peripherally inserted central catheter (PICC) can be used for TPN if placed in the superior vena cava. Many problems can occur with PICC lines, however. They are noted for migration, thrombophlebitis, and clotted catheters. Many patients have discomfort from holding their arm straight to keep the catheter from kinking and the infusion running.

8. How can infection risks be minimized?

Using strict aseptic technique can reduce the incidence of infections. Frequent hand washing is the single most important prevention against infection, though this is forgotten by many health care personnel. Using sterile technique and luminar flow hood to mix the TPN solution also lowers the infection rate. When inserting and accessing the central line, sterility must be maintained. Opening into the hubs and using the ports of the TPN line for drawing blood or giving drugs should be kept to a minimum.

9. What metabolic complications might you expect to see in the acute patient just starting TPN?

Short-term Metabolic Complications	Long-term Metabolic Complications
Electrolytes imbalance	Hepatic dysfunction
Glucose intolerance	Elevated triglycerides
Respiratory failure	Essential fatty acid deficiency

10. How should patients receiving TPN be managed and monitored in order to avoid these metabolic complications?

Glucose. Many factors may influence glucose, including increased stress levels, malnutrition, septicemia, diabetes, and drugs, but controlling the blood sugar is still the primary objective. Slowly advancing the rate (25 ml/hr) of the TPN solution with hypertonic glucose will allow progressive pancreatic adaptation to the dextrose load. Capillary blood glucose should be monitored every 4–6 hours. Starting an insulin drip or decreasing the infusing dextrose load may be necessary to control blood sugars. Keep the blood sugar in the range of 100–150 mg/dl but, in all cases less than 200 mg/dl. Some authors advocate even tighter control with target blood sugar values in the range of 80–110 mg/dl. If blood sugars cannot be controlled, the TPN solution should not be advanced.

Electrolytes. Upon starting TPN, electrolyte levels should be obtained daily and corrected. Once the TPN solution is at the maximum rate, monitoring the electrolytes depends on the condition of the patient. If the patient is critical, electrolytes should be monitored daily; if stable, then twice weekly or even just weekly. Correction of electrolytes in the TPN solution should be approached with caution. Any changes made in the TPN solution must be good for 24 hours before changing the TPN solution again. In most cases, it is best to leave the electrolytes in TPN unmodified and correct electrolyte or fluid abnormalities with separate intravenous fluids. Of course, this depends on the particular problem.

Respiratory Failure. Respiratory failure occurs in malnourished patients who are overfed glucose calories. Excess glucose produces fat. This in turn produces excess carbon dioxide production, which increases the work required to eliminate carbon dioxide. To prevent this syndrome, especially in the respiratory-compromised patient, avoid overfeeding and give 30% of the caloric requirements as fat. In all cases, give no more than 5–7 mg/kg/min of glucose.

Hepatic Function. Hepatic dysfunction should be considered with moderate increases in alkaline phosphatase and amino transferase. Liver enzymes should be monitored at least weekly. If an elevation occurs, cholecystitis should be suspected, and the TPN rate should be decreased or readjusted.

Triglycerides. Triglyceride levels should be monitored at least weekly if lipids are infused. If levels over 400 mg/dl occur, lipids should be cut back or preferably discontinued.

Essential Fatty Acid Deficiency. Because the body cannot produce essential fats, this complication results from inadequate fat intake. Even if most of the calories are from glucose, enough lipids should be given to provide 6–8% of calories.

11. What is the refeeding syndrome and how is it treated?

With initiation of TPN, a rapid shift of water, electrolytes, vitamins, and glucose moves into the cells. In a patient who is depleted to begin with, this can cause deficits in the extracellular fluid. This is known as refeeding syndrome. The major symptoms include glucose intolerance, lethargy, confusion, weakness, and coma. A high level of dextrose solutions given to malnourished patients may shift excess fluid to dependent parts of the body. Potassium, phosphorus, and magnesium shift into the intracellular fluid, lowering serum levels. Characteristically, refeeding syndrome is observed in the first 24–48 hours of TPN. In the depleted patient, initiation of TPN should begin at 25 cc/hr and should be advanced gradually to full nutritional needs over 48–72 hours, while serum electrolytes, glucose, blood urea nitrogen (BUN), and creatinine are monitored and symptoms are examined.

12. Can hyperglycemia be prevented?

The pancreas produces an increased level of insulin with the dextrose infusion, but there is a time lag and a limit to the amount of insulin produced. TPN solutions should be started relatively slowly and increased over 48–72 hours to full rate. The initial infusion rate should be no more than 25–50 ml/hr and perhaps lower if the patient has a previous history of glucose intolerance. The initial rate should be maintained for 12–24 hours and then increased slowly to the final rate. Blood sugars should be monitored with accuchecks every 4–6 hours. The blood sugar should be maintained below 200 mg/dl, preferably in the range of 120–180 mg/dl. The addition of 20–30 units/L of insulin will often prevent hyperglycemia, but if it is necessary to give more than that, it should be given as a separate insulin drip infusion. After the glucose level is stable, more insulin can be added to the TPN solution.

The increasing trend toward moderate fat TPN is encouraging in this regard. If 30–40% of calories are given as fat and another 20% as protein, then the amount of glucose necessary to meet the patient's needs is greatly reduced. To formulate a solution containing 1 calorie per milliliter, it is only necessary to use 15% glucose.

13. Is it appropriate to add insulin to TPN solutions?

Yes, it is useful to add insulin to the TPN solution to control the blood sugar. Insulin is fully compatible with TPN solutions. Some of the insulin will be absorbed by the glass or plastic bottle, the tubing, and the filter, but the dose can be adjusted to compensate. However, if the amount of insulin required by the patient is greater than 50 units per liter or so, using insulin in the TPN may not be safe. The patient with insulin resistance or a high insulin requirement for other reasons should be managed with an insulin drip separate from the TPN solution (see question 12).

14. What is rebound hypoglycemia and is it preventable?

This syndrome results from the acute discontinuation of the TPN solution. This typically happens when patients are sent for tests and the TPN solution runs out or when the central venous line is abruptly lost. Either way, the infusion is discontinued abruptly. Whether or not insulin is contained in the TPN, the patient will be left with an elevated insulin concentration. With the discontinuation of the solution, the dextrose level drops, but the serum level of insulin remains elevated. This can be prevented by giving 10% dextrose by a peripheral vein for several hours after the TPN has been discontinued.

15. What complications might occur from not treating hyperglycemia?

Hyperglycemia leads to osmotic diuresis. If the tubular maximum of glucose is exceeded, the glucose passes out through the distal tubules, carrying water with it. The excretion of free water may cause the development of hyperglycemic, hyperosomotic, nonketotic dehydration, which may lead to coma and even death. This sequence of events may occur within 48 hours and sometimes within 24 hours.

Another problem may result from poor use of carbohydrates, if they are given in excess. Carbohydrates are converted to energy and fat, and carbon dioxide is released in the process. This increases the work of breathing and may be a factor in failure to wean a patient from the ventilator.

16. What are the main electrolytes used in TPN? Are there maximum concentrations?

Sodium, potassium, acetate, and chloride are compatible in all TPN solutions. Calcium and phosphorus as additives may precipitate depending on the solution's pH, type of calcium salt (calcium chloride should not be used), temperature, and type and amount of amino acid product. Usually the addition of magnesium is given as magnesium sulfate; thus the calcium should not be given as a chloride salt, because calcium sulfate precipitates rather quickly.

	STANDARD CONCENTRATIONS	MAXIMUM CONCENTRATIONS
Sodium (Na)	35–50 mEg/L	
Potassium (K)	30–40 mEg/L	
Chloride (Cl)	35–50 mEg/L	
Acetate	140–160 mEg/L	
Calcium (Ca)	5 mEg/L	15 mEg/L
Magnesium (Mg)	5–10 mEg/L	20 mEg/L
Phosphorus (Phos)	12–15 mm/L	20 mEg/L

17. What are the common additives for electrolyte salt forms for TPN solutions?

Sodium: Sodium chloride, sodium acetate, sodium phosphate, sodium lactate
Potassium: Potassium chloride, potassium acetate, potassium phosphate
Calcium: Calcium chloride, calcium gluconate
Magnesium: Magnesium sulfate
Sodium bicarbonate should not be used as an additive because of the reactions of the bicarbonate with other ions. Instead, sodium or potassium acetate or sodium lactate can be used as a substitute for sodium bicarbonate.

18. Can metabolic acidosis be attributed to the TPN solution?

Acidosis can result from TPN solutions in two ways. Metabolic acidosis can be caused by the amino acid solution, which has an increased number of cationic amino acids that in turn produce free hydrogen ions. This type of metabolic acidosis generally occurs with renal or pulmonary compromised patients. Using a mixture of increased anionic amino acids compared with cationic amino acids will reduce the risk of this type of metabolic acidosis.

The second type of metabolic acidosis can be attributed to excessive chloride infusion. Excessive chloride infusion increases the glomerular filtration of chloride ions, which are reabsorbed with sodium in the renal tubules. This can product a hyperchloremic acidosis.

BIBLIOGRAPHY

1. A.S.P.E.N. Board of Directors: Guidelines for the use of parenteral and enteral nutrition in adult and pediatric patients. JPEN 17:1SA–52SA, 1993.
2. Civetta JM, Taylor RW, Korby RR: Critical Care, 2nd ed. Philadelphia, J. B. Lippincott, 1992.
3. Grant JP: Handbook of Total Parenteral Nutrition, 2nd ed. Philadelphia, W. B. Saunders, 1992.
4. Rombeau JL, Caldwell MD: Clinical Nutrition Parenteral Nutrition, 2nd ed. Philadelphia, W. B. Saunders, 1993.
5. Ross VM, Orr PA: Prevention of infections related to central venous catheters. Crit Care Nurse Q 20:79–88, 1997.
6. Schroper WB: Ultrasound-guided control venous access. Nutr Clin Pract 16:280–283, 2001.
7. Van den Berghe G, Wouters P, Weskers F, et al: Intensive insulin therapy in the critically ill patient. N Engl J Med 345:1359–1367, 2001.

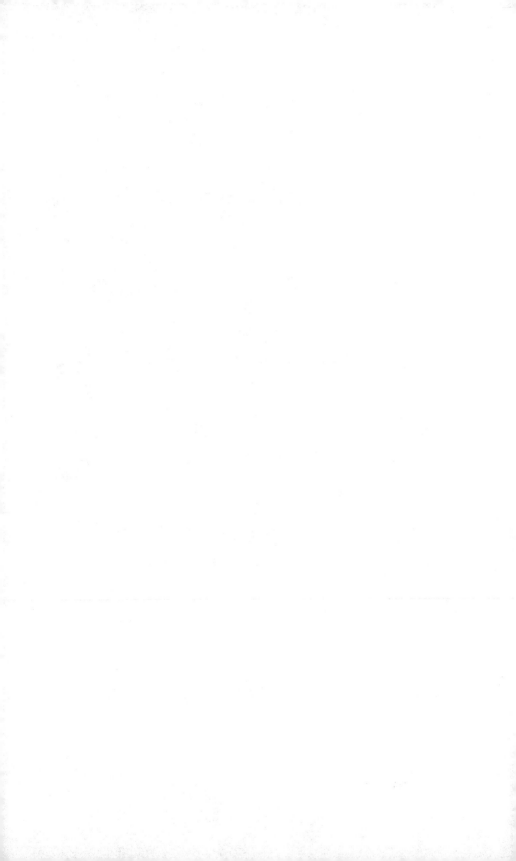

42. DRUG–NUTRIENT INTERACTIONS

David S. Seres, MD, CNSP, Cynthia L. Lieu, PharmD, BCNSP,
and Danielle L. Petrocelli, BS, PharmD

1. What are the possible interactions between food and drugs?

Foods and specific nutrients can affect the dissolution, absorption, pharmacodynamics, metabolism, and excretion of drugs. Similarly, drugs can alter the same processes as they relate to nutrients. Often this effect is the mechanism of action for a particular drug, such as the effect of the antineoplastic methotrexate, which blocks the metabolism of folate. In such cases, we do not refer to the action as a drug–nutrient effect per se. Although such "desirable" effects are not discussed in this chapter, they should be considered a part of the subject.

2. Has the definition of food changed recently?

Because the Food and Drug Administration now classifies "supplements" as foods, a number of substances with pharmacologic activities, including herbs, herbal extracts, and purified substances, must now be considered along with the items usually defined as foods. The importance of this distinction, or lack thereof, is evident when studies show that up to 50% of surgical patients take supplements of one kind or another. Of patients taking herbs or other supplements in one preoperative study, 27% were taking substances that inhibit coagulation, 12% were taking substances that affect blood pressure, 9% were taking substances that cause sedation, 5% were taking substances that have cardiac effects, and 4% were taking substances that alter electrolytes.

3. How does food affect the absorption of drugs?

Different components of food can affect gastric pH and emptying time, the secretion of fluids and enzymes, gastrointestinal motility, mesenteric and hepatic portal blood flow, and bile flow rate. Such changes can alter the rate of absorption, the extent of absorption, or both.

4. What are the major components of a diet that can affect drug absorption?

Fat and protein are the dietary components most likely to affect intestinal absorption of medications. The list of affected medications is quite lengthy. Because of our increased awareness of this problem, most pharmacies have reference materials describing this particular set of interactions. Patients should be cautioned to check with their pharmacist on the timing of meals and medication ingestion.

5. What other components of a diet can affect drug absorption?

In addition to fat and protein, pH, electrolyte content, and fiber can affect drug as well as mineral absorption. For instance, calcium and iron are best absorbed in an acidic environment.

6. What components of a diet can affect the metabolism or excretion of drugs?

The list of components in the diet that can affect drug metabolism is long and includes substances that can alter the rate of metabolism and/or the rate of urinary excretion of various medications. One example of this type of interaction is the induction of oxidative metabolism of drugs such as theophylline by charcoal-broiled foods. Flavonoids in citrus fruits, fatty acids content, protein and specific amino acid content, herbs, spices, vitamins, and minerals are just some of the other nutrients that can exert an effect on drug metabolism. High doses of vitamin C may reduce the renal clearance of acidic drugs such as acetylsalicylic acid and barbituric acid. Due to the huge numbers of these interactions, a specific list of the more important ones is included in Table 1.

Table 1. Food–Nutrient Interactions with Drugs

MEDICATION(S)	DIET, MEAL, NUTRIENT, OR CONDITION	POTENTIAL INTERACTION
Alendronate, risedronate	Food, beverages (including sparkling or mineral water, coffee, tea, juice) medications, antacids, vitamins	Significant reduction of absorption of medication, high risk of treatment failure. Medication should be swallowed with at least 6–8 oz of plain water only before first meal of the day, and no food or other fluids should be consumed for at least 30 minutes to 1 hour after taking medication.
Didanosine, indinavir, zalcitabine, isoniazid, rifampin, captopril, peridopril, ampicillin, erythromycin (stearate and enteric-coated formulations), melphalan	Food	Reduced absorption and bioavailability of medication; risk of treatment failure. Medication should be taken on an empty stomach.
Lovastatin, macrodantin, nelfinavir, ritonavir, saquinivir, ganciclovir, clofazimine	Food	Increased absorption and bioavailability of medication (desired). Medication should be taken with food.
Itraconazole	Food	Capsules: increased bioavailability, improved clinical response. Liquid/solution: should be taken on an empty stomach.
	Achlorhydria	Reduced absorption of itraconazole. Counteract by coadministration of acidic beverage, such as cola, to increase bioavailability.
Misoprostol, quinidine sulfate	Food	Reduced absorption rate and peak plasma concentration of medication without affecting bioavailability. Medication should be taken with food or after a meal to decrease incidence of adverse effects while maintaining desired drug effect.
Penicillamine	Food, milk, multivalent cations (e.g., calcium, magnesium, iron, zinc)	Reduced bioavailability of penicillamine. Take on empty stomach.
Azithromycin	Food	Capsules and suspension: reduced bioavailability of azithromycin. Take on empty stomach. Tablet bioavailability not affected by food intake.
Nifedipine	Food	Capsules or tablets: reduced peak plasma concentration of nifedipine without affecting bioavailability, with reduced risk of adverse effects. Sustained-release preparations: increased bioavailability; increased hypotensive effect. Modified-release: Adalat CC should be taken on an empty stomach.

(*Table continued on next page.*)

Table 1.   Food–Nutrient Interactions with Drugs (Continued)

MEDICATION(S)	DIET, MEAL, NUTRIENT, OR CONDITION	POTENTIAL INTERACTION
Isotretinoin	Food	Increased bioavailability of isotretinoin when taken with or shortly after a meal. Take with a consistent relationship to meals, titrate dosage to desired drug effect and adverse effects.
Griseofulvin	Food	Increased bioavailability of griseofulvin with fat-containing meal, higher with high-fat vs. low-fat meal; not increased when taken with carbohydrates or protein; risk of treatment failure when taken in fasted state.
Cyclosporine, tacrolimus, sirolimus, carbamazepine	Food	Fluctuations in concentration, interindividual variation. Take with consistent relationship to meals to avoid adverse fluctuations in concentrations.
Ketoconazole	High fat meal	Increased bioavailability of ketoconazole.
	High carbohydrate meal	Decreased bioavailability of ketoconazole.
Atrovaquone	Fat containing meal	Increased bioavailability of atrovaquone. Treatment more consistently achieved when administered with food or nutrition supplement with moderate fat content.
Theophylline	Food	Absorption variable, depending on product and formulation. Check manufacturers' recommendations for specific products.
Sustained-release theophylline	High fat meal	Sudden release of theophylline ("dose dumping") → increased theophylline level, possible toxicity.
Theophyllline	High-protein/low carbohydrate diet	Increased hepatic clearance of theophylline, lower blood levels of theophylline.
Tetracyclines, fluoroquinolones (e.g., norfloxacin, ciprofloxacin, enoxacin, gatifloxacin, levofloxacin)	Multivalent cations (e.g., calcium, magnesium, iron, zinc, aluminum) in milk, dairy products, antacids, multivitamin/mineral products, supplements, sucralfate, enteral nutrition supplements and tube feedings	Reduced absorption and bioavailability of medication due to chelation. Avoid coadministration, take 1 hour before meal/supplement or 2 hours after meal/supplement.
Digoxin	Bran fiber, pectin-containing foods (apples, pears), fiber supplements	Decreased digoxin absorption and bioavailability due to binding by fibers; may require dosage adjustment; risk of treatment failure.
Lovastatin	Fiber	Decreased lovastatin absorption; risk of treatment failure.
Levodopa	High fiber diet	Increased bioavailability of levodopa.

(Table continued on next page.)

Table 1.   Food–Nutrient Interactions with Drugs (Continued)

MEDICATION(S)	DIET, MEAL, NUTRIENT, OR CONDITION	POTENTIAL INTERACTION
Levodopa *(cont.)*	High protein diet (2 gm/kg/d)	Reduced effect of levodopa, altered drug distribution, competitive inhibition for carrier across blood brain barrier.
	Pyridoxine (vitamin B6)	Reduced effectiveness of levodopa.
MAO inhibitors (phenelzine, tranylcy-promine, procarbazine)	Tyramine containing foods: Aged cheese, sour cream, yogurt; aged, dried, fermented, salted, smoked and pickled meats and fish; beer, ale, champagne, wine, sherry, liqueurs; avocados, bananas, figs, raisins, over-ripe fruits, papaya products (including meat tenderizers), beans (fava, soy and soy products), spinach, tomatoes, protein extracts, yeast (and extracts), caffeine containing foods (coffee, tea, cola, chocolate)	See question 12 for range of reactions.
Lithium	Sodium or salt	High sodium intake: increased lithium excretion, decreased serum lithium level. Low sodium intake: decreased lithium excretion, increased serum lithium level, risk of lithium toxicity.
Warfarin	Vitamin K containing foods	Decreased effectiveness. See question 9.
CNS depressants, antihista-mines, antidepressants, antipsychotics, muscle relaxants, narcotics, metaclopramide	Alcohol	Increased sedation; may cause respira-tory depression.
Metronidazole, procarba-zine, griseofulvin, cefamandole, cefotetan, cefmetazole, cefoperazone, chlorpropamide	Alcohol	Disulfiram (Antabuse)-like reactions; may be life-threatening.
Phenytoin	Enteral nutrition supplements or tube feedings	Reduced phenytoin bioavailability, high risk of treatment failure. Possible toxicity when feeding is discontinued without phenytoin dosage adjustment.
Theophylline	Methylxanthines, especially caffeine	Increased theophylline level and half-life; increased risk of theophylline side effects.
Cyclosporine	d-alpha-tocopheryl-polyethy-lene-glycol-1000 succinate (TPGS), a water-soluble form of vitamin E	Increased cyclosporine absorption.

(Table continued on next page.)

Table 1. Food–Nutrient Interactions with Drugs (Continued)

MEDICATION(S)	DIET, MEAL, NUTRIENT, OR CONDITION	POTENTIAL INTERACTION
Levothyroxine	Calcium carbonate	Decreased levothyroxine absorption with concomitant administration of levothyroxine and calcium carbonate. May result in hypothyroidism. Can be minimized by spacing administration times.
Thiazide diuretics	Sodium, chloride, potassium, magnesium, calcium	Increased excretion of sodium, chloride, potassium and magnesium; decreased calcium excretion.
Loop diuretics	Potassium, magnesium, and calcium	Increased excretion of potassium, magnesium, and calcium.
Potassium-sparing diuretics, ACE inhibitors	High intake of potassium-rich foods (e.g., banana, spinach); excessive use of potassium-containing salt substitutes	Hyperkalemia, cardiac arrhythmias.
Cisplatin	Magnesium	Increased excretion of magnesium.
Amphotericin B	Potassium, magnesium	Increased excretion of potassium and magnesium.
Cholestyramine, colestipol, mineral oil laxatives, orlistat	Fat soluble vitamins	Reduced absorption, increased excretion of fat soluble vitamins → possible fat soluble vitamin deficiency.
Phenytoin	Folic acid	Decreased folate level, possible folate deficiency; folic acid supplementation may change the pharmacokinetics of phenytoin, decrease serum phenytoin levels, with possible seizure breakthrough.
Isoniazid	Pyridoxine (vitamin B6)	Vitamin B-6 deficiency.
Acetylsalicylic acid, barbituric acid, acidic drugs	High doses of vitamin C	Reduced renal clearance of acidic drugs.
Cyclosporine	Potassium, magnesium	Hyperkalemia, hypomagnesemia.
Valproic acid	Carnitine	Decreased carnitine level, carnitine deficiency, encephalopathy, death; reversal of symptoms with carnitine supplementation.
HMG-CoA reductase inhibitors	Coenzyme Q10 (ubiquinone)	Decreased level of coenzyme Q10.

7. Can drugs cause fat malabsorption?

Bile acid sequestrants and some laxatives may induce fat malabsorption. Orlistat (Xenical), which is marketed for weight loss, exerts its effect by inducing fat malabsorption. Malabsorption of fat may induce diarrhea and deficiencies of vitamins A, D, E, and K and beta carotene.

8. Can foods and drugs cause osteoporosis?

Medications that increase the risk of osteoporosis by a variety of mechanisms include aluminum-containing antacids, glucocorticoids, excessive thyroid replacement, long-term heparin therapy, chronic lithium therapy, chemotherapy, anticonvulsants, tetracycline, furosemide, cyclosporine, and gonadotropin-releasing hormone agonists.

While technically a nutrient–nutrient interaction, it is important to note that chronic ingestion of carbonated beverages, particularly diet cola, has been implicated in the genesis of premature osteoporosis in young women. Diets that increase renal excretion of acids have been
shown to increase urinary calcium excretion. Diets that are high in sodium, protein, phosphates,
vitamin A, caffeine, and alcohol and low in calcium and vitamin D are also considered risk factors for osteoporosis.

9. Does warfarin interact with components of the diet?

Warfarin works by blocking the synthesis of vitamin K-dependent clotting factors. High
amounts of vitamin K overwhelm the effects of warfarin and cause blood thinning to be ineffective at previously effective doses. Patients must be counseled to eat a normal well-balanced diet
while maintaining a *consistent* amount of vitamin K in the diet. Drastic dietary changes may alter
the amount of warfarin needed for proper anticoagulation therapy. The daily requirement for vitamin K is about 1 μg/kg of body weight. Patients who regularly consume foods high in vitamin K
may require a larger dose of warfarin than expected to achieve adequate anticoagulation.

Partial List of Foods High in Vitamin K

Mayonnaise	Kale leafs
Canola, salad, and soybean oil	Lettuce
Broccoli	Mustard greens
Brussels sprouts	Parsley
Cabbage	Spinach leafs
Collard greens	Turnip greens
Endive	Watercress
Green scallions	Liver
Coriander	Enteral supplements (e.g., Ensure, Osmolite)

In addition, seaweed and sushi containing seaweed can interact with warfarin and decrease
the international normalized ratio (INR). For a more complete listing, see referenced websites.

10. Many medications are used to delay clotting, including anticoagulant medications (e.g., warfarin, heparin) and antiplatelet medications (e.g., dipyridamole, ticlopidine, clopidogrel, and aspirin). Are there any herbs or vitamins that may interact with these medications?

Many herbs and vitamins have effects on blood clotting and may increase bleeding risk and
prolong measurements of clotting function, such as prothrombin time and INR. Examples include
chamomile, danshen, dong quai, fenugreek, feverfew, fish oil, garlic, ginger, ginkgo, papaya extract (papain), St. John's wort, tumeric (curcumin), and vitamin E. Some herbs, such as coenzyme
Q10 (ubiquinone), ginseng, and green tea, may decrease the effectiveness of anticoagulants.

11. Can grapefruit juice and other citrus fruits cause changes in drug metabolism?

Several constituents of grapefruit inhibit the metabolism and increase the bioavailability of a
long list of medications by blocking both the cytochrome P450 3A4 (CYP3A4) isoenzyme and
P-glycoprotein. The importance and prevalence of the interactions between dietary substances
and various isoenzymes of cytochrome P450 and P-glycoprotein are becoming better understood.
It is expected that many more drug–drug, drug–herb, and drug–nutrient interactions involving
these enzymes will be described.

Many substances in citrus, including flavonoids (naringin and naringenin) and fumaro-
coumarins (bergapten and 6',7'-dihydroxybergamottin) may be active in these respects. Cytochrome P-450 3A4 is present in both the intestinal wall and the liver and is responsible for the
metabolism of many medications; however, it appears that only CYP3A4 associated with the gut
is affected by the components in grapefruit. Intestinal P-glycoprotein pumps these drugs out of

the cell and back into the intestine. Blocking these enzymes, therefore, increases the absorption of the medications from the gut and decreases their breakdown in the liver. The end result is an increase in blood levels of these medications and an increased risk of toxicity. The risk of toxicity resulting from this interaction can be quite severe. Death has been reported in a patient due to terfenadine toxicity as a result of grapefruit juice consumption concomitantly with terfenadine.

The content of the above substances varies among different grapefruit juice batches, making it impossible to determine if one is safer than another. Recent studies have shown that as little as 5 ounces of grapefruit juice or eating one grapefruit is enough to cause a drug interaction. The effects can last up to 3–7 days after the last glass of grapefruit juice.

Grapefruit is not the only fruit that inhibits the cytochrome P-450 3A4 system. New evidence suggests that seville oranges, tangelos, and limes have similar effects. Marmalades made from grapefruit peel may also have the potential to cause a drug interaction. Alternative therapy should be given if the patient is unwilling to give up grapefruit, grapefruit juice, or the other implicated fruits.

Partial Listing of Potential Drug Interactions with Grapefruit

Benzodiazepines (diazepam, midazolam, triazolam)

Caffeine

Calcium channel blockers (amlodipine, felodipine, nifedipine, nimodipine, nisoldipine, nitrendipine, pranidipine, but no interactions with diltiazem or verapamil)

Amiodarone

Cisapride

Carbamazepine

Clomipramine

Immunosuppressants (cyclosporine, tacrolimus, sirolimus)

HMG-CoA reductase inhibitors/statins (atorvastatin, cerivastatin, lovastatin, simvastatin)

Methylprednisolone

Itraconzaole

Saquinavir

Buspirone

Sertraline

Methadone

Sildenafil

Ethinyl estradiol

Terfenadine

Dextromethorphan

Extended-release tablets

12. Why do people taking antidepressants of the monoamine oxidase inhibitor (MAOI) class need to be so careful with their diet?

Tyramine, an amino acid with potent vasopressor activity, is found in various foods. Tyramine contained in foods is normally metabolized by the enzyme monoamine oxidase (MAO) found in the gut and the liver. By inhibiting the activity of monamine oxidase, MAOIs inhibit the breakdown of tyramine. Ingestion of as little as 6 mg of tyramine may produce a significant reaction, regardless of the dose or duration of therapy of the MAOI. The reactions may be mild, with slight elevations in blood pressure and flushing, or lead to a severe hypertensive crisis. A hypertensive crisis may be characterized by some or all of the following symptoms: occipital headache that may radiate frontally, palpitations, neck stiffness or soreness, nausea, vomiting, sweating (sometimes with fever and sometimes with cold, clammy skin), dilated pupils, and pho-tophobia. Either tachycardia or bradycardia may be present and can be associated with constrict-ing chest pain.

Patients treated with MAOIs should avoid high-protein foods that have undergone protein breakdown by aging, fermentation, pickling, smoking, or bacterial contamination. Patients should avoid cheeses (especially aged varieties), pickled herring, beer or wine (including nonal-coholic varieties), liver, yeast extract (including brewer's yeast in large quantities), dry sausage (including Genoa salami, hard salami, pepperoni, and Lebanon bologna), pods of broad beans (fava and soy beans), meat extracts, and yogurt. Excessive amounts of caffeine and chocolate may also cause hypertensive reactions.

Patients need to avoid tyramine-containing foods for several days before starting therapy and for two weeks after therapy is discontinued. A period of 2 weeks is required to restore normal amine metabolism after withdrawal of MAOIs, presumably because of the time necessary for the resynthesis of monoamine oxidase.

13. What special considerations must be taken into account when medications are adminis-tered with enteral tube feeding?

1. Drugs administered through feeding tubes can cause tubes to clog.

2. The amount of time that the enteral feeding needs to be turned off and the volume of fluid required for flushing to administer certain medications must be factored into the feeding plan.

3. Long-acting medications, for the most part, cannot be broken into small components or dissolved without destroying the matrix that is responsible for the desired slowing of absorption. As a result, the entire dose is absorbed at the time of administration as opposed to slowly over the period of time indicated. Therefore, enteric-coated, sustained-release, or controlled-release med-ication formulations should not be crushed and administered through feeding tubes.

4. Certain medications should not be given while enteral feedings are being administered. Carbamazepine, phenytoin, ciprofloxacin, norfloxacin, hydralazine, sucralfate, warfarin, lev-odopa, and levothyroxine are the most common examples of medications that are significantly less well absorbed when given with feeds; feeds should be held before and after administration of these medications. (It should be noted that when administered with tube feedings, ofloxacin is less bioavailable than when administered with water, but it is significantly more bioavailable than ciprofloxacin when either is administered with enteral feedings.)

5. Medications in liquid form are easier to administer through a feeding tube since they do not have to be crushed. However, these medications are commonly flavored with sorbitol, a non-absorbed sugar that is a common cause of osmotic diarrhea in tube-fed patients.

14. What herbs may have interactions with medications for glucose control?

A number of herbs and supplements are known to have the potential to reduce blood glu-cose and thereby reduce the need for insulin and increase the risk for hypoglycemia. Examples include aloe, bilberry, chromium, cinnamon, coenzyme Q10, fenugreek, garlic, ginger, gin-seng, and karela or bitter melon (*Momordica charantia*). Glucosamine may increase insulin re-sistance and raise blood glucose. Since insulin secretion is chromium-dependent, a chromium deficient patient receiving chromium supplementation has a reduced requirement of supple-mental insulin.

15. Can herbs interact with cardiovascular medications?

Glycyrrhizic acid in true licorice may cause high blood pressure, hypokalemia, and edema. The hypokalemia may predispose patients to arrhythmias and digoxin toxicity if severe enough. However, most licorice found on the market these days is artificially flavored or flavored with anise.

Ma huang (ephedra) emulates epinephrine. It increases blood pressure, causes palpitations, and may induce arrhythmias. It has recently come under scrutiny as the possible cause of a sig-nificant number of fatalities.

16. Is it true that St. John's wort is safe?

St. John's wort (*Hypericum perforatum*), due to its popularity and the large number of drugs with which it may interact, is one of the herbs causing the most concern with regard to safety. Coadministration of St. John's wort significantly reduces the concentration of cyclosporine and tacrolimus. In some cases, this effect has resulted in acute rejection of a transplanted heart, liver, kidney, or pancreas. The effectiveness of oral contraceptives may also be compromised, leading to unintended pregnancy. Furthermore, St. John's wort may prolong the effects of anesthesia and reduce the therapeutic efficacy of multiple drugs. St John's wort exerts some serotonin re-uptake inhibition, which, when combined with an MAOI, may result in serotonin syndrome. Constituents of St. John's wort have demonstrated mild monoamine oxidase inhibitory effects. There is one case report of a hypertensive crisis after a patient consumed aged cheeses and red wine.

17. Why does St. John's wort interact with so many medications?

St. John's wort is found in herbal products used for the treatment of depression, anxiety, sleep disorders, and menstrual disorders. St. John's wort appears to induce CYP3A4 activity in the intestine and liver and intestinal P-glycoprotein expression. When taken with certain medications, St. John's wort has the potential to impair absorption and increase metabolism of the medication, reducing the serum drug concentration and leading to suboptimal therapeutic effect. A partial listing of the medications that may be affected can be found in Table 2.

Table 2. Herbal Interactions with Drugs

HERBAL OR OTHER SUPPLEMENT	MEDICATION(S)	POTENTIAL EFFECT(S) OF INTERACTION
Brewer's yeast	MAO inhibitors	Hypertensive crisis
Chamomile	Warfarin	Increase bleeding, increase bruising
Chromium	Anti-diabetic agents	Decrease blood glucose, decrease need for insulin, decrease required dosage of antidiabetic agent, hypoglycemia
Cinnamon	Antidiabetic agents	Decrease blood glucose, decrease need for insulin, decrease required dosage of antidiabetic agent, hypoglycemia
Danshen (*Salvia miltiorrhiza*)	Digoxin	May result in falsely elevated or lowered serum digoxin concentrations depending on method of measurement; can be eliminated by monitoring free digoxin concentration
	Warfarin	Increase INR; increase bleeding, increase bruising
Dong quai (*Angelica sinesis*)	Warfarin	Increase INR; increase bleeding, increase bruising
Echinacea	Hepatotoxic medications: anabolic steroids, amiodarone, methotrexate, ketoconazole, anesthetics	Theoretical increase in risk for hepato-toxicity; no cases reported
Fenugreek (*Trigonella foenum graecum*)	Anticoagulants, antiplatelet agents, NSAIDs	Increase INR; increase bleeding, increase bruising
Fenugreek	Antidiabetic agents	Decrease blood glucose, decrease need for insulin, decrease required dosage of antidiabetic agent, hypoglycemia
Feverfew	Anticoagulants, antiplatelet agents, NSAIDs, warfarin	Increase bleeding

(Table continued on next page.)

Table 2.   Herbal Interactions with Drugs (Continued)

HERBAL OR OTHER SUPPLEMENT	MEDICATION(S)	POTENTIAL EFFECT(S) OF INTERACTION
Garlic (*Allium sativum*)	Saquinavir	May reduce squinavir concentration
	Antidiabetic medications	May increase serum insulin levels → decrease blood glucose, decrease need for insulin, decrease required dosage of antidiabetic agent, hypoglycemia
	Anticoagulants, antiplatelet agents, NSAIDs	Increase INR; increase bleeding, increase bruising
Gamma linolenic acid (GLA): found in borage oil, evening primrose oil	Anticonvulsants	Decrease seizure threshold
Ginger	Anticoagulants, antiplatelet agents, NSAIDs	Increase bleeding, increase bruising
Ginkgo biloba	Thiazide diuretic	Hypertension
	Anticonvulsants	Precipitate seizures; increase anticonvulsant dosage requirement
	Anticoagulants, antiplatelet agents, NSAIDs	Increase INR, PT; increase bleeding, increase bruising
Ginseng (Siberian ginseng)	Digoxin	Falsely increases digoxin assay level
	Phenelzine	Insomnia, headache, irritability, tremor, mania-like symptoms
	Warfarin	Decrease INR; decrease anticoagulant effect
	Antidiabetic medications	Decrease blood glucose, decrease need for insulin, decrease required dosage of antidiabetic agent, hypoglycemia
Glucosamine	Antidiabetic medications	Increase insulin resistance, increase blood glucose
Grapefruit	See question 11	
Green tea	Warfarin	Decrease INR, decrease anticoagulant effect
Kava (*Piper methysticum*)	CNS depressants: sedatives, sleeping pills, benzodiazepines, barbiturates, antipsychotics, alcohol	Increase sedation, lethargy, disorientation, semicomatose state
	Medications to treat Parkinson's disease	Exacerbation of Parkinson's disease
Kelp	Thyroid hormone	Hyperthyroidism
Licorice	Digoxin, loop diuretics	Pseudoaldosteronism activity may cause hypokalemia (increasing risk of digoxin toxicity)
Ma huang (ephedra)	Antihypertensive agents	Antagonize effects of antihypertensive medications
	MAO inhibitors, methylxanthines, decongestants, stimulant drugs, caffeine	Enhanced sympathomimetic effects, hypertension, tachycardia, myocardial infarction, stroke, sudden death
	Cardiac glycosides, halothane	Arrhythmias

(Table continued on next page.)

Table 2. Herbal Interactions with Drugs (Continued)

HERBAL OR OTHER SUPPLEMENT	MEDICATION(S)	POTENTIAL EFFECT(S) OF INTERACTION
St. John's wort (*Hypericum perforatum*)	MAO inhibitors (phenelzine)	May bind to brain MAO receptors; hypertensive crisis, convulsion, death
	SSRIs	Serotonin syndrome: headache, sweating, dizziness, agitation, nausea, weakness, fatigue, lethargy, incoherence, akasthesia, hyperreflexia, hypertension, tachycardia
	Sertraline	Mania, dizziness, nausea, vomiting, headache, epigastric pain, anxiety, confusion, restlessness, irritability
	Piroxicam, tetracycline	Enhance photosensitivity
	Oral contraceptives	Breakthrough bleeding, irregular menstrual bleeding, and pregnancy
	Cyclosporine, tacrolimus	Decrease drug concentration, increase risk of transplanted organ rejection
	Digoxin, indinavir, nevirapine, amitriptyline, simvastatin, midazolam, theophylline	Decrease drug concentration, reduced therapeutic efficacy
	Warfarin	Increase INR; increase bleeding, increase bruising
Valerian	CNS depressants, benzodiazepines, barbiturates, other sedative-hypnotics, alcohol	Increase sedation
	Thiopental, pentobarbital	Prolongs thiopental- and pentobarbital- induced sleep
Vitamin E	Anticoagulants, antiplatelet agents, NSAIDs	Increase INR, PT; increase bleeding, increase bruising
Yohimbine	Antidepressants, antihypertensives, sympathomimetics, MAO inhibitors, caffeine, ephedrine, ma huang, St. John's wort	Acts as an alpha-2 antagonist, which may cause increased hypertensive effects

MAO = monoamine oxidase, INR = international normalized ratio, PT = prothrombin time, SSRIs = selective serotonin reuptake inhibitors.

18. What herbal products should be discontinued prior to diagnostic procedures or surgery?

The American Society of Anesthesiologists (ASA) recommends that patients discontinue all herbal therapies at least 2–3 weeks before surgery because of the potential for significant morbidity resulting from interactions among herbs, prescription drugs, and the administration of anesthetics. As mentioned above, St. John's wort may prolong the effects of anesthesia, causing delayed emergence as well as possibly reducing the concentration and therapeutic efficacy of multiple drugs.

Many herbs and supplements have the potential to increase bleeding or inhibit coagulation. Examples include coenzyme Q10, danshen, dong quai, fenugreek, feverfew, garlic, ginger, ginkgo, ginseng, vitamin E, and fish oil. In fact, part of the salutary effect of fish oil in the diet comes from its ability to cause measurable platelet inhibition similar to aspirin.

In addition to St. John's wort, several herbs, including valerian and kava kava, increase the sedative effect of anesthesia. Ma huang (ephedra) mimics epinephrine, causing an increase in blood pressure, heart rate, and the potential for serious arrhythmias.

Because hepatotoxic effects may be associated with its persistent use, echinacea may have the potential to increase the risk for hepatotoxicity when compromises in hepatic function or blood flow occur due to anesthetic agents. However, this concern is only theoretical; there have been no reported cases.

Patients physically dependent on valerian may experience benzodiazepine-like withdrawal with abrupt discontinuation. The dose of valerian should be tapered starting several weeks before surgery, or patients should continue taking valerian up to the day of surgery and take benzodiazepines if withdrawal symptoms develop during the postoperative period.

19. This is starting to get complicated. How does someone stay informed about all of these interactions?

At the end of this chapter is a list of websites devoted to these issues. Some cover herb–drug interactions, whereas others cover drug–nutrient interactions. Many pharmacies maintain lists of these interactions, but patients need to be told to ask for information. Clinicians must make a habit of asking patients about their use of over-the-counter products, herbal products, vitamins, minerals, and other supplements. Clinicians should check to make sure that these supplements do not interfere with prescribed medications, reminding patients who take prescription medications to check to see that their supplements do not interfere with medications.

BIBLIOGRAPHY

1. Ang-Lee MK, Moss J, Yuan CS: Herbal medicines and perioperative care. JAMA 286:208–216, 2001.
2. Dipiro JT, Talbert RT, Yee GC, et al: Pharmacotherapy: A Pathophysiologic Approach, 4th ed. New York, McGraw-Hill, 1999.
3. Evans AM: Influence of dietary components on the gastrointestinal metabolism and transport of drugs. Ther Drug Monit 22(1):131–136, 2000.
4. Fugh-Berman A, Ernst E: Herb-drug interactions: Review and assessment of report reliability. Br J Clin Pharmacol 52:587–595, 2001.
5. Kane GC, Lipsky JJ: Drug-grapefruit juice interactions. Mayo Clin Proc 75:933–942, 2000.
6. Lacy CF: Lacey Drug information Handbook, 9th ed. 2001–2002.
7. Maka DA. Murphy LK: Drug-nutrient interactions: A review. AACN Clinical Issues 11:580–589, 2000.
8. Maskalyk J: Grapefruit juice: Potential drug interations. Can Med Assoc J 167:279–280, 2002.
9. Miller LG: Herbal medicinals: Selected clinical considerations focusing on known or potential drug-herb interactions. Arch Intern Med 158:2200–2211, 1998.
10. Monhassel M: Alternative medicine. Implications for clinical practice. Pharmacist May–June, 2000.
11. Penrod LE, Allen JB, Cabacungan LR: Warfarin resistance and enteral feedings: 2 case reports and a supporting in vitro study. Arch Phys Med Rehabil 82:1270–1273, 2001.
12. Schmidt LE, Dalhoff K: Food-drug interactions. Drugs 62:1481–1502, 2002.
13. Scott GN, Elmer GW: Update on natural product—drug interactions. Am J Health-System Pharm 59:339–347, 2002.
14. Skidmore-Roth L: Mosby's Handbook of Herbs and Natural Supplements. St. Louis, Elsevier Science, 2001.
15. Smolinske, S: Dietary Supplement Adverse Reactions and Interactions, 2000 Update. Pharmacy Practice News. February, 2000.

Selected Websites

National Center for Complementary and Alternative Medicine, The National Institutes of Health: http://nccam.nih.gov
Natural Pharmacist: http://www.tnp.com
Office of Dietary Supplements, National Institutes of Health: http://dietary-supplements.info.nih.gov
Pharmacist's Letter: http://www.pharmacistletter.com

43. NURSING CARE OF THE PATIENT RECEIVING TOTAL PARENTERAL NUTRITION

Vicki M. Ross, MSN, RN, Pamela A. Orr, BSN, RN, and Marie Ann T. Lansangan, BSN, RN

1. What is the purpose of nursing care for the patient receiving total parenteral nutrition (TPN)?

Nursing care ensures the adequate and safe delivery of TPN. This includes the safety and care of the catheter and delivery system, the proper administration of the TPN itself, and the continued reassessment of the patient to minimize complications (see Chapter 41, Complications of TPN).

2. What is the best method of determining adequate delivery of TPN?

Accurate intake and output records remain the best method of ensuring that TPN has been given. Comparison of actual intake with the desired rate of fluid administration enables the clinician to detect deficits. Daily weights, while useful, are less reliable. They provide a useful monitor of fluid status in critically ill patients. Day-to-day fluctuations in weight do not reflect changes in lean body mass, but rather changes in water and sodium.

3. Does TPN require special solution bags and infusion tubing?

One or multi-liter glass or plastic containers may be safely used to store or administer TPN solutions. Glass or plastic allows visualization of the solution for large pieces of particulate matter or solution instability. Bags or bottles containing particulate matter or thin yellow or white lines that do not disappear with rotation of the solution should be considered unsafe and discarded immediately.

It is well documented that lipid emulsions leach the plasticizer DEHP (diethylhexylphthalate) from the solution container. Because of safety concerns, bags containing DEHP should not be used for long-term storage of parenteral solutions which contain lipids.

4. What are desirable features for TPN infusion pumps?

The best infusion pump is one that includes safety features and addresses the needs of specific patient populations. Some desirable safety features are an occlusion or low-flow alarm, a high-flow alarm, an AC/DC conversion with a low-battery alarm, a hold and call-back alarm, and a patient lockout system.

The occlusion or low-flow alarm lowers the risk of central venous catheter tubing occlusion by alerting the nurse when the infusions are near completion or a kinking in the catheter tubing has occurred. High-flow alarms indicate high infusion rates, which might occur with intravenous tubing pulling from the pump. Some pump tubing is designed to automatically shut off when disconnected from the pump. In the event the tubing malfunctions, a high-flow alarm prevents large amounts of TPN from being infused into the patient. AC/DC conversion allows infusion pumps to run with wall electricity or battery. If pumps are not equipped with AC/DC conversions and low-battery alarms, TPN may be stopped when the patient is transported or the pump is unplugged for long periods. Hold buttons permit stopping the TPN for a few seconds to a few minutes without turning off the TPN. The call-back alarm alerts the nurse that the infusion is off and reduces the risk of catheter clotting or forgetting to start the TPN again.

Infusion pumps should be easy to use but not so easy that a confused patient might alter TPN infusion rates. Lockout features or special procedures that prohibit confused patients or visitors from altering TPN rates are ideal.

In addition to safety features, pump characteristics should match the needs of the healthcare providers and patients. Acutely ill patients in the intensive care unit may require a reliable continuous infusion pump, while patients in rehabilitation units will require portable pumps with programmable features to enable cycling of the TPN.

5. Should filters be used with TPN?

Because TPN may contain particulate matter not visualized by the naked eye and because TPN solutions are a growth media for bacteria and fungi, filters should be used. The ideal filters prevent air, particulate matter, bacteria, and fungi from reaching the patient without impeding the delivery of drugs and nutrients. Small filters (0.22 micron) will trap smaller-sized particulate matter but cannot be used with lipid-containing formulations. Lipids must be administered below the filter. If the lipid is mixed with the other components, as in three-in-one formulations, a 1.2-micron filter can be used.

In-line filters are best. Compared to detachable filters, in-line filters reduce line manipulation and potential contamination. The only disadvantage is that the cost of in-line filters may be slightly higher than attachable filters due to the special tubing required and the need to change the entire tubing if problems occur with the filter.

6. What types of catheters are used for TPN?

The following types of CVCs are used for the infusion of TPN:

1. Central venous catheters for short-term use are placed at the bedside or under fluoroscopy.

2. Peripherally inserted central catheters (PICCs) are also placed at the bedside or in the clinic or under flouroscopy and can be used for weeks or months.

3. Long-term tunneled catheters, such as the Hickman, Broviac, or Groshong, are usually placed in the operating room. These are ideal for home TPN.

4. Subcutaneously placed ports, such as Port-a-cath, are also placed in the operating room. They require special noncoring needles to prevent port damage when accessing the central venous catheter. Ports are best if the central line is accessed occasionally, not daily or continuously; for that reason are generally used for TPN.

A variety of catheter lumens, sizes, and composition types are on the market today. Catheters must be long enough for the tip to reach the area of the superior vena cava and right atrium and contain enough lumens to dedicate one lumen for the administration of TPN. Central venous catheters must be pliable enough to withstand infusion pump pressures without perforating, but not so stiff as to be thrombogenic to the vessel.

7. What vein is preferable for administering TPN?

Due to their hypertonicity, TPN solutions should never be administered via peripheral veins. The tip of the central venous catheter should be in an area of high blood flow, which is usually in the superior vena cava (SVC), or the inferior vena cava (IVC) at the junction of the right atrium. Insertion sites for central venous catheters vary. Subclavian or internal jugular approaches are often used for placement of temporary central venous catheters. Femoral approaches may be used in emergencies, but not routinely due to the increased risk of infections and thrombosis. Failures of femoral catheters to reach the SVC or IVC increase the risk of thrombosis with the infusion of hypertonic fluids. Antecubital veins are used for initial insertion of PICCs, and catheters are threaded up the upper extremity veins to the SVC.

Long-term catheters, such as the Hickman, Broviac, or Groshong, usually exit the body on the chest while the catheter tip is in the SVC or proximal right atrium.

8. Should central venous catheters be changed on a routine basis?

Unlike peripheral venous catheters, central venous catheters do not need to be changed on a regular basis.

In the maintenance of CVCs, decisions regarding the frequency of catheter replacement are substantially more complicated. Some investigators have shown duration of catheterization to be a risk factor for infection, and routine replacement of CVCs at specified intervals has been advocated as a measure to reduce infection. However, more recent data suggest that the daily risk of infection remains constant and show that routine replacements of CVCs, without a clinical indication, do not reduce the rate of catheter colonization.

If a catheter infection is suspected, then the central venous catheter should be changed and cultures obtained. CVCs should always be discontinued when no longer necessary.

9. How fast can the rate of the TPN infusion be increased?

It is possible to rapidly increase the rate of TPN to target levels within 24 hours in normal or mildly malnourished patients. Begin at a rate of 25 to 50 ml/hour, and increase by 25–50 ml/hour, within 48–72 hours, and increase to the target rate. However, for severely malnourished patients, slower rates are safer. Large amounts of dextrose infused over the first 24 to 48 hours may be harmful. Initiate TPN at a slow rate to deliver approximately 1–2 mg/kg/min of dextrose (equivalent to about 100 to 200 gm/day). If electrolytes and glucose are within normal limits, continue to increase by 1–2 mg/kg/min per day to the maximum rate. If glucose or electrolyte values are not within normal limits, correct the glucose and replenish the electrolytes before increasing the rate of the TPN. The use of TPN solutions containing only 15% glucose, in which 30% to 40% of calories are supplied as fat, speeds up the process considerably. (See Chapter 41 for further discussion of refeeding syndrome.)

Initiation and adjustment of TPN infusion rates should take into account the nutritional status of the patient and their caloric requirements. For example, a patient with adequate nutrition prior to initiating TPN is less likely to experience the shifts in electrolytes when compared to a patient who has been without nutrition for weeks.

In general, it is safe to increase TPN infusions to maximum rate over 48–72 hours. This allows time to assess the patients' tolerance of dextrose loads and the repletion of electrolytes and fluids if necessary.

10. It is safe to initiate TPN in patients with hyperglycemia?

TPN therapy should not be initiated until serum glucose levels are below 200 mg/dl. Lowering serum glucose levels in critically ill patients usually requires an insulin drip. Once the serum glucose is controlled, TPN may be initiated. In addition to insulin therapy, lower concentrations of dextrose and higher percentages of fat may be used in TPN formulations to control serum glucose levels.

Insulin drips are ideal and most accurate for controlling glucose in critically ill patients. If insulin drips are not possible, sliding scale insulin (SSI) may be used to calculate the amount of insulin to be added to the TPN. SSI is not recommended for the treatment of hyperglycemia. However, two-thirds of the previous day's SSI can be added every 24 hours to the TPN to control the glucose. For example, for a patient who received 18 units of SSI on the previous day, 12 units of insulin would be added to the TPN.

When TPN is initiated, patients with known glucose intolerance are particularly at risk for developing hyperglycemia. This includes patients with diabetes mellitus, severely stressed or septic patients, and patients receiving corticosteroid therapy. Obtain capillary blood glucose, at least by bedside determination, at least every four to six hours in these patients to assess tolerance of the dextrose from the TPN infusion. As hyperglycemia causes fluid and electrolyte complications and immunologic dysfunction, do not increase TPN infusion rates until glucose levels are consistently below 200 mg/dl.

11. What precautions are required when beginning lipid emulsions?

Prior to initiating lipid emulsions, it is important to check triglyceride levels, which should be < 400 mg/dl. Lipid clearance is considered adequate if serum triglyceride levels are maintained at < 400 mg/dl (4.5 mmol/L) during continuous lipid infusion and < 200 mg/dl (2.5 mmol/L) 4 hours after infusion.

Use of lipids is contraindicated in the management of patients with abnormal lipid metabolism such as hyperlipidemia, lipid nephrosis, or hypertriglyceridemia-induced pancreatitis. Caution should be practiced for use of lipids in immunosuppressed patients during critical illness (i.e., < 1 g/kg/day). Patients with severe egg allergies may not tolerate lipids because of the egg phospholipid contained in the fat emulsion.

Lipids or fat emulsions provide non-protein calories and prevent essential fatty acid depletion. Fat emulsions also provide rich media for the growth of bacteria and fungi. Scrupulous hand washing prior to handling lipids is imperative to reduce the risk of touch contamination. Lipid emulsions hung alone are best administered over an extended period of time that does not exceed 12 hours. When lipids are infused alone, discard all bottles and tubing after 12 hours. Three-in-one TPN countainers and tubing should be changed every 24 hours.

Lipids may be infused into the TPN line downstream from the filter, or above 1.2 micron filter, which is large enough to pass the lipid emlsion particles. No other drugs should be infused into a line containing lipids or TPN.

12. What type of care is required to insert central venous catheters?

Use sterile technique when inserting central venous catheters. Remove all unnecessary equipment and dressings from the area prior to opening the sterile central venous catheters packs. Prior to draping patients, suction tracheostomies and change wound dressings to avoid contamination of sterile fields. Inform patients that large sterile drapes will cover their face and body. Sedate patients if necessary, to reduce anxiety.

Assist the physician or nurse inserting central venous catheters to reduce risks of catheter/field contamination as the physician reaches for equipment. Anyone placing or directly assisting with insertion of central venous catheters should wear sterile gown, gloves, mask, and cap. All other persons in the room should wear at least a mask and cap. (See Chapter 40, Venous Access.)

13. What type of care is required on dressing the exit site of central?

Once a central venous catheter is inserted, cover with a sterile dressing. There is some latitude in the type of dressing which can be used (gauze or transparent), but a dressing must be used. A sterile dressing, changed often enough to maintain sterility, must be kept over the exit site. In general, occlusive dressings can be kept in place longer than non-occlusive dressings. X-ray confirmation of placement should be done prior to infusing TPN.

Despite numerous studies, no product for antisepsis or dressing has proved to have consistent superiority in reducing the number of central venous catheter infections. Chlorhexidine combined with 70% isopropyl alcohol has shown shome promise for skin decontamination, and is now available in convenient, easy-to-use form. Iodophors such as povidone-iodine are typically used for skin decontamination, and as an ointment for continued antibacterial activity. Gauze or transparent film dressings may be used to cover the site and stabilize the catheter.

Suturing the central venous catheter prevents accidental dislodgment of catheters. If sutures break, secure the central venous catheter with tape or dressing and contact the physician or surgeon to resuture the catheter in place. As the excess portion of central venous catheters remains outside the body, note any changes in catheter length and report them to the physician immediately. If movement of the catheter tip outside the vessel wall is suspected, TPN should be stopped until an x-ray has been obtained and placement confirmed. Because central venous catheters are associated with high rates of infection, hands must be washed scrupulously prior to handling them. Keep handling and manipulation of catheters and hubs to a minimum. Use aseptic technique when assessing or handling hubs and ports.

14. What type of care is required for discontinuation of central venous catheters?

Discontinue central venous catheters when TPN is no longer necessary or a complication, such as catheter sepsis, is suspected. To prevent air emboli, lower the head of the bed and ask patients to exhale slowly as the catheter is pulled out, to increase intrathoracic pressure. Cover the exit site with a sterile dressing and assess the patient for signs for respiratory distress or bleeding.

15. What physical signs should be monitored when a patient is receiving TPN?

Weigh the patient daily and maintain accurate intake and output records to assess fluid status. Assess gastrointestinal function and the ability to consume and absorb nutrition orally.

When patients are able to consume and absorb adequate amounts of nutrition orally, TPN should be discontinued. Assess central venous catheters sites for signs of increasing erythema or drainage. Change central venous catheters to a new site if a site infection develops. Obtain accurate temperature every four to eight hours in addition to pulse, respiratory rate, and blood pressure to assess for impending signs of infection. Obtain capillary blood glucose every four to six hours to assess tolerance of dextrose.

16. What is nitrogen balance?
Patients excrete nitrogen as a waste product. As patients become catabolic, nitrogen excretion increases. The goal in nutritional support is to maintain a positive nitrogen balance by providing more nitrogen intake than the amount that is excreted. To measure nitrogen, an accurate 24 hour urine collection is required. The amount of nitrogen excreted in the urine, corrected for non-urinary losses, is subtracted from the amount of nitrogen delivered in the form of protein (protein is approximately 16% nitrogen) to derive the nitrogen balance. One goal of nutritional support is to maintain a positive nitrogen balance (see Appendix I).

17. What laboratory studies should be monitored when a patient is receiving TPN?
Prior to initiating TPN, laboratory values to assess renal and liver function and nutritional status should be drawn. This would include sodium, potassium, chloride, carbon dioxide, glucose, blood urea nitrogen, creatinine, magnesium, phosphorus, cholesterol, triglycerides, total bilirubin, ALT, AST, albumin and prealbumin.

As TPN is initiated and the rate increased, electrolytes, including magnesium and phosphorus, should be obtained daily. Nutritional markers and lab for renal and liver function should be obtained at least two to three times per week in hospitalized patients. Obtain serum glucose or capillary blood glucose determinations every four to six hours.

18. Can blood work be drawn from the central venous catheters?
Due to the increased risk of infections when manipulating TPN lines and catheters, it is preferable not to draw blood from central venous catheters. If blood is drawn from central venous catheters, aspirate at least 5 to 10 ml of blood to avoid erroneous lab results. Blood cultures should be drawn peripherally. If blood is drawn from central venous catheters, clearly mark the label and requisition with "blood drawn from central venous catheter."

19. Can patency of central venous catheters be maintained with routine saline flushes?
Although the efficacy of using saline to maintain patency in peripheral catheters is established, use of saline to maintain patency in central catheters is less certain. Flush central venous catheters with enough heparin to fill the catheter (unless contraindicated). Typically, this requires 0.5 to 1.0 ml. for temporary catheters and 1.0 to 5.0 ml. for longer tunneled catheters. Protocols for dilution and frequency of heparin flushes differ. Heparin dilutions for central venous catheter flush range from 100 to 1000 units per ml. Temporary catheters typically require heparin flushes three to four times per day. Tunneled catheters, depending upon their design, can be flushed once or twice a week, or even monthly (Groshong catheters). Implanted ports must be flushed monthly. To avoid drug interactions, always flush first with saline and then with heparin after administering medications.

20. What are the points of entrance for organisms causing TPN associated infections?
Organisms causing central venous catheter associated infections may arise from infusion bags, but the most common sites are tubing hubs, stopcocks, skin at the insertion site, side ports, and other infections in the body. Hematogenous seeding of catheters occurs when organisms in other parts of the body attach and multiply on the intravascular portion of the catheter, or the fibrin sheath surrounding it. Reducing other nosocomial infections such as urinary tract infections and pneumonia can also reduce the number of catheter-associated infections.

Preventive methods include mixing TPN under laminar flow hoods by experienced pharmacists, adherence to protocols for changing bags and tubing, and dedicating one lumen of central venous catheters for TPN. Good hand washing cannot be overemphasized. Stopcocks on TPN lines should be avoided and hub manipulation kept to a minimum. Use aseptic technique when accessing central lines. Maintain clean, dry dressings over exit sites.

21. What are the recommendations for patients with fever?

When a previously afebrile patient spikes a temperature, the central venous catheter must be considered as a possible source for the infection. One method of diagnosing central venous catheter associated infections is to draw blood cultures from a peripheral site and obtain the intercutaneous section and tip of the catheter for cultures. If all sources yield the same organisms, the central venous catheter is considered the source of the infection. Unfortunately, this process requires discontinuing or changing the central venous catheter to obtain catheter sections for culture. Catheter-associated infections cannot be completely excluded in any other way. Once a patient becomes febrile, the catheter must be regarded with suspicion, even if another source is clearly identified, because it may become secondarily infected. If the blood culture is positive, the catheter should be removed, since the likelihood is high that it will become secondarily infected.

22. What is the safest method for discontinuing TPN?

Although research has not supported the existence of rebound hypoglycemia in adult patients when TPN is discontinued, the safest method for discontinuing TPN is to taper the rate of the infusion over two to four hours. If TPN must be stopped abruptly and there is concern about preventing hypoglycemia in the patient, 10% dextrose can be hung and capillary blood glucose obtained two hours later.

BIBLIOGRAPHY

1. American Dietetic Association: Nutrition Support. Manual of Clinical Dietetics, 6th ed. Chicago, American Dietetic Association, 2000, p 622.
2. Centers for Disease Control and Prevention: Guidelines for the prevention of intravascular catheter-related infections. MMWR 51(RR-10):6–9, 2002.
3. Gottschlich M: The Science and Practice of Nutrition Support. Kendall/Hunt, Iowa, Aspen, 2001, pp 211–251.
4. Rombeau J, Rolandelli R: Clinical Nutrition: Parenteral Nutrition, 3rd ed. Philadelphia, W.B. Saunders, 2001.
5. Shikora S, Martindale R, Schwaitzberg S: Nutritional Considerations in the Intensive Care Unit. Dubuque, IA, Kendall/Hunt, 2002.
6. Shuster MH: Parenteral nutrition. In Hennessy K, Orr M (eds): Nutrition Support Core Curriculum, 3rd ed. Silver Spring, MD, Aspen, 1997.

44. HOME PARENTERAL NUTRITION

Alyce F. Newton, MS, RD

1. What are the indications for home parenteral nutrition (HPN)?
In addition to having a dysfunctional gastrointestinal tract, candidates for home parenteral nutrition (HPN) must meet criteria for safe administration. The home environment must be assessed for safe delivery of intravenous nutrition, including a working telephone, running water for hand washing and cleaning preparation areas, electricity, and a working refrigerator large enough to store parenteral solutions at the appropriate temperature. Patients and/or caregivers should be able to follow instructions to administer and monitor the tolerance to HPN. The patient and/or caregiver must understand the risks, benefits, and costs of parenteral nutrition before initiating HPN.

2. What preparation is required in order to discharge a patient on HPN?
- The referring physician, who maintains the primary care of the patient, places a referral for HPN.
- If the referral is from the hospital, the nutrition support team members and/order discharge planners contact the infusion provider with referral information. The discharge planners or the home infusion provider evaluates the patient's reimbursement for HPN. Reimbursement for HPN is provided by third-party payers (insurance companies) and Medicare/Medicaid. All HPN-reimbursement requirements should be completed prior to discharge. Social workers may also be involved to identify and coordinate payment of services related to HPN.
- Patient/caregiver education should begin as soon as the patient is identified as a candidate for HPN. The HPN provider and/or nursing provider at home should continue this.

3. What are the guidelines for choosing a HPN provider?
Ideally, the HPN provider (also called infusion provider) should be located in acceptable proximity to the patient. The HPN provider should have experienced personnel, including pharmacists, nurses, and dietitians. Nursing may be provided by the HPN provider by a nursing agency. Although the HPN patient should be medically stable, problems may arise and the HPN provider should be available 7 days per week, 24 hours per day. The experience and expertise of the HPN provider are an important component in the success of the HPN experience.

The realities of managed care are that most insurance companies have contracts with one or more HPN providers and choice may be limited. However, it is appropriate to review the credentials of the provider. Although variable, states often grant certificates and/or licensure to infusion providers and home care agencies. Medicare also certifies certain nursing and home health agencies.

4. What type of intravenous access is appropriate for HPN?
The type and placement of central venous catheters (CVC) should be based on patient preference, experience of the person inserting the catheter, and length of therapy. A central venous catheter is required for HPN due to the osmolality of PN and the duration of the HPN therapy. Often catheters are composed of a silicone or polyurethane material to reduce fibrin sheath development, platelet aggregation, and thrombus formation. Tunneled catheters with Dacron cuffs anchored in the subcutaneous tissue, such as the Groshong, Hickman, and Broviac catheters, have a lower risk of infection and less potential for dislodgment.

Peripherally inserted central catheters (PICC) lines are often used for HPN therapy that is expected to last more than 2 months. Implanted ports, which are often used for chemotherapy, may also be used for the administration of HPN. Weekly port needle changes are required for HPN infusion. Noncoring needles are required for accessing implanted ports (see Chapter 40). In summary, if the therapy is short-term (weeks to months) and the patient has adequate antecubital veins, the PICC catheter is best. For long-term use (months to years), the tunneled central venous catheters (CVC) may be the best choice.

5. Describe the role of the caregiver. How do patients and caregivers handle the demands of HPN?

Caregivers may or may not be related to the patient. They assist the patient with the preparation, administration, and monitoring of the HPN. Safe and effective administration of HPN requires adherence to strict procedures. The patient and caregiver(s) are responsible for the administration of the HPN as ordered by the physician as well as the identification and prevention of complications. Patients and caregivers often complain of feelings of depression and fatigue related to the time and energy HPN requires and may benefit from the skills of a psychologist or qualified therapist.

6. Are "standard" PN formulas appropriate for home use?

Hospitals use standard PN formulas to decrease errors, costs, and waste. The standard PN solution may not deliver the patient's exact nutrient requirements, but the HPN provider should be able to individualize the optimal solution for the HPN patient.

7. What should be included in the monitoring of a patient receiving HPN?

HPN monitoring should include assessments of the vascular access device, metabolic monitoring, and weekly assessments of weight, strength, and the ability to perform activities of daily living.

Monitoring guidelines for patients receiving home parenteral nutrition[8]

Chemistry profile: electrolytes, glucose, carbon dioxide (CO_2), blood urea nitrogen (BUN), creatinine, total protein, albumin, triglycerides, calcium, phosphorus, magnesium	√	√	√
Liver function tests: total bilirubin, alkaline phosphatase, lactate dehydrogenase (LDH), serum glutamic-oxaloacetic transaminase (SGOT), serum glutamic-pyruvic transaminase (SGPT), prothrombin time (PT)	√	√	√
Complete blood count with differential	√	√	√
Depending on underlying disease condition: zinc, vitamin B12, iron studies, copper	√		

Changes in oral intake and gut function should be evaluated on a routine basis. Adjustment to HPN changes in home environment and psychosocial problems related to or affecting the delivery of HPN must also be addressed. Electrolytes, renal function, and liver function should be evaluated weekly, then monthly when stable. Nutritional markers, including vitamin and mineral levels, may be checked annually or as required for long-term HPN patients.

8. What is "cycled" HPN?

In the acute care setting, PN solutions are usually administered continuously. Although this technique can also be done in the home, most patients benefit from the mental well-being that comes from disconnection from the PN for part of the day. Cycling allows the patient to deliver the HPN solutions over 8–16 hours, typically overnight. The regimen usually includes a tapering of the rate over 1–2 hours at the beginning and/or end of the infusion, with maximum rate in the middle of the infusion. For example, the home infusion pump may be set for 2000 ml over 12 hours, and the rate is automatically set at 91 ml/hr for the first hour, 181 ml per hour for 10 hours, and 91 mil per hour for the last hour. The theory is that the pancreas does not react quickly to abrupt changes in the dextrose load and that the insulin persists after the infusion is stopped. This theory has been questioned recently, along with the need to taper. However, tapering rates among cycled PN patients remains a common practice. The majority of HPN patients use ambulatory infusion pumps with backpacks.

9. Which central venous catheters (CVC) may be inserted at home?
The majority of the central venous catheters are inserted in a controlled setting by the physician. In certain states, however, the Nurse Practice Act permits the home insertion of a PICC line by a qualified registered nurse using sterile and aseptic technique. Radiology confirmation of central placement is required before use of the catheter. Interventional radiologists may place PICC lines using ultrasound in the radiology suite when bedside placement is difficult or not possible.

10. What information or skills are necessary for patients and caregivers before initiating HPN?
It is helpful is patients and caregivers understand their vital role in the administration of the HPN therapy. Daily nursing visits may be authorized only for the first 3 days, then decrease to once per week. Patients and caregivers need to know about the risks and benefits of parenteral nutrition, the use of aseptic technique, and storage and admixture techniques for HPN. Following home instruction, they should be able to demonstrate their understanding of safe disposal of needles and sharps, the preparation of the HPN solution along with the addition of multivitamins and other patient additives, and the use and care of infusion pumps and tubing. It is important to assess the patient and caregiver's knowledge of the infusion periodically during the HPN therapy.

11. What are the most common complications of HPN?
HPN patients may experience the same insertion, metabolic, mechanical, and infectious complications as hospitalized PN patients. Insertion complications include catheter tip malposition, hemothorax, pneumothorax, brachial plexus injury, hematoma, air embolism, and subcutaneous emphysema. Mechanical complications include catheter-induced thrombosis, central venous thrombosis, catheter clogging, and catheter damage. Metabolic complications include fluid and electrolyte imbalances and blood glucose disturbances. The cycled HPN patient is more likely to experience dehydration than a patient receiving continuous infusion, especially during periods of increased gastrointestinal output or decreased oral supplementation of fluids. Hyperglycemia is the most common metabolic complication and is usually related to dextrose content of the PN. Recent literature has indicated that stringent glucose control (glucose ≤ 110 mg/dl) is associated with reduced mortality and morbidity (reduced polyneuropathy of critical illness, bacteremia, inflammation and anemia) in the acute care setting. Long-term metabolic complications of HPN include liver disease, metabolic bone disease, micronutrient depletion, and micronutrient toxicity disorders. The most common cause for readmission to hospital for patients receiving HPN is the underlying disease, and catheter-related infections.

12. What is refeeding syndrome?
Malnourished patients who were previously without feeding either enterally or parenterally for a prolonged period and who receive their total caloric needs on initiation of PN may develop refeeding syndrome. This syndrome can become a medical emergency if cardiac arrhythmias occur, caused by electrolyte imbalances. Hypophosphatemia, hypomagnesemia, and hypokalemia may occur following excessive infusion of dextrose with inadequate mineral replacement. Clinically, the patient should be monitored for shortness of breath, weakness, dizziness, muscle spasms, tetany, peripheral edema, and pulmonary congestion.

13. Can PN be started in the home?
Careful patient selection is the key to successful initiation of PN in the home, especially when it might be desirable to avoid hospitalization or a prolonged discharge-planning period.

Medically stable patients, without risk of refeeding syndrome, are preferred. If severe dehydration or metabolic or electrolyte abnormalities exist, the patient should be hospitalized to start PN. In some cases, a pre-PN hydration infusion with electrolytes may help normalize blood levels prior to the infusion of PN and prevent refeeding syndrome.

14. What are the most effective methods of reducing the risk of infection in patients receiving HPN?

One of the most effective methods is scrupulous hand washing. Teach patients and caregivers to wash hands with soap and water before handling the HPN solutions or catheters. Maintenance of clean, dry catheter sites and the use of aseptic technique when accessing catheter hubs can also reduce the risk of catheter infections. Early recognition of signs and symptoms of infection can prevent the removal of the CVC. Teaching patients to take their temperatures daily and to notify their physician of temperature elevation or tenderness, erythema, or drainage at the insertion site is important in avoiding catheter related infections.

15. What are the financial considerations in HPN?

Even for the well-insured patient, the first concern is: How much am I going to have to pay for all of this? Copayments and deductibles may cause out-of-pocket expenses to rise rapidly. Consideration must be given to lifetime maximum benefits, which may become exhausted within a few years. Although patients may feel well enough to return to work, the disease process or fatigue may require them to cut back hours. Patients are likely to have higher absenteeism than is covered by sick time or vacation. Changing jobs or seeking employment after initiating HPN therapy may result in an improved income but may change insurance benefits. Many patients eventually find it necessary to seek public assistance, disability status, or Medicare coverage. Caregivers and family members are often put into financial risk because of joint responsibility for debt, higher absenteeism, or the need to reduce household income to obtain assistance.

16. How does Medicare reimburse for HPN?

Medicare Part B reimburses for HPN under the prosthetic device category. In other words, providing HPN solutions into the vein creates an "artificial alimentary tract." HPN is covered for the individual with a permanent, severe disorder of the gastrointestinal tract that does not allow absorption of adequate nutrients to maintain body weight or functional ability. When a disorder is defined as permanent, it does not preclude any chance of recovery; it requires only the need for PN for at least 90 days. The primary physician is required to submit an initial certification of medical necessity (CMN) and to recertify the need for HPN after 6 months. Additional documentation may be required for patients with a diagnosis that falls outside the identified Medicare categories: if calories are provided outside the range of 20–35 calories/kg/day; if protein is provided outside the range of 0.8–1.5 gm/kg/day; if lipids are in excess of 15 units (1 unit = 250 ml) of a 20% solution per month or 30 units (500 ml) of a 10% unit per month; or if special parenteral formulas are ordered. If the coverage requirements for HPN are met, the HPN solutions, administration supplies, and pumps will be covered.

Public assistance programs and private insurance companies often use guidelines similar to Medicare in determining coverage. Payment methods and approval by the appropriate third-party payers must be determined before discharging patients home on PN.

17. What arrangements are needed before patients travel with HPN?

Once patients are stabilized on the HPN regimen, traveling with their solutions becomes a possibility. For trips of 1 week or less, patients may carry their own HPN in a refrigerated or iced container. For trips longer than 1 week, arrangements may be made to ship the necessary solutions. It is also helpful for patients and caregivers to carry a detailed medical history, physician and nutrition support team phone numbers, and names and phone numbers of local resources when possible.

18. What is the Oley Foundation?

The Oley Foundation connects people receiving HPN for emotional support, encouragement, information sharing, and continuing education about their therapy. *The Lifeline Letter*, published by the Oley Foundation and free to all persons receiving HPN, provides real-life stories written by HPN recipients and current, practical medical information. The Oley Foundation was established in 1983 and is supported by grants and donations.

19. What is ASPEN?

The American Society for Parenteral and Enteral Nutrition (ASPEN) is an organization composed of health care professionals from medicine, nursing, pharmacy, dietetics, and nutrition science. ASPEN publishes two journals: Journal of Parenteral and Enteral Nutrition (JPEN), an international journal of nutrition and metabolic support and Nutrition in Clinical Practice (NCP). Articles are peer-reviewed with practical solutions in clinical nutrition. JPEN is published bimonthly and includes preeminent research papers in clinical nutrition, specialized nutrition support, patient care, education, and research. NCP is published bimonthly and includes invited reviews of nutrition support related topics, clinical dilemmas, and solicited manuscripts on clinical patient care topics. ASPEN can be contacted at <www.nutritioncare.org>.

BIBLIOGRAPHY

1. ASPEN Board of Directors: Guidelines for use of parenteral and enteral nutrition in adult and pediatric patients. JPEN 26:1SA–138SA, 2002.
2. Grant J: Recognition, prevention, and treatment of home total parenteral nutrition central venous access complications. JPEN 26:S21–S28, 2002.
3. Howard L, Heaphey L, Fleming CR, et al: Four years of North American registry home parenteral nutrition outcomes data and their implications for patient management. JPEN 15:384–393, 1991.
4. Reddy P, Malone M: Cost and outcomes analysis of home parenteral and enteral nutrition. JPEN 22:302–310, 1998.
5. Smith C: Quality of life in long-term parenteral nutrition patients and their family caregivers. JPEN 17:501–506, 1993.
6. Vanek V: The ins and outs of venous access, Part II. Nutr Clin Pract 17:142–155, 2002.
7. Van den Berghe G, et al: Outcome benefit of intensive insulin therapy in the critically ill: Insulin dose versus glycemic control. Crit Care Med 31:359–366, 2003.
8. Ireton-Jones C, DeLegge M, Epperson L, Alexander J: Management of the home parenteral nutrition patient. Nutr Clin Pract 18:310–317, 2003.

IX. Enteral Nutrition

45. INDICATIONS FOR ENTERAL NUTRITION

Theresa A. Fessler, MS, RD, CNSD,
Carol Ireton-Jones, PhD, RD, LD, CNSD, FACN, and Howard L. Kremer, MD

1. What is enteral nutrition?
According to the American Society for Parenteral and Enteral Nutrition (ASPEN), enteral nutrition involves the nonvolitional delivery of nutrients by tube into the GI tract.

2. Who is a candidate for enteral nutrition support?
A patient with a functional GI tract who either will not, cannot, or should not eat for medical reasons, and who is malnourished or is at risk for developing malnutrition. Enteral nutrition should be considered in any patient who has had or is expected to have no or inadequate nutritional intake for a period of 7–14 days.

3. Who is at risk for malnutrition?
- A patient who will have no or inadequate nutritional intake for > 7 days
- A patient who has had unintentional weight loss of ≥ 10% of body weight within the last 6 months or ≥ 5% within 1 month, or whose weight is 20% below ideal body weight (IBW)
- Patients with chronic disease or increased metabolic requirements who are not able to take in adequate nutrition
- In the neonate, infant, or child, low birth weight, acute weight loss of ≥ 10%, inadequate growth or weight gain, and weight for age or weight for height < third percentile on growth charts
- Patients who have undergone recent surgery, critical illness, or trauma

4. What are some common situations in which enteral feeding may become necessary in the acute-care hospital setting?
Trauma, major surgery, ventilator dependence, severely impaired mental status, severe dysphagia, coma, and cachexia with chronic disease. Inability to eat adequately or lack of appetite along with malnutrition is a reason to use enteral feedings as a substitute for, or to supplement, oral intake. Diseases that lead to cachexia are cancer, AIDS, inflammatory bowel disease, chronic obstructive pulmonary disease, anorexia nervosa, and chronic starvation.

5. What are the advantages of feeding a patient enterally as compared with using parenteral nutrition?
The *ASPEN Practice Guidelines Indications for Specialized Nutrition Support* state that enteral nutrition should generally be used in preference to parenteral nutrition. If the gut is functional, using the intestine is appropriate unless medically contraindicated. Two meta-analyses of enteral vs. parenteral nutrition have produced different results. No documented evidence supports the belief that enteral nutrition is more physiologic than parenteral nutrition. In comparing outcomes of enteral and parenteral nutrition, data suggest that parenteral nutrition results in a higher risk of infection, partly due to a higher rate of hyperglycemia, rather than a frank decrease in infection due to enteral nutrition. Clearly, enteral nutrition is less expensive than parenteral nutrition. Hyperglycemia is less likely in enterally fed patients. Complications can be decreased in enteral patients when care is provided by an experienced and skilled staff.

6. How soon after trauma or surgery can enteral feedings be initiated?

This depends on the route of administration. Small bowel motility resumes in 4–6 hours after surgery. Gastric motility resumes in 24–72 hours. Colonic ileus may last as long as 5 days post-operatively. Feeding into the small intestine with enteral or easily absorbed formulas can be started immediately after surgery. Only if there has been surgery on the small bowel or in the retroperitoneum does one need to be more cautious, and even then feedings can be initiated within 48–72 hours. Feeding into the stomach can usually start within 2–4 days.

7. Are enteral feedings contraindicated in patients with hypoalbuminemia?

No. Enteral feeding is appropriate and has been shown to be well tolerated in patients with low albumin levels. Several previous studies have suggested a relationship between hypoalbuminemia and tube-feeding–related diarrhea. However, these studies have uniformly failed to prove the relationship and have not clearly identified other risk factors for diarrhea in those patients. Despite statements to the contrary, there is no proven cause-and-effect relationship between low serum albumin levels and diarrhea in enterally fed patients.

8. Are nausea and vomiting contraindications to enteral feeding?

Although the feeding initially should be decreased or stopped if these symptoms occur, slow continuous feedings instead of bolus feedings, and isotonic rather than hypertonic formulas, are more likely to be tolerated. Antinausea medications and drugs that stimulate gut motility may be helpful. In addition, postpyloric and jejunal feeding tubes make enteral feeding possible when gastric feedings are not tolerated.

9. Is diarrhea a contraindication to enteral feeding?

Generally, no. Unless a patient has an underlying intestinal or digestive disorder, significant nutrient absorption still occurs in the small bowel during periods of diarrhea. Standard definitions for diarrhea are lacking. Patients and nursing staff use the term in a subjective manner that does not necessarily correlate with actual high-volume stool output. Diarrhea is multifactorial and often results from infection, GI disorders, or enterally administered medications.

Infectious causes, such as *Clostridium difficile*, should be ruled out. Physicians also order stool tests for fecal lactoferrin or fecal leukocytes to assess for infection or inflammatory process. Fecal fat can be tested to rule out maldigestion and malabsorption, which may occur in pancreatic exocrine insufficiency, deficiency of bile salts, or bacterial overgrowth. Disorders of intestinal mucosa may also cause malabsorption, such as inflammatory bowel disease or ischemia. Diarrhea can also occur in situations of inadequate bile acid reabsorption, as in patients with ileal resection, in which case bile acid-binding medications may help.

Medications may cause diarrhea in many situations. Liquid medications used for tube fed patients very often contain sorbitol, a sugar alcohol that causes osmotic diarrhea when it reaches the colon. Enteral administration of magnesium, potassium, and phosphate salts can also cause loose stools. Medication lists should also be checked to ensure that a patient is not receiving laxatives or stool softeners, which may have been needed at one time, but were not discontinued. Lactulose, chemotherapy drugs, and antibiotics are other common causes of diarrhea.

Fiber is often added to nutrition regimens to help promote the development of formed stools; however, there is little clinical research in this area, and the effects of fiber vary for each individual. Bacterial fermentation of fiber produces short-chain fatty acids in the colon, which help to stimulate colonic absorption of water and electrolytes; thus it has theoretical advantages. Some patients have more formed stools after addition of fiber, whereas others complain of flatulence, bloating, and worsened diarrhea. If GI disease processes are identified and treated and if medication and infectious causes are ruled out, antidiarrheal medications can be used and enteral feedings continued as tolerated.

10. Should enteral feedings be limited or avoided in a critically ill patient who is hemodynamically unstable?

No, but the subject is controversial. The reduction in splanchnic blood flow in patients who are hypotensive or on vasopressor drugs may interfere with normal gut function. Some clinicians consider this a contraindication to enteral feeding, whereas others use enteral feeding and believe it is beneficial in such patients. If a patient must lie flat or in a prone position, it is prudent to avoid the use of enteral feeding until the patient is stable enough to elevate the head of the bed at least 30°. *ASPEN Practice Guidelines* recommend that in cardiac surgery patients enteral feeding should not be initiated until the patient is hemodynamically stable. If a patient has vascular disease that causes obstruction of blood flow to the intestines, enteral feeding can worsen ischemia and should be avoided.

In their reviews of the literature, Zaloga and colleagues and McClave and Chang recommend that enteral feedings proceed with caution, but only after fluid resuscitation and restoration of adequate perfusion pressure. Feedings may be started at a low rate, 25–30 ml/hour, and the patient should be monitored carefully for signs of intolerance such as abdominal distention, pain, vomiting, or increased gastric drainage. If signs of feeding intolerance occur, radiology tests should be done to look for dilation or the presence of air in the intestines or in the peritoneal space as well as laboratory blood tests for white blood cell count, lactate, and metabolic acidosis.

11. Is inflammatory bowel disease a contraindication to enteral feeding?

No. Enteral feeding is preferred for patients with Crohn's disease and ulcerative colitis, unless the patient has a high-output enterocutaneous fistula, severe diarrhea, or obstruction.

12. Why are some diabetic patients intolerant to nasogastric feedings and what can be done to promote tolerance?

Diabetic patients often have gastroparesis, a condition in which gastric emptying is delayed because of impaired neurologic function. These patients may experience nausea, vomiting, early satiety, and possibly insulin reactions if food remains in the stomach for too long. High gastric residuals (> 200 cc) or vomiting with initiation of enteral feeding are signs of this problem.

Prokinetic drugs, such as metoclopramide or cisapride, may help stimulate gastric emptying. The use of jejunostomy tubes or nasojejunal or gastrojejunal tubes can facilitate enteral feeding in the patient with severe gastroparesis.

13. How does a health care provider determine whether or not a patient with a stroke or head injury requires tube feedings?

If the patient has a functional gut and is unresponsive or too lethargic to eat adequately, and if the patient's condition warrants aggressive or supportive measures, tube feeding is appropriate. If the patient is alert enough to eat orally, a swallowing evaluation or esophageal motility study might be advisable. If dysphagia and significant aspiration risk exists or if the patient lacks a gag reflex, enteral tube feeding is the recommended form of nutritional support.

14. Is tube feeding appropriate in every patient with a functional gut who cannot eat orally?

No. The benefits of providing nutrition support should outweigh any harm or suffering to the patient. If there is no reasonable chance that a patient will improve or recover, and if "quality of life" is determined to be lacking, the situation should be discussed with the patient, or with the patient's family members or legal guardian if applicable, to determine the appropriateness of nutritional support. Some patients prefer that certain life-prolonging procedures not be done in situations in which no hope for recovery or improvement exists. For the patient who cannot communicate, legal guardianship may become necessary for medical decisions. Advanced directives are helpful in determining whether nutrition support should be initiated or continued in end-stage illness or other terminal situations.

15. What are some contraindications to enteral feeding?

Enteral feeding should not be used in situations in which the GI tract is not functional. Specifically, enteral feeding will not be tolerated in such conditions as intractable vomiting, paralytic ileus, intestinal perforation, intestinal obstruction, ischemic bowel, severe diarrhea, severe gastrointestinal hemorrhage, high-output enterocutaneous fistulas, severe enterocolitis, severe malabsorption, and acute intestinal pseudo-obstruction (Ogilvie's syndrome).

Insufficient absorptive capacity of the GI tract will also preclude the use of enteral feeding. Patients who have had resection of a significant amount of small bowel will be unlikely to tolerate enteral feedings or unable to absorb adequate nutrients enterally. Patients undergoing high-dose chemotherapy, radiation treatments, and bone marrow transplant procedures will be unlikely to tolerate enteral feedings because of the damaging effects of these procedures on intestinal mucosa.

Patients who have had massive intestinal resection often require parenteral nutrition indefinitely. Patients with less than 100 cm of small bowel distal to the ligament of Treitz who do not have a colon cannot subsist on enteral or oral feeding alone. If the patient still has a colon, as little as 50 cm of small bowel may be enough to maintain nutritional status on oral and/or enteral nutrition if the patient has had enough time to allow the bowel to adapt. Medications to reduce gastric acid and secretions and antidiarrheal drugs may be necessary.

16. Is enteral feeding appropriate in acute pancreatitis?

Yes. Enteral feedings into the jejunum at, and preferably distal to, the ligament of Treitz are the appropriate way to feed patients with acute pancreatitis who are malnourished or expected to be without adequate nutrition for 5–7 days. Jejunal enteral feedings have been successful in both mild and severe acute pancreatitis. Enteral nutrition is contraindicated only in situations of nonfunction of the intestinal tract, such as ileus, intestinal obstruction, intestinal perforation, or high-output enterocutaneous fistula. Pancreatic enzyme replacement or low fat elemental or semi-elemental enteral feedings may be needed if steatorrhea occurs with feeding. (see Chapter 26).

17. Is enteral feeding contraindicated in hyperemesis gravidarum?

No. Nasogastric feedings have been successful in many patients with hyperemesis during pregnancy. There are fewer reports of successful postpyloric feedings in hyperemesis gravidarum. Enteral nutrition should be initiated at a low rate, continuously, and preferably using an isotonic formula. Parenteral feeding would be necessary only if enteral and oral feeding is not tolerated in sufficient amounts to achieve appropriate weight gain and fetal growth.

BIBLIOGRAPHY

1. ASPEN Board of Directors and the Clinical Guidelines Task Force: Guidelines for the use of parenteral and enteral nutrition in adult and pediatric patients. JPEN 26(Suppl):46SA–50 SA, 61SA–63SA, 68SA–74SA, 90SA–94SA, 2002.
2. Benya R, Layden T, Mobarhan S: Diarrhea associated with tube feeding: The importance of using objective criteria. J Clin Gastroenterol 13:167–172, 1991.
3. Duggan C, Nurko S: "Feeding the gut": The scientific basis for continued enteral nutrition during acute diarrhea. J Pediatr 131:801–808, 1997.
4. Eisenberg P: An overview of diarrhea in the patient receiving enteral nutrition. Gastroenterol Nurs 25:95-104, 2002.
5. Kalfarentzos F, Kehagias J, Mead N, et al: Enteral nutrition is superior to parenteral nutrition in severe acute pancreatitis: Results of a randomized prospective trial. Br J Surg 84:1665–1669, 1997.
6. McClave SA, Chang W: Feeding the hypotensive patient: Does enteral feeding precipitate or protect against ischemic bowel?. Nutr Clin Pract 18:279–284, 2003.
7. McClave SA, Greene LM, Snider HL, et al: Comparison of the safety of early enteral vs parenteral nutrition in mild acute pancreatitis. JPEN 21:14–20, 1997.
8. Patterson ML, Dominguez JM, Lyman B, et al: Enteral feeding in the hypoalbuminemic patient. JPEN 14:362–365, 1990.
9. Reese JL, Means ME, Hanrahan K, et al: Diarrhea associated with nasogastric feedings. Oncol Nurs Forum 23:59–66, 1996.
10. Russell MK, Andrews MR, Brewer CK, et al: Standards for specialized nutrition support: adult hospitalized patients. Nutr Clin Pract 17:384–391, 2002.
11. Wagner BA, Worthington P, Russo-Stieglitz KE, et al: Nutritional management of hyperemesis gravidarum. Nutr Clin Pract 15:65–76, 2000.
12. Williams MS, Harper R, Magnuson B, et al: Diarrhea management in enterally fed patients. Nutr Clin Pract 13:225–229, 1998.
13. Windsor ACJ, Kanwar S, Li AGK, et al: Compared with parenteral nutrition, enteral feeding attenuates the acute phase response and improves disease severity in acute pancreatitis. Gut 42:431–435, 1998.
14. Yoder AJ, Parrish CR, Yeaton P: A retrospective review of the course of patients with pancreatitis discharged on jejunal feedings. Nutr Clin Pract 17:314–320, 2002.
15. Zaloga GP, Roberts PR, Marik P: Feeding the hemodynamically unstable patient: a critical evaluation of the evidence. Nutr Clin Pract 18: 285–293, 2003.

46. TYPES OF ENTERAL NUTRITION

Theresa A. Fessler, MS, RD, CNSD

1. What sources of protein, carbohydrate, and fat are used in enteral formulas?

Protein. Casein is usually the primary protein source, or a mixture of casein and soy protein isolate. Other sources are lactalbumin, egg white solids, pureed beef, and dry milk. Some specialty formulas contain partially hydrolyzed protein: polypeptide fragments or di- and tri-peptides from the protein sources and also from whey, meat, or collagen. "Elemental" and specialty formulas may contain crystalline L-amino acids.

Carbohydrate. Glucose polymers such as maltodextrins, glucose oligo- and polysaccharides, and corn syrup. Modified food starch, starch, sucrose, dextrins, and maltose may also be used.

Fat. Polyunsaturated fatty acids from one or a combination of oils. Corn, safflower, sunflower, soybean, and canola oils. Some formulas also contain medium-chain triglyceride (MCT) oil. Some specialty formulas may contain "structured" lipids, which are reesterified triglycerides containing both long- and medium-chain fatty acids. Omega-3 fatty acids from fish oils are also included in some formulas.

2. Are enteral formulas nutritionally complete?

Most standard polymeric enteral formulas contain all known essential nutrients, with the exception of fiber and phytochemicals, which are found in whole foods. Most formulas provide at or above the recommended dietary allowances for vitamins and minerals when sufficient quantity to provide energy needs is given. Specialty formulas may be deficient in certain nutrients as appropriate for certain disease states. Additional water is usually added to nutrition regimens as formula alone does not provide adequate hydration.

3. How can the types of enteral feedings be classified?

Enteral products can be classified according to various criteria. Products are most commonly divided into classifications based on formula content and intended use. Other possible classification criteria are caloric density, nitrogen content, disease state specificity, or palatability for oral use. Even the simplest categories overlap, and a given product may fit into multiple classifications. Enteral feedings are usually divided into the categories of "standard formulas," "modular components," and "specialty formulas."

4. What are the benefits of using standard formulas?

Standard formulas are appropriate for stable, hospitalized patients and for those on long-term enteral nutrition support. They provide approximately 1000–1060 calories and 34–44 gm of protein per liter. The standard polymeric formulas are usually well tolerated. They are isotonic and lactose-free while providing essential nutrients in appropriate balance. They can be administered into the stomach, duodenum, or jejunum. Formulas can be individualized to particular patient requirements by using modular components in the nutrition regimen, if necessary. Because they are less costly than specialty products, they can be used at low rates to establish feeding tolerance before switching to more expensive specialty formulas.

Some concentrated products may be considered "standard" because they are nutritionally complete and appropriate for long-term bolus, gravity, or pump feedings by patients in the home care setting. Many patients and clinicians prefer concentrated formulas for long-term use because the patient can infuse the required quantity of formula more quickly and conveniently than with a dilute formula and provide remaining fluid needs with additional water flushes throughout the day. Typical concentrated standard formulas contain 1200–1500 calories and 55–68 gm of protein per liter.

5. Why do some enteral formulas contain fiber?

Fiber is generally used to help promote bowel regularity, especially for patients who receive long-term enteral feeding. Soluble fiber has been known to increase transit time in the colon and may promote the development of formed stools. Insoluble fiber may decrease transit time in the colon and increase fecal mass, thus promoting bowel regularity. Soluble fiber ferments in the colon, producing short-chain fatty acids, which are nutrients for colon mucosal cells and can have a trophic effect on mucosa and decrease the risk of bacterial translocation. Soluble fiber is thought to delay glucose absorption for better glucose control for diabetic patients. However, fiber can increase flatulence and distention, which may cause significant discomfort for some patients.

Although fiber has been categorized as soluble and insoluble in recent years, this distinction depends on methods of analysis and does not necessarily determine which benefits a certain fiber has. Because some soluble and insoluble fibers can share the same types of physiologic effects, classification is likely be changed to one that groups fibers based on their health benefits.

If a fiber-containing product is not available at an institution, a separate fiber supplement can be mixed with water and administered into the feeding tube. Care should be taken to provide adequate free water with fiber to avoid intestinal obstruction. Also, tubes should be flushed afterward to prevent clogging.

6. What types of fiber are used in enteral formulas?

Soy polysaccharide is a commonly used fiber source because of its solubility and because it has only a small effect on the viscosity of the formula. Soy polysaccharide contains both soluble and insoluble fibers. Other fibers currently used in enteral formulas are microcrystalline cellulose, carboxymethyl cellulose, partially hydrolyzed guar gum, gum arabic (acacia), and oat fiber. One manufacturer uses fruits and vegetables as the fiber source for its blenderized product.

7. What kind of formula can be used for a patient with a milk allergy?

True milk allergy is caused by a reaction to one of the proteins in milk. A formula should be used that does not contain milk protein. As noted above, most formulas contain casein. Whey and lactalbumin also come from milk and can be problematic in an allergic patient. Soy-based or other formulas without casein are indicated for patients with true milk allergy. Milk allergy should not be confused with lactose intolerance.

8. What formulas should be used in lactose-intolerant patients?

Standard formulas can be used without difficulty. Most enteral formulas and oral supplements are lactose free, even though they may contain casein. Milk-based products that contain lactose should be avoided, such as instant breakfast drink mix and formulas with dry milk solids.

Lactose, which is the sugar found in milk, is not well tolerated by patients who lack the enzyme lactase in the intestinal brush border. Because the lactose is not digested in the small intestine, it is broken down by colonic bacterial enzymes into monosaccharides and then to acids. Gas production, osmotic diarrhea, and irritation of the colon occur. The patient complains of flatulence, bloating, and diarrhea. Most such patients simply avoid milk and milk products. If it is important that the patient drink milk, a product that digests lactose is available to add to milk. This makes it possible for lactose-intolerant patients to drink milk without gastrointestinal side effects.

9. When should concentrated enteral formulas be used?

A formula is considered to be concentrated if it provides 1.5–2 calories per milliliter. The major advantage is fluid restriction. Fluid restriction is sometimes necessary in conditions such as renal failure, liver failure, congestive heart failure, pulmonary edema, complications of head injury, or the syndrome of inappropriate antidiuretic hormone (SIADH). Use of a concentrated formula can provide all nutrients in only 1000–1200 ml per day.

A concentrated formula might also be used in a situation of hypermetabolism, in order to provide a large amount of nutrients in a limited volume. For orally fed patients, with extreme weakness, early satiety, or anorexia, concentrated oral supplements are used to provide as much nutrition as possible in a limited volume.

10. What is the purpose of high protein or "high nitrogen" formulas?

High protein formulas are designed for use in hypermetabolic patients to deliver a maximal amount of protein to help with healing and to minimize nitrogen losses. Patients with trauma, head injury, spinal cord injury, pressure ulcers, burns, cellulitis, and other wounds benefit from high protein formulas. High protein formulas are also appropriate for obese critically ill or stressed patients who are on hypocaloric high protein nutrition regimens. High protein formulas are contraindicated in nondialyzed renal patients with azotemia and in patients with severe hepatic encephalopathy that is unresponsive to pharmacotherapy.

The term *high nitrogen* (HN), as listed in some product names, is used to mean high protein simply because amino acids, of which protein is made, contain nitrogen. An average of 1 gm of nitrogen is contained in every 6.25 gm of dietary protein. A patient's dietary nitrogen intake, along with laboratory measurement of urinary nitrogen, can give clinicians an idea of protein status and needs.

11. Why and in what situations are special renal formulas necessary?

Patients with advanced chronic renal failure who are not yet dialyzed are typically restricted in intake of water, electrolytes, and protein. Renal formulas were designed to minimize accumulation of water in the body as well as accumulation of electrolytes and urea nitrogen in the bloodstream. Renal formulas contain restricted amounts of potassium, sodium, magnesium, and phosphorus. Some are lower in vitamin A and all are lower in vitamin D than standard formulas because of altered metabolism in renal failure.

For patients who are dialyzed regularly, restrictions in fluid, electrolytes, and protein can be relaxed. In fact, it is important that malnourished and stressed catabolic patients receive adequate protein because of high metabolic needs as well as amino acid losses during dialysis. Patients on hemodialysis and peritoneal dialysis require higher amounts of protein that may not be provided by current renal formulations. For those who receive continuous arteriovenous or venovenous hemodialysis (CAVHD or CVVHD), protein and electrolyte restrictions typically are not needed, and standard or high-protein enteral products can be used.

Renal formulas are useful for fluid and electrolyte restriction but have some disadvantages. They are more expensive than standard products, and additional protein is often necessary, using a separate protein supplement. Renal formulas are high in fat, at 35% to > 45% of total calories.

12. Are diabetic formulas better than standard formulas in achieving glucose control?

Special formulas for glucose intolerance are designed with less carbohydrate, more fat, and added fiber. These formulas provide 34–40% of calories as carbohydrate, 40–45% as fat, and 17–20% as protein. Initial studies that showed effectiveness were done in healthy patients who drank the product. The amount of carbohydrate is the most significant factor in blood glucose control. Although fat and fiber may slow gastric emptying and fiber is thought to delay glucose absorption in the gut, the clinical effectiveness of these factors is not well documented. The necessity or effectiveness of these formulas compared with standard formulas in enterally fed diabetic patients has yet to be established. Many hospitals do not carry special diabetic formulas because of the lack of sufficient proof that they are truly effective.

13. What are hepatic formulas and when is their use appropriate?

Hepatic formulas were designed to restrict protein, fluid, and sodium for patients with liver failure. They contain a higher percentage of branched-chain amino acids (BCAA) and a lower amount of aromatic amino acids than standard formulas. They also are high in carbohydrate and low in total fat, with a larger percentage of fat from medium-chain triglyceride (MCT) oil.

Serum BCAAs are decreased below normal in patients with hepatic failure, whereas levels of aromatic amino acids are increased. This abnormality has been believed to be the cause of hepatic encephalopathy. Thus a product that contains higher amounts of BCAA has a theoretical advantage. In cholestatic liver disease, there is less production of bile acids, and some patients with alcoholic liver disease may have exocrine pancreatic insufficiency, limiting the digestion of dietary fats. MCT oil requires less bile acids and lipase for digestion; thus it is better utilized in patients with fat malabsorption.

Most patients with liver disease are severely malnourished and need adequate protein for repletion. Protein restriction and use of specialized hepatic formulas are not indicated unless the patient has acute hepatic encephalopathy that is not responsive to pharmacotherapy. The effectiveness of hepatic formulas on clinical outcome is still uncertain, and there is no consensus among clinicians on their use. Disadvantages include very high carbohydrate content and considerably higher cost than standard formulas.

14. What is the rationale for a specialized pulmonary formula?

Pulmonary formulas are designed with lower amounts of carbohydrate and a higher percentage of calories from fat (40–55%) than standard formulas. They are moderately fluid-restricted, with 1.5 calories/ml. Pulmonary formulas are intended for use in patients with respiratory failure who are on mechanical ventilation and for patients with chronic obstructive pulmonary disease or respiratory problems associated with cystic fibrosis.

The purpose of the lower carbohydrate formulation is to decrease carbon dioxide (CO_2) production, resulting in a lower respiratory quotient (RQ). RQ is the ratio of CO_2 produced to oxygen consumed in metabolism. Fat has a lower RQ (0.7) than carbohydrate (1.0). The theory is that a lower RQ decreases CO_2 retention and decreases CO_2 production to facilitate weaning from the ventilator.

Due to lack of adequate studies, the possible clinical benefit of this formula has not been established. Overfeeding of total calories, regardless of formula type, causes an increase in CO_2 production and delays ventilator weaning. When overfeeding is avoided, percentage of calories from fat has not been found to be a significant factor. It is more important to avoid excessive calorie administration than to provide a specialty formula for ventilated patients; thus routine use of specialty pulmonary formulas is not recommended.

15. What is the significance of elemental formulas?

Elemental formulas contain protein that has been partially hydrolyzed to peptides or totally hydrolyzed to free amino acids. Most elemental formulas are low or very low in total fat and contain MCT oil as a significant percentage of the fat content. They are used in clinical situations in which rapid absorption from the small bowel is desired, such as in exacerbation of inflammatory bowel disease, malabsorption, or short bowel syndrome. Because of their low viscosity, they are sometimes used for patients who have needle catheter jejunostomy tubes, because these very small-bore tubes are more likely to clog with polymeric formulas.

Free amino acids were once thought to be better absorbed in patients with malabsorption or severe stress, but further studies have shown that peptides of varying chain length are better absorbed. Although elemental formulas are marketed for use in stressed patients, clinical evidence of significant advantages compared with polymeric formulas is lacking in most situations.

Very low fat elemental formulas that contain MCT oil are sometimes used for patients who do not tolerate polymeric formulas, such as those with pancreatitis and pancreatic exocrine insufficiency. Because medium chain fatty acids are not transported in chyle and do not contribute significantly to the triglyceride content of lymphatic fluid, MCT-containing formulas are sometimes used for patients with chylous ascites, chylothorax, and lymphatic obstruction or other defects in lymphatic transport.

16. What are immune-enhancing formulas? In what situations might their use be beneficial?

Formulas containing arginine, glutamine, nucleotides, and omega three fatty acids have been developed with the intent of improved immune response in critically ill septic, trauma, surgical, and burn patients. The amino acids arginine and glutamine and nucleotides (components of nucleic acids) have been associated with enhanced cellular immune function. Nucleotides and glutamine also function in growth of intestinal mucosal cells. Omega three fatty acids modulate the inflammatory response as they are precursors to certain prostaglandins and leukotrienes that are less inflammatory and do not suppress immune function, whereas large amounts of omega-six fatty acids can be proinflammatory and immunosuppressive.

Studies have compared immune-enhancing formulas with standard formulas in elective surgery, critically ill intensive care, and critically ill trauma and burn patients. Formulas containing omega three fatty acids have been shown to decrease length of time on ventilator support for patients with acute respiratory distress syndrome. Elective surgery patients on immunonutrition have decreased infectious complications and shorter length of hospital stay with no adverse effect on mortality. The effect of immunonutrition in other critically ill patients is less clear. Some reviewers suggest a trend toward increased mortality with use of immunonutrition compared with standard formulas in certain subgroups of severely septic patients.

At the time of this writing, the use of immunonutrition is controversial and should be done with careful consideration of each patient's clinical situation. A clear understanding of the clinical effects of each individual immunonutrient is not possible because of differences in study designs, patient populations, amounts of formula actually administered, control formulas, and the amounts of each immunonutrient in the different formulas available. Further research in this area will be helpful.

17. What is glutamine and why is it supplemented in some formulas?

Glutamine is the most abundant free amino acid in the body. While it can be synthesized in the body, it may be conditionally essential in stress states. It is the major amino acid involved in interorgan metabolism. During stress, glutamine uptake from intestine and transport from muscle and lung tissue may increase, as may cellular requirements for glutamine. Glutamine is an important fuel for intestinal mucosa and may help in maintaining mucosal growth and repair. It is also reported to decrease the incidence of bacteremia in animal studies. Glutamine is added to some formulas designed for stressed patients and is sometimes used for patients with intestinal damage. Clinical benefits of enteral glutamine supplementation in humans have not been proven (see Chapter 33, Glutamine and Arginine).

18. What are "modular" feedings? In what situations are they useful?

Modular feedings are components that provide just one macronutrient—protein, carbohydrate, fat, or fiber. They are used in situations in which one or more nutrients must be restricted and/or when additional calories or protein is required. Modular feedings can be administered as boluses in feeding tubes (mixed with water, if in powder form) or mixed into formulas, foods, and drinks. Additional calories can be provided by modular fat or carbohydrate sources. Water itself can be considered a modular nutrient also. Water flushes are typically ordered to provide adequate hydration, because enteral formulas do not contain adequate water to meet fluid requirements in most stable patients. Some commonly available modular feedings are described below.

Protein. Protein powders are made with intact protein, usually casein or whey. Some are made with egg white. Protein powders provide approximately 3-4 grams of protein per tablespoon, or 6 gm per scoop (scoop included with product). Amino acid supplements are also available in powdered form, such as glutamine and arginine.

Carbohydrate. Glucose polymers or maltodextrins are available in either powdered or liquid form. They contribute to osmolality, but not as much as simple sugars. A glucose polymer product currently on the market provides 23 calories per tablespoon, or 3.8 calories/gm.

Fat. Vegetable oils provide polyunsaturated fatty acids, which require normal digestive and absorptive capacity. Regular safflower, corn, or soybean oil provides 8 calories/ml. A commercially available 50% safflower oil emulsion provides 4.5 calories/ml. MCT oil contains fatty acids primarily of 8 and 10 carbon atoms in length and is useful for patients who are unable to digest or absorb regular dietary fats. MCT oil requires less digestion by pancreatic lipase or bile salts. Medium chain fatty acids are transported directly to the liver for oxidation and not carried by the lymphatic system, as long chain fatty acids are. MCT oil provides 7.7 calories/ml.

Fiber. Various fiber supplements are on the market. Fiber can be mixed with water and bolused into feeding tubes. Tubes should be flushed after fiber administration to help prevent tube clogging. Extra care should be taken with small bore feeding tubes.

19. How are oral supplements different from products made for tube feeding?
Oral nutritional supplements are intended for patients who have poor appetite or who have difficulty eating enough regular foods to obtain adequate nutrition. Products made for oral use contain flavoring and more simple sugars than products developed for enteral use only. Oral products have a higher osmolality than standard enteral formulas. Oral products are packaged in single-serving cans or boxes for convenience. They can also be used for bolus tube feedings into the stomach.

BIBLIOGRAPHY

1. Allen EM, van Heeckeren DW, Spector ML, et al: Management of nutritional and infectious complications of postoperative chylothorax in children. J Pediatr Surg 26:1169–1174, 1991.
2. American Society for Parenteral and Enteral Nutrition, Board of Directors: The ASPEN Nutrition Support Practice Manual. Silver Spring, MD, American Society for Parenteral and Enteral Nutrition, 1998.
3. ASPEN Board of Directors and the Clinical Guidelines Task Force: Guidelines for the use of parenteral and enteral nutrition in adult and pediatric patients. JPEN 26 (Suppl):52SA–56 SA, 63SA–68SA, 78SA–80 SA, 88SA–93SA, 2002.
4. Beale RJ, Bryg DJ, Bihari DJ: Immunonutrition in the critically ill: A systematic review of clinical outcome. Crit Care Med 27:2799–2805, 1999.
5. Burge JC, Goon A, Choban PS, et al: Efficacy of hypocaloric total parenteral nutrition in hospitalized obese patients: A prospective, double-blind randomized trial. JPEN 18:203–207, 1994.
6. Celona-Jacobs N, Lipson DA, Unger LD, et al: Improvement of chronic chylous pleural effusion using a restricted fat diet and medium chain triglycerides in a patient with congenital lymphangiectasia. Nutr Clin Pract 15:127-129, 2000.
7. Dickerson RN, Boschert KJ, Kudsk KA, et al: Hypocaloric enteral tube feeding in critically ill obese patients. Nutrition 18:241–246, 2002.
8. Fabbri A, Magrini N, Bianchi G, et al: Overview of randomized clinical trials of oral branched-chain amino acid treatment in chronic hepatic encephalopathy. JPEN 20:159–164, 1996.
9. Gadek JE, DeMichele SJ, Karlstad MD, et al: Effect of enteral feeding with eicosapenaeoic acid, gamma-linolenic acid, and antioxidants in patients with acute respiratory distress syndrome. Crit Care Med 27:1409–1420, 1999.
10. Galban C, Montejo JC, Mesejo A, et al: An immune-enhancing enteral diet reduces mortality rate and episodes of bacteremia in septic intensive care unit patients. Crit Care Med 28:643–648, 2000.
11. Heyland DK, Novak F: Immunonutrition in the critically ill patient: More harm than good? JPEN 25(Suppl):S51–S54, 2001.
12. Jurkovitch GJ: Outcome studies using immune-enhancing diets: Blunt and penetrating torso trauma patients. JPEN 25(Suppl):S14–S17, 2001.
13. Kopple JD: The nutrition management of the patient with acute renal failure. JPEN 20:3–12, 1996.
14. Macias WL, Alaka KJ, Murphy MH, et al: Impact of the nutritional regimen on protein catabolism and nitrogen balance in patients with acute renal failure. JPEN 20:56–62, 1996.
15. Marchesini G, Bianchi G, Rossi B, et al: Nutritional treatment with branched-chain amino acids in advanced liver cirrhosis. J Gastroenterol 35(Suppl):7–12, 2000.
16. Marlett JA, McBurney MI, Slavin JL: Position of the American Dietetic Association: Health implications of dietary fiber. J Am Diet Assoc 102:993–1000, 2002.
17. Martindale RG, Cresci GA: Use of immune-enhancing diets in burns. JPEN 25(Suppl):S24–S26, 2001.
18. McClave SA: The effects of immune-enhancing diets (IEDs) on mortality, hospital length of stay, duration of mechanical ventilation, and other parameters. JPEN 25(Suppl):S 44–S49, 2001.
19. McCowan KC, Bistrian BR: Immunonutrition: Problematic or problem solving? Am J Clin Nutr 77:764–770, 2003.
20. Oltermann MH, Rassas TN: Immunonutrition in a multidisciplinary ICU population: A review of the literature. JPEN 25(Suppl):S30–S34, 2001.
21. Russell MK, Charney P: Is there a role for specialized enteral nutrition in the intensive care unit? Nutr Clin Pract 17:156–168, 2002.
22. Sax HC: Effect of Immune enhancing formulas (IEF) in general surgery patients. JPEN 25(Suppl):S19–S22, 2001.
23. Schloerb PR: Immune-enhancing diets: products, components, and their rationale. JPEN 25(Suppl):S3–S7, 2001.
24. Talpers SS, Romberger DJ, Bunce SB, et al: Nutritionally associated increased carbon dioxide production. Excess total calories versus high proportion of carbohydrate calories. Chest 102:551–555, 1992.
25. Van den Berg B, Stam H: Metabolic and respiratory effects of enteral nutrition in patients during mechanical ventilation. Intens Care Med 14:206–211, 1988.

47. ENTERAL ACCESS

Mark H. DeLegge, MD, FACG

1. Why is enteral access important?

Enteral feeding, fluids, and many medications cannot be delivered in patients who cannot or will not eat without the presence of enteral access. The clinician who practices nutritional support must have knowledge of enteral access tubes, the variety of placement techniques, their indications, and their complications.

2. What are the types of enteral access devices?

Enteral access tubes provide a means through which nutrients, water, or medications can be delivered to the gastrointestinal tract. The majority of these tubes are made of soft materials, such as polyurethane or silicone. Most feeding tubes have a diameter range of 8–24 fr. (2.6–8 mm). These measurements are of the external diameter of the tubes. The actual internal diameter of the feeding tubes can be much smaller. Enteral feeding tubes may be divided into two categories: short-term access tubes (required for 4 weeks or less) or long-term tubes (required for > 4 weeks).

3. What should be used for short-term enteral access?

Short-term access tubes are oro/nasogastric or oro/nasojejunal feeding tubes. Some clinicians believe that the prolonged use (> 1 week) of a nasogastric or nasojejunal feeding tube can lead to the development of otitis, sinusitis, and fever. These same clinicians believe in the use of orogastric and orojejunal tubes to prevent such complications. Both oroenteric and nasoenteric tubes are subject to early failure secondary to clogging or displacement.

4. How are nasoenteric or oroenteric tubes placed?

Placement of an oro/nasogastric tube is generally accomplished at the bedside. These tubes often have an enclosed stylet to stiffen the tube for forward passage. After tube lubrication, the patient's head is flexed forward. The tip of the gastric tube is passed into the oral or nasal cavity. The patient is asked to sip water as the tube is passed forward, generally to a length of 55–60 cm. If the patient has a depressed level of consciousness, the gastric tube must be advanced without the benefit of the patient assisting by swallowing.

Placement of an oro/nasojejunal tubes is more difficult. Passage to the gastric cavity is accomplished as described above. The patient is then placed, if possible, on the left side while the tube is advanced slowly. The jejunal feeding tube is slowly rotated clockwise as the tube is advanced to its final location. Pharmacologic means of stimulating gastric muscle contractions, such as intravenous metoclopramide or erythromycin, may be used to assist in jejunal tube passage from the stomach to the small intestine, although their effectiveness remains controversial.

5. Are there other methods to assist in the passage of oro/naso feeding tubes?

When bedside placement of oro/naso feeding tubes is unsuccessful, either endoscopic or fluroscopic methods can be used to assist successful feeding tube passage. With endoscopy, the physician is able to visualize directly the stomach and small bowel as the feeding tube is pushed or pulled into position. With fluoroscopy, the feeding tube may be advanced into position as its forward progress is monitored by fluroscopic visualization.

6. How do you check for adequate placement of oro/nasoenteric feeding tubes?

Before feeding, the tip of a gastric or jejunal feeding tube must be confirmed to be in proper position to prevent associated complications, especially tube feeding-related aspiration. The many methods proposed for confirming the location of a feeding tube tip include auscultation of a bolus of air passed through the tube, color of fluid withdrawn from the tube, or checking the pH of material aspirated through the tube. None of these methods should be relied on to initiate tube feeding. Only radiographic confirmation of the tube tip location should be used to confirm its exact location.

7. When should you use a nasojejunal tube vs. a nasogastric tube?

Nasojejunal tubes are much more difficult to place into the small intestine than a nasogastric tube is to place into the stomach. This difficulty may result in a significant delay in initiating tube feedings in patients who require a nasojejunal feeding tube. Nasojejual feeding tubes should be used only in patients who have gastroparesis, an intolerance to gastric feedings, a significantly altered gastric anatomy that prevents adequate feeding, or significant risk for tube-feeding aspiration.

8. What are the complications of naso- and oroenteric feeding tubes?

Complications of nasoenteric tubes include otitis, sinusitis, pharyngitis, nasopharyngeal ulceration, tube clogging, and early displacement, usually from the patient removing the feeding tube. Occasionally, the tip of the feeing tube may cause small bowel or gastric ulcerations. Oroenteric tubes are subject to the same complications as nasoenteric tubes except for a presumptive decrease in both otitis and sinusitis.

9. How are naso- and oroenteric feeding tubes secured?

Because of the frequency of displacement of oro/nasoenteric tubes, securing them to a patient's nose or face is important. Many institutions simply tape an oroenteric tube to the side of a patient's face or to the endotracheal tube if the patient is also intubated. Nasoenteric tubes are frequently attached to the nose with tape or a commercially available adhesive bandage. Some clinicians sew the nasoenteric tube to the nasal septum, although this technique is not recommended because of the potential trauma to the nasal septum. Other clinicians use a bridle; a small (5-fr) tube passed through one nare, around the nasopharynx, and out the opposite nare, allowing the feeding tube to be tied into position.

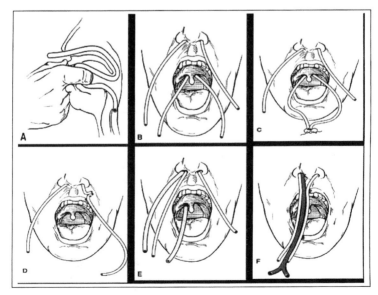

Bridling nasoenteric tubes. (Reprinted with permission from Dr. Stephan McClave, University of Louisville Medical Center.)

10. What is used for feeding tube occlusion?

Feeding tube occlusion can occur with any feeding tube and is usually secondary to medications or tube feeding. The proven method of feeding tube clearance consists of instillation of warm water into the tube and gentle agitation by slowly pushing and pulling the warm water with an attached 30- to 60-cc syringe. The use of pancreatic enzymes mixed with sodium bicarbonate may assist in the dissolving of tube-feeding precipitate No other fluid (e.g., Coca-Cola, cranberry juice, or meat tenderizer) has been shown to be effective in clearing a clogged feeding tube. In extreme circumstances, a small brush on a catheter, such as an endoscopic retrograde cholangiopancreatography (ERCP) cytology brush, may be used to clear small diameter feeding tubes (8–14 fr). Larger diameter feeding tubes (16–28 fr) may be cleared with commercially available percutaneous endoscopic gastrostomy (PEG) brushes.

11. What are long-term enteral access devices?

Long-term enteral access devices include PEG tubes, percutaneous endoscopic gastric/jejunostomy (PEG/J), direct percutaneous jejunostomy (DPEJ), surgical gastrostomy, and surgical jejunostomy. These feeding tubes generally range in size from 8 fr to 28 fr, with the smaller diameter tubes used for jejunal access and the larger diameter tubes used for gastric access. PEG tubes and surgical gastrostomies are used for gastric access. Percutaneous endoscopic gastro/jejunostomy, DPEJ, and surgical jejunostomy are used for small bowel access. Percutaneous endoscopic feeding tubes (PEG, PEG/J, and DPEJ) are placed in the endoscopy suite or at the patient's bedside under conscious sedation with an endoscope. Surgical feeding tubes are usually placed in the operating room. In the PEG/J procedure, a PEG tube (18–28 fr) is placed into the stomach and a separate jejunal feeding tube (9–12 fr) is passed through the PEG tube into the small intestine. This approach allows the clinician to feed the patient through the jejunal tube and concurrently decompress the patient through the gastric tube. A DPEJ tube can be 10–24 fr in size and is placed with an endoscope directly into the small bowel. There is no opening to the stomach. If gastric decompression is necessary, a separate gastrostomy or PEG tube should be placed.

Percutaneous Endoscopic Gastro/Jejunostomy Systems (PEG/J)*

PEG TUBE SIZE	CORRESPONDING JEJUNAL TUBE SIZE
28 fr	12 fr
24 fr	12 fr
22 fr	9 fr
20 fr	9 fr
18 fr	9 fr

* These systems allow concurrent jejunal feeding and gastric decompression.

12. What are the complications of PEG, PEG/J, and DPEJ tubes?

Percutaneous endoscopic gastrostomies, PEG/J, and DPEJ are associated with complications related to the feeding tube passing through the abdominal wall into the stomach or small intestine, or to the endoscopic procedure itself.

Aspiration. Intraprocedure oropharyngeal aspiration is common during PEG, PEG/J, or DPEJ placement, although usually not life-threatening. Pneumonia may develop. It may be treated with antibiotics.

Colocutaneous fistula. During PEG placement, the feeding tube may be passed through the colon prior to entering the stomach. This may lead to peritoneal infection or stool leakage around the PEG site on the abdominal wall. More commonly, this complication is not noticed until the original PEG tube is removed, and a replacement balloon tip PEG tube is passed back through the same PEG site at the patient's bedside. The tip of the replacement PEG tube finds its way back into the colon but cannot find the opening (fistula) from the colon back into the stomach. After tube feedings are reinitiated, diarrhea and dehydration develop as the tube feeding is instilled directly into the colon. To fix this complication, the feeding tube needs to be completely removed and a new PEG tube placed at a separate site. Occasionally, surgical repair of the fistula is required.

Skin infection/wound breakdown. Other complications of PEG, DPEJ, or PEG/J placement are related to infection or breakdown of the PEG or DPEJ wound site. The use of antibiotics prior to the PEG, PEG/J, or DPEJ procedure reduces the development of skin site infections. After PEG, PEG/J, or DPEJ placement, an external bolster is placed over the feeding tube and moved toward the abdominal skin surface. This bolster is usually in a bar or disc design. External bolsters must be placed in loose proximity to the abdominal skin surface. Tight apposition leads to blood flow compromise, wound infection, and wound breakdown, allowing gastric contents to spill onto the abdominal skin surface with the development of infection, erosions, and ulcerations. If wound breakdown occurs, a barrier cream should be applied to the surrounding abdominal wall skin surface. Occasionally, an ostomy pouch needs to be placed over the wound to capture gastric secretions. The patient should also be placed on an acid-suppressing medication to minimize abdominal wall skin damage from gastric acid. Placing a larger replacement tube into the PEG, PEG/J, or DPEJ tract causes further tract breakdown. Sometimes, the feeding tube must be completely removed and a new feeding tube placed at a different site on the abdominal wall.

Buried bumper. Occasionally, the internal bolster of the feeding tube becomes buried in the abdominal wall. This leads to pain, peri-PEG or peri-DPEJ tube leakage, and difficulty with infusing formula through the tube. Treatment requires removing the PEG or DPEJ tube and placing a new tube through the same or a new site on the abdominal wall.

Early displacement. One of the gravest complications of PEG, PEG/J, or DPEJ tube placement is early displacement of the feeding tube. At this point, the gastric or jejunal wall and the abdominal wall have not healed together to form a tract from the outside of the patient to the stomach or small intestine. Leakage of gastric or small bowel contents into the peritoneal cavity may occur with the development of peritonitis. More ominously, a clinician may pass a replacement PEG or DPEJ tube at the bedside. Because the tract has not healed together, the feeding tube may pass directly through the tract into the peritoneal cavity rather than into the stomach or small bowel. The initiation of tube feedings quickly leads to peritonitis and sepsis. With the placement of surgical gastrostomies or jejunostomies, the small bowel or stomach is sewn to the abdominal wall. In such cases, early feeding tube displacement does not lead to the stomach or small bowel falling away from the abdominal wall. However, gastrostomy and jejunostomy site infections and peritubular leakage are more common with these surgical procedures. In addition, surgical gastrostomies and jejunostomies are usually placed in the operating room with general anesthesia.

13. How are PEG, PEG/J, and DPEJ site infections prevented?

Percutaneous feeding-tube skin site infections can be prevented by the use of preprocedure intravenous antibiotics and a clean surgical technique during placement of the feeding tube. Once the tube is in place, the first week of feeding tube wound site care is very important. The wound should be clear of blood, secretions, and other contaminants. This goal may be accomplished by the use of hydrogen peroxide for cleansing the feeding tube site and a gauze sponge placed over the wound daily during the first week. The gauze sponge should be a notched or tracheostomy sponge placed over the external bumper of the PEG tube. Placing the sponge between the external bumper and the abdominal wall leads to tissue compression and potential breakdown of the wound. Subsequently, the wound may be cleansed with soap and water and covered as needed for protection of the wound or to prevent gastric or small bowel leakage onto the patient's clothes.

14. What is a gastric residual? How should it be utilized?

A gastric residual is the amount of fluid (secretions, medications, and tube feedings) in the gastric cavity at any point in time. Typically, residuals are checked on an intermittent basis, such as every 8 hours when continuous feedings are used and before each feeding when bolus feedings are used. A 60-cc syringe is attached to the end of the PEG or gastrostomy tube, and all fluid within reach of the tip of the tube is withdrawn. If the residual is less than 200 cc, the residual is placed back into the stomach and tube feeding is continued. If the residual is between 200 and

400 cc, the residual is placed back into the stomach and rechecked in 2 hours. Feedings are held. In 2 hours, if the residual remains greater than 200 cc or if the original residual was greater than 400 cc, the feedings should be held and the physician called. A decision may be made to reduce the rate or amount of tube-feeding infusion, to add a gastric motility pharmacologic agent, or to place a jejunal feeding tube to bypass the stomach. If the rechecked residual is less than 200 cc, tube feedings can be restarted. Small bowel residuals are generally not checked. If the feeding tube has a small diameter (12 fr or less), frequent checking for small bowel residuals may lead to feeding tube occlusion with a precipitate of tube feeding or medication.

15. How can the risk of tube-feeding aspiration be minimized?
The risk of tube-feeding aspiration with gastric feedings may be minimized by the placement of a jejunal feeding tube. Options include a PEG/J to allow gastric decompression and jejunal feeding, a DPEJ, or surgical jejunostomy. In addition, the head of the patient's bed should be raised at 30° or greater. Gastric feedings should be frequently checked (at least every 8 hours) to monitor for signs of gastric intolerance of tube feedings. A promotility pharmacologic agent may aid with gastric emptying.

16. When should a percutaneous endoscopic gastrojejunostomy (PEG/J) tube be placed?
A PEG/J tube should be placed when a patient requires jejunal feeding for less than 6 months. It is also an appropriate enteral tube system for the patient who requires both jejunal feeding and gastric decompression, such as the patient with gastroparesis and tube-feeding aspiration. These tubes are not appropriate for long-term (> 6 month) jejunal feeding because they are subject to jejunal tube clogging, kinking, and migration or displacement of the jejunal feeding tube tip from the small intestine into the stomach.

17. When should a DPEJ tube be placed?
A DPEJ should be placed in patients who require jejunal feeding for greater than 6 months. In such patients, if gastric decompression is also necessary, a separate PEG or surgical gastrostomy tube can be placed.

18. What are the indications for radiologic PEG, PEG/J, or PEJ placement?
Fluroscopic placement of feeding tubes is usually performed by an interventional radiologist. The radiologist can provide access to either the stomach or small intestine. These feeding tubes usually have a diameter of 10–16 fr. If the radiologist wants to access the small intestine, the feeding tube is placed through the stomach into the small bowel and not directly through the abdominal wall into the small intestine. Patients who physically cannot tolerate general anesthesia or conscious sedation are good candidates for fluroscopically placed feeding tubes. Patients who cannot have endoscopy because of oral or esophageal obstruction are also good candidates. In some medical centers, the radiologist is the expert in enteral access because of experience with the procedures.

19. What are the indications for surgical gastrostomy or jejunostomy tube placement?
Surgical gastrostomy and jejunostomy are usually performed in the operating room. If a patient is going to the operating room for another procedure, such as a tracheostomy, the feeding tube should be placed during the same anesthesia session. In addition, if anatomy makes placement of an endoscopic or radiologic feeding tube technically impossible, placement of surgical feeding tubes is appropriate.

BIBLIOGRAPHY

1. DeLegge MH: Enteral access—the foundation of feeding. J Parent Ent Nutr 25(S):S8–S13, 2000.
2. DiSario JA, Baskin WN, Brown RD, et al: Endoscopic approaches to enteral nutrition support. Gastrointest Endosc 57:901–908, 2002.
3. Fleming CR, Kirby DF, DeLegge MH: American Gastroenterological Association technical review on tube feeding for enteral nutrition. Gastroenterology 108:1282–1301, 1995.
4. Kirby DF, Kudsk KA: Obtaining and maintaining access for nutrition support. In Kudsk KA, Pritchard C (eds): From Nutrition Support to Pharmacologic Nutrition. Berlin, Springer-Verlag, 2000, pp 125–137.

48. HOME ENTERAL NUTRITION

Carol Ireton-Jones, PhD, RD, LD, CNSD, FACN, Mark H. DeLegge, MD, FACG, and Melinda Pine, RD, LD, CNSD

1. Who should receive home enteral support?

Home enteral nutrition support should be used in patients who cannot meet their nutrient requirements by oral intake and who are able to receive therapy outside of an acute care setting (ASPEN Guidelines for Parenteral and Enteral Nutrition Support). The indications for home enteral nutrition support are the same as those for the use of enteral nutrition support in the hospital in that the gastrointestinal tract should be functional. Home enteral nutrition is often used for people requiring longer-term or life-time nutrition support with diagnoses such as swallowing disorders secondary to stroke or neuromuscular illness, head and neck cancers, or gastroparesis. The patient's and caregiver's ability to be trained and perform the tasks associated with home enteral feeding as well as financial status and home environment should be evaluated before sending a patient home.

2. When should the home nutrition plan be determined?

The home nutrition support plan should be developed as a part of the discharge planning. This plan includes evaluation of the home environment and education of the patients and caregiver. Reimbursement for the home enteral formula and supplies should be determined before planning for home enteral feeding because it can be a challenge and the financial burden of providing for the enteral formula and supplies may lie completely with the patient. Therefore, the nutrition care plan may need to be revised to include community resources or an alternative to returning home.

3. What type of gastrointestinal access should you use for a patient with a high aspiration risk?

Feeding tubes placed in the small intestine are most appropriate, whether they are percutaneously or surgically placed jejunostomy or gastrojejunostomy (GJ) tubes. The least risk of aspiration from enteral feeding is via a dual tube system with a large-bore gastrostomy for gastric drainage and a smaller, longer tube passed to the small bowel (GJ). Continuously infused feedings to the small intestine help to decrease the risk of aspiration because the natural barriers of the lower esophageal and pylorus sphincter help reduce reflux. This method has increased expense and restricts patient mobility.

Surgically placed jejunostomy tubes are satisfactory for most patients, but they are subject to major drawbacks (see question 4). Gastrostomy tubes are the least satisfactory because gastroesophageal reflux is common even in normal patients.

4. When should a jejunostomy be used as opposed to a gastrostomy?

Although a tube can be placed through a gastrostomy and threaded into the jejunum using endoscopic techniques, true jejunostomies must usually be done surgically. A loop of bowel is brought up to the abdominal wall, a tube is placed through the abdominal wall into the jejunum, and the jejunum is then attached to the abdominal wall to prevent it from pulling away from the tube. These procedures are subject to complications, particularly small bowel obstruction, leakage, and dislodgment of the tube with leakage into the peritoneal cavity. Jejunostomy tubes may now be placed by endoscopy (PEJ). Because these jejunal tubes are larger, they are less likely to occlude. Jejunal tubes may be replaced at the bedside with balloon tubes, using only 3–5 ml of water or air in the balloon. Jejunostomy tubes may be used with an enteral pump. Jejunostomy tubes may be quite difficult to use at home, but in the patient who cannot tolerate gastric feedings, jejunostomy may be essential.

5. What feeding options are best for a highly motivated patient who wants to maintain a somewhat normal lifestyle?

Although a select group of motivated young adult and adolescent patients may learn to intubate themselves daily using small-bore nasogastric feeding tubes, most active people of all ages prefer a low-profile gastrostomy. They can use bolus or intermittent feedings, which can be accomplished easily using clean technique.

6. What type of feeding is best for a patient whom you want to transition from the enteral feeding program to an oral diet?

Cyclic tube feeding at night provides less interference with oral intake at meals during the day. Early satiety, appetite suppression, and gastric fullness are symptoms experienced during attempts to increase oral intake while the patient is receiving a continuous infusion of nutrients.

7. What are the chronic effects of permanent enteral therapy?

The longer patients are on a home feeding program, the more independent they become in managing their own care and the less it affects their daily activities. Long-term enteral nutrition may often improve the management of other chronic comorbid disease in appropriate populations.

8. How much time do you have to replace a gastrostomy tube that has come out or become dislodged?

Only a few hours because the ostomy site begins to close. Home enteral feeding patients should be informed of this fact and instructed to clean and replace the previous tube until a placement tube is available. When followed by a home care company, the patient should be able to call the company directly. If not, a call to the physician is warranted.

9. Can a leaking feeding tube be fixed?

A leaking tube is probably the most common problem with gastrostomies. Preventive care is important. The stoma sites should be cleaned daily with a 50% solution of hydrogen peroxide and water or with simple soap and water. After initial placement, approximately 1–2 cm should be left between the external bumper of the feeding tube and the abdominal well. This margin avoids tissue pressure necrosis and subsequent tube site leakage and infection. Commercially available devices can be used to control movement of the tube to prevent enlargement of the ostomy site.

Tubes that leak should be considered abnormal, and a surgeon or gastroenterologist should do an evaluation. Often an enterostomal therapist, who is a nurse with specialty training, may be able to help resolve the problem. Changing the tube to a large tube to control the leak rarely works.

Leaking jejunostomy tubes should be subjected to the same regimen. The use of aggressive acid suppression with proton pump inhibitors can reduce gastric secretions and assist in ostomy closure. Antibiotics are indicated if an infection is present. Occasionally the PEG tube needs to be removed and subsequently replaced after the ostomy has closed completely. A leak from a jejunostomy may indicate a more serious problem early after initial placement. The bowel may separate from the abdominal wall, which then causes the tube to migrate into the peritoneal cavity. This migration can lead directly to peritonitis, especially if feedings are continued without paying attention to the leak.

10. How should you treat an obstructed feeding tube at home?

The best approach to tube obstruction is prevention. When acidic material mixes with formula, coagulation may occur. Flushing before and after gastric residual checks prevents gastric secretions from adhering to the tube lumen, decreasing the risk of tube obstruction. Soft, pliable, small-bore feeding tubes and a slow rate of formula infusion have a high incidence of obstruction. Water remains the most effective choice for irrigating feeding tubes. If water fails, pancreolipase may be an effective alternative, although it is not always easy to obtain. Care of the tube should stress:

- Flush the feeding tube with at least 30 ml of water every 4–6 hours during continuous feedings, before and after each intermittent feeding, and before and after checking gastric residuals.
- Use drugs in liquid form if possible; if not, thoroughly crush the pills and dissolve them in 15–30 ml water.
- Do not crush sustained-release or enteric-coated meds. Alternate medications need to be obtained if the patient cannot swallow or gastric absorption or digestion is inadequate.
- If the tube becomes obstructed, flush with water.

In some cases, physicians have passed a 19-gauge, long-line catheter or endoscopic cytology brush through the tube lumen to break up the obstruction. This procedure is effective and relatively safe—in trained hands.

11. Are water flushes necessary to prevent dehydration in patients receiving home enteral nutrition?

Patients receiving home enteral nutrition are at risk for dehydration, especially if they have a decreased level of consciousness. Care should be taken to ensure that total fluid needs are met from free water in formula and multiple flushes throughout the day. Most commercial formulas contain 1 kcal/ml, with approximately 84% free water or 840 ml of free water per liter. Normal fluid requirements for adults are 30–35 ml/kg body weight. Fluid needs should be calculated with appropriate additions if fluid losses are excessive fluid losses (e.g., from diarrhea or fistula). Then fluid needs should be compared with fluid provided by the enteral formula to ensure that the patient receives adequate free water intake. Concentrated formulas pose a greater risk of dehydration because they have lower percentages of free water. An average 2 kcal/ml enteral formula is approximately 70% free water. Use of concentrated formulas requires attention to fluids needs and may require additional provision of free water intermittently.

12. What is the most appropriate way to manage enteral feeding complications such as diarrhea constipation in enteral patients at home?

Home enteral patients often receive little follow-up after discharge. Therefore, when complications arise, it may be difficult for the patient to know whom to contact for assistance in managing diarrhea or other complications such as constipation. Again, the key is education before discharge about potential complications and written materials for patients to keep with them post discharge. If the patient has a home care company that has clinical staff or a clinical dietitian, the patient can contact the home care company for assistance. The patient should contact the primary physician if there is no clinical contact from the company providing the enteral feeding and/or supplies.

Most cases of diarrhea can be prevented or controlled. Common causes are pharmacologic agents (61%); *Clostridium difficile* infection (17%), which is more commonly seen in hospitalized patients than those at home; and intolerance to the feeding formula or administration technique. Medications that are hyperosmolar, contain sorbitol, or are used in elixir form can cause diarrhea; for example, a patient receiving magnesium-containing antacids and ibuprofen or acetaminophen in elixir form is highly likely to experience diarrhea.

Attention to clean technique at home and proper storage of enteral feeding formula as well as temperature of the formula can alleviate problems with diarrhea. Fiber-containing formulas may be helpful in some cases, although controversy exists about the type and amount of fiber required for optimal bowel function. Antidiarrheal medications may be helpful after all other causes have been ruled out. In a patient with an albumin less than 2.0 gm/dl, small bowel wall edema may develop, interfering with the ability to absorb nutrients. Therefore, a specialized formula may be necessary to enhance absorption to ensure adequate protein and kcal intake.

If a home enteral nutrition patient reports constipation, the first therapy should be to increase fluid intake. Switching formulas, adding bulk-forming agents, and using enemas may be attempted if simple fluid additions do not solve the problem; however, these therapies require more time and intervention. The more mobile patients are, the less likely they are to develop constipation.

13. How do you manage patients with high residual volumes?

Checking for residual volumes is usually done in home enteral patients who are obtunded or at risk for elevated gastric residuals. It is required when patients experience nausea, vomiting, bloating, or abdominal pain. This assessment should be done prior to a bolus feeding but may be done at any time in a patient on continuous feeding. A residual greater than 200 ml warrants overall evaluation of patient status. Withhold the enteral feeding 30–60 minutes, and recheck gastric residual. If it remains greater than 200 ml, the physician should be contacted. Ambulation is usually quite helpful and can produce immediate results. When continued high residuals are experienced, reduce the rate to an amount that has been previously tolerated. Prokinetic agents may be necessary but should be used only temporarily. If gastroparesis is diagnosed, a small intestine feeding is required.

14. What is needed for routine monitoring in a home enteral nutrition patient?

After discharge from the hospital, utilizing a home care agency with clinical staff that monitors home enteral patients is important. Because many home enteral patients receive their feeding supplies and formulas from a durable medical equipment company, clinical staff is not available; therefore, no clinical monitoring is provided. The physician or hospital nutrition support specialist should follow the patient within the first 14 days after discharge to ensure that the home enteral nutrition regimen has been implemented properly and that the patient and caregiver are completing the implementation and storage processes accurately. Routine monitoring should include intake data of formula and fluid, weight, and presence of any signs of intolerance. In addition, goals of therapy should be established and evaluated on an ongoing basis.

15. How do patients receive reimbursement for the home enteral nutrition support regimen?

Reimbursement is a major issue in home enteral nutrition. There are three methods by which a patient may receive reimbursement for home enteral nutrition support: a commercial payer, a governmental agency such as Medicare or Medicaid, or self pay. Commercial payers (i.e., insurance companies) reimburse for enteral nutrition based on the employer's requests when the insurance is purchased. Often the enteral supplies (i.e., feeding tube, enteral pump, and supplies for feeding) are included in the reimbursement, but the enteral formula is not included because it is referenced as "food" that the patient would purchase routinely. This practice varies by payer and insurance plan. Medicaid reimbursement is determined on a state-by-state basis, varying in amount reimbursed.

Medicare does reimburse for home enteral nutrition; however, Medicare recipients must be enrolled in Medicare Part B and meet stringent criteria. For Medicare to reimburse for enteral feeding, the patient must require it for 90 days or a lifetime. In addition, the patient must meet diagnosis criteria indicating a physiologic reason that the mouth must be bypassed (dysphagia) for the patient to receive enteral nutrition to maintain weight and strength commensurate with overall health status. Furthermore, the physician must document on a certificate of medical necessity (CMN) that the home enteral nutrition support is permanent, existing for 90 days at the onset of therapy. If an enteral pump is necessary, documentation should be included to demonstrate that gravity or bolus administration was tried and intolerance noted. Reimbursement from Medicare is not available for patients who have anorexia or for supplementation through oral means.

BIBLIOGRAPHY

1. ASPEN: Standards for home nutrition support. Nutr Clin Pract 7:65–89, 1992.
2. Ireton-Jones C: Home enteral nutrition from the provider's perspective. JPEN 26:S8–S9, 2002.
3. Ireton-Jones C: Homecare. In Gottschlich M, Matarese L (eds): Nutrition Support: A Clinical Guide, 2nd ed. Philadelphia, W.B. Saunders, 2003, pp 301–314.
4. Kohn C, Keithley JK: Techniques for evaluating and managing diarrhea in the tube fed patient. Nutr Clin Pract 2:250–257, 1982.
5. Mancuard SP, Stegall KS: Unclogging feeding tubes with pancreatic enzyme. JPEN 14(2):198–200, 1990.
6. McCrea JD, Lysen L, Mello L, et al: Position of the American Dietetic Association: Nutrition monitoring of the home parenteral and enteral patient. J Am Diet Assoc 89:263–265, 1989.

7. Metheny N, et al: Effect of feeding tube properties and three irrigants on clogging rates. Nurs Res 37:165–169, 1988.
8. Raymond JL, Farjood L: Adding Fiber to enteral formulas: yes or no? J Am Diet Assoc 93:527, 1993.
9. Shuster MH, Mancino JM: Ensuring successful home tube feeding in the geriatric population: Geri Nurs 2:67–82, 1994.

APPENDIX I. NUTRITION-RELATED FORMULAS AND CALCULATIONS

Carol Ireton-Jones, PhD, RD, LD, CNSD, FACN, and Charles W. Van Way III, MD

1. Energy expenditure equations

Harris-Benedict equations

For males:

HBEE = 66.47 + 13.75 × wt (kg) + 5.0 × ht (cm) – 6.76 × age (yr)

For females:

HBEE = 655.1 + 9.56 × wt (kg) + 1.85 × ht (cm) – 4.68 × age (yr)

where HBEE = kcal/day, wt = actual body weight in kg, ht = height in cm, age = current age in years.

Factors to account for daily energy expenditure in normal persons:

- Light activity: HBEE × 1.1
- Moderate activity: HBEE × 1.2–1.3
- Heavy activity: HBEE × 1.4–1.5

Factors to account for daily energy expenditure in ill or injured patients:

- Mild stress (ex: post operative): HBEE × 1.1
- Moderate stress (ex: moderate injury or infection): HBEE × 1.2–1.3
- Severe stress (ex: multiple system organ failure): HBEE × 1.4–1.5

Ireton-Jones equations

For spontaneously breathing patients:

IJEE(s) = 629 – 11(A) + 25(W) – 609 (O)

For ventilator-dependent patients:

IJEE (v) = 1784 – 11(A) + 5(W) + 244(S) + 239(T) + 804(B)

where IJEE = kcal/day, s = spontaneously breathing, v = ventilator-dependent, A = age (yr); W = actual body weight (kg); S = sex (male = 1, female = 0); T = diagnosis of trauma (present = 1, absent = 0); B = diagnosis of burn (present = 1, absent = 0); O = obesity > 30% above IBW from 1959 Metropolitan Life Insurance tables or BMI > 27 (present = 1, absent = 0).

2. Conversion of kilocalories (kcal to kilojoules (kj)

$$kJ = 4.15 \times kcal$$
$$kcal = 0.24 \times kJ$$

Kilojoules are used frequently, especially in the research literature, instead of kilocalories.

3. Calorie content of macronutrients (protein, carbohydrate, dextrose, and fat)

PROTEIN	CARBOHYDRATE	DEXTROSE	FAT
4 kcal/gm	4 kcal/gm	3.4 kcal/gm (dextrose is in the hydrous form with one molecule of water per molecule of glucose yielding less energy)	9 kcal/gm

4. Body surface area

$$BSA = H^{0.725} \times W^{0.425} \ 3 \ 7.184 \times 10^{-3}$$

where **BSA** is a body surface area in square meters; **W** is weight in kilograms; and **H** is height in centimeters.

5. Body mass index

$$BMI = \left(\frac{W}{(H)^2} \right)$$

BMI is body mass index in kilograms
per square meter
H is height in centimeters, **W** is weight in kilograms

6. Ideal body weight
Hamwi formula
Males: 106 pounds for 5 feet of height + 6 pounds for each inch above 5 feet
Females: 100 pounds for 5 feet of height + 5 pounds for each inch above 5 feet

7. Respiratory quotient

$$RQ = \left(\frac{V_{CO_2}}{V_{O_2}} \right)$$

RQ is the respiratory quotient.
V_{CO_2} and V_{O_2} are the carbon dioxide production and the oxygen consumption, respectively.

8. Urea nitrogen appearance rate and nitrogen appearance rate
The calculation of the urea appearance rate is based on the fact that urea, a small molecule, is freely distributed over the total body water.

$$UAR = (BUN_a - BUN_b) \times W \times 0.67 \times 10^{-2} + UUN$$

UAR is urea appearance rate in grams per day.
BUN_a and BUN_b are the BUN at the beginning and end of the 24 hour period, in milligrams per deciliter. The factor 10^{-2} converts from mg/dl to gm/liter.
W is the body weight in kilograms; (**W** × **0.67**) approximates the total body water.
UUN is the urine urea nitrogen over the 24 hours.
To convert from the urea appearance rate to the nitrogen appearance rate, multiply by 1.25:

$$NAR = 1.25 \times UAR$$

NAR is the nitrogen appearance rate in grams per day.

9. Fluid requirements for daily maintenance

Body weight	Fluid Requirements
Up to 10 kg	100 ml/kg
> 10 kg to 20 kg	1000 ml + 50 ml/kg for each kg > 10 kg
> 20 kg	1500 ml + 20 ml/kg for each kg > 20 kg

Adult rule of thumb: 30–35 ml/kg
Extraordinary fluid losses should be taken into account (i.e., ostomy losses, fistula drainage, fever) and added to the daily maintenance fluid requirements. Fluid status should also be evaluated to avoid fluid overload in sensitive patients.

10. Calcium correction factor for low serum albumin
Serum total calcium can be evaluated only with a concomitant evolution of serum albumin because calcium is about 50% bound to serum albumin. A low serum albumin may cause a decrease in serum calcium but have no effect on serum ionized calcium.
Determine serum albumin and serum calcium. If serum albumin is low, subtract current number from 4.0. Add this number to the serum calcium to determine the actual serum calcium.
Example: serum albumin = 2.8 gm/dl and serum calcium = 7.8 mg/d
4.0 – 2.8 = 1.2
Add 1.2 to serum calcium of 7.8 = 9.0 mg/dl or no deficit.

11. Nitrogen balance calculation

Nitrogen balance = nitrogen intake (from all sources) – nitrogen output

Nitrogen* intake (oral, enteral, and parenteral)

minus

Nitrogen output (derived from a 24-hour urine urea nitrogen (UUN gm/24 hours) + 4 grams accounting for non-urine nitrogen losses)

equals

Nitrogen balance

Positive nitrogen balance indicates adequate nutrition support.

Negative nitrogen balance indicates inadequate nutrition support.

*6.25 gm protein = 1 gm of nitrogen

12. Urinary nitrogen secretion and catabolic level

UUN excretion	Catabolic Level
< 5	Normal
5–10	Mild
10–15	Moderate
> 15	Severe

Pursell TA, Turner W: Pocket Manual of Intensive Nutritional Care. Philadelphia, BC Decker, 1990.

APPENDIX II: NUTRITION-RELATED TABLES

Carol Ireton-Jones, PhD, RD, LD, CNSD, FACN, and Charles W. Van Way III, MD

Table 1. Recommended Dietary Allowances*

CATE-GORY	AGE (YR)	WEIGHT (KG)	WEIGHT (LB)	HEIGHT (CM)	HEIGHT (IN)	PRO-TEIN (G)	VITA-MIN A (µG)	VITA-MIN D (µG)	VITA-MIN E (MG α-TE)	VITA-MIN K (µG)	VITA-MIN C (MG)	THIA-MIN (MG)	RIBO-FLA-VIN (MG)	NIA-CIN (MG NE)	VITA-MIN B6 (MG)	FO-LATE (µG)	VITA-MIN B12 (MG)	CAL-CIUM (MG)	PHOS-PHO-RUS (MG)	MAGNE-SIUM (MG)	IRON (MG)	ZINC (MG)	IO-DINE (µG)	SELE-NIUM (µG)
Infants	0.0–0.5	6	13	60	24	13	375	7.5	3	5	30	0.3	0.4	5	0.3	25	0.3	400	300	40	6	5	40	10
	0.5–1.0	9	20	71	28	14	375	10	4	10	35	0.4	0.5	6	0.6	35	0.5	600	500	60	10	5	50	15
Children	1–3	13	29	90	35	16	400	10	6	15	40	0.7	0.8	9	1.0	50	0.7	800	800	80	10	10	70	20
	4–6	20	44	112	44	24	500	10	7	20	45	0.9	1.1	12	1.1	75	1.0	800	800	120	10	10	90	20
	7–10	28	62	132	52	28	700	10	7	30	45	1.0	1.2	13	1.4	100	1.4	800	800	170	10	10	120	30
Males	11–14	45	99	157	62	45	1000	10	10	45	50	1.3	1.5	17	1.7	150	2.0	1200	1200	270	12	15	150	40
	15–18	66	145	176	69	59	1000	10	10	65	60	1.5	1.8	20	2.0	200	2.0	1200	1200	400	12	15	150	50
	19–24	72	160	177	70	58	1000	10	10	70	60	1.5	1.7	19	2.0	200	2.0	1200	1200	350	10	15	150	70
	25–50	79	174	176	70	63	1000	5	10	80	60	1.5	1.7	19	2.0	200	2.0	800	800	350	10	15	150	70
	51+	77	170	173	68	63	1000	5	10	80	60	1.2	1.4	15	2.0	200	2.0	800	800	350	10	15	150	70
Females	11–14	46	101	157	62	46	800	10	8	45	50	1.1	1.3	15	1.4	150	2.0	1200	1200	280	15	12	150	45
	15–18	55	120	163	64	44	800	10	8	55	60	1.1	1.3	15	1.5	150	2.0	1200	1200	300	15	12	150	50
	19–24	58	128	164	65	46	800	10	8	60	60	1.1	1.3	15	1.6	150	2.0	1200	1200	280	15	12	150	55
	25–50	63	138	163	64	50	800	5	8	65	60	1.1	1.3	15	1.6	150	2.0	800	800	280	15	12	150	55
	51+	65	143	160	63	50	800	5	8	65	60	1.0	1.2	13	1.6	150	2.0	800	800	280	10	12	150	55
Pregnant						60	800	10	10	65	70	1.5	1.6	17	2.2	400	2.2	1200	1200	320	30	15	175	65
Lactat-ing	1st 6 months					65	1300	10	12	65	95	1.6	1.8	20	2.1	250	2.6	1200	1200	355	15	19	200	75
	2nd 6 months					62	1200	10	11	65	90	1.6	1.7	20	2.1	250	2.6	1200	1200	340	15	16	200	75

* From Food and Nutrition Board, National Research Council, National Academy of Sciences: Recommended Dietary Allowances, 10th ed. Washington, DC, National Academy Press, 1989. As cited in Mahan LK, Escott-Stump S (eds): Krause's Food, Nutrition, and Diet Therapy, 9th ed. Philadelphia, WB Saunders, 1996.

Table 2. Milliequivalents and Milligrams of Electrolytes*

TO CONVERT MILLIGRAMS TO MILLIEQUIVALENTS

1. Divide milligrams by atomic weight and then multiply by the valence

$$\frac{\text{Milligrams}}{\text{Atomic weight}} \times \text{valence} = \text{milliequivalents}$$

MINERAL ELEMENT	CHEMICAL SYMBOL	ATOMIC WEIGHT	VALENCE
Chlorine	Cl	35.4	1
Potassium	K	39	1
Sodium	Na	23	1
Calcium	Ca	40	2
Magnesium	Mg	24.3	2
Sulfur	S	32	
Sulfate	SO_4	96	2

TO CONVERT SPECIFIC WEIGHT OF SODIUM TO SODIUM CHLORIDE

1. Multiply by 2.54

    Example: 1,000 mg sodium × 2.54 = 2,540 mg sodium chloride (2.5 g)

TO CONVERT SPECIFIC WEIGHT OF SODIUM CHLORIDE TO SODIUM

1. Multiply by 0.393

    Example: 2.5 g sodium chloride = 2.5 × 0.393 = 1,000 mg sodium

MILLIGRAMS	SODIUM VALUES (MILLIEQUIVALENTS)	GRAMS OF SODIUM CHLORIDE
500	21.8	1.3
1,000	43.5	2.5
1,500	75.3	3.8
2,000	87.0	5.0

* Adapted from Mayo Clinic Diet Manual, 4th ed. Philadelphia, WB Saunders, 1971. Cited in Mahan LK, Escott-Stump S (eds): Krause's Food, Nutrition, and Diet Therapy, 9th ed. Philadelphia, W.B. Saunders, 1996.

Table 3. BMI Categories

Underweight = < 18.5
Normal weight = 18.5–24.9
Overweight = 18.5–24.9
Obesity = BMI of 30 or greater

Table 4. Calculation of Body Weight in Pounds for Particular Body Mass Index Values

BODY MASS INDEX	19	20	21	22	23	24	25	26	27	28	29	30	35	40
HEIGHT (IN)						BODY WEIGHT (LB)								
58	91	95	100	105	110	115	119	124	129	134	138	143	167	191
59	94	99	104	109	114	119	124	128	133	138	143	148	173	198
60	97	102	107	112	118	123	128	133	138	143	148	153	179	204
61	100	106	111	116	121	127	132	137	143	148	153	158	185	211
62	104	109	115	120	125	131	136	142	147	153	158	164	191	218
63	107	113	118	124	130	135	141	146	152	158	163	169	197	225
64	110	116	122	128	134	140	145	151	157	163	169	174	203	233
65	114	120	126	132	138	144	150	156	162	168	174	180	210	240
66	117	124	130	136	142	148	155	161	167	173	179	185	216	247
67	121	127	134	140	147	153	159	166	172	178	185	191	223	255
68	125	131	138	144	151	158	164	171	177	184	190	197	230	263
69	128	135	142	149	155	162	169	176	182	189	196	203	237	270
70	132	139	146	153	160	167	174	181	188	195	202	209	243	278
71	136	143	150	157	165	172	179	186	193	200	207	215	250	286
72	140	147	155	162	169	177	184	191	199	206	213	221	258	294
73	144	151	159	166	174	182	189	197	204	212	219	227	265	303
74	148	155	163	171	179	187	194	202	210	218	225	233	272	311
75	152	160	168	176	184	192	200	208	216	224	232	240	279	319
76	156	164	172	180	189	197	205	213	221	230	238	246	287	328

Table 5. Calculation of Body Mass Index from Height in Inches and Weight in Pounds

BODY MASS INDEX (KG/M²)

HEIGHT (IN) \ WEIGHT (LB)	90	95	100	105	110	115	120	125	130	135	140	145	150	160	170	180	190	200	210	220	230	240	260	280	300
58	19	20	21	22	23	24	25	26	27	28	29	30	31	34	36	38	40	42	44	46	48	50	54	59	63
59	18	19	20	21	22	23	24	25	26	27	28	29	30	32	34	36	38	40	43	45	47	49	53	57	61
60	18	19	20	21	22	23	23	24	25	26	27	28	29	31	33	35	37	39	41	43	45	47	51	55	59
61	17	18	19	20	21	22	23	24	25	26	27	27	28	30	32	34	36	38	40	42	44	45	49	53	57
62		17	18	19	20	21	22	23	24	25	26	27	28	29	31	33	35	37	38	40	42	44	48	51	55
63		17	18	19	20	20	21	22	23	24	25	26	27	28	30	32	34	36	37	39	41	43	46	50	53
64			17	18	19	20	21	22	22	23	24	25	26	28	29	31	33	34	36	38	40	41	45	48	52
65			17	18	18	19	20	21	22	23	23	24	25	27	28	30	32	33	35	37	38	40	43	47	50
66				17	18	19	19	20	21	22	23	23	24	26	27	29	31	32	34	36	37	39	42	45	49
67					17	18	19	20	20	21	22	23	24	25	27	28	30	31	33	35	36	38	41	44	47
68					17	18	18	19	20	21	21	22	23	24	26	27	29	30	32	34	35	37	40	43	46
69						17	18	18	19	20	21	21	22	24	25	27	28	30	31	33	34	36	38	41	44
70						17	17	18	19	19	20	20	21	23	24	26	27	29	30	32	33	35	37	40	43
71							17	17	18	19	20	20	21	22	24	25	27	28	29	31	32	34	36	39	42
72							17	17	18	18	19	20	20	22	23	24	26	27	29	30	31	33	35	38	41
73								17	17	18	19	19	20	21	22	24	25	26	28	29	30	32	34	37	40
74									17	18	18	19	19	21	22	23	24	26	27	28	30	31	33	36	39
75										17	18	18	19	20	21	23	24	25	26	28	29	30	33	35	38
76											17	18	18	20	21	22	23	24	26	27	28	29	32	34	37
77											17	17	18	19	20	21	23	24	25	26	27	29	31	33	36
78												17	17	19	20	21	22	23	24	25	27	28	30	32	35
79													17	18	19	20	21	23	24	25	26	27	29	32	34
80																									

Table 6. Calculation of Body Weight in Kilograms for Particular Body Mass Index Values

BODY MASS INDEX	19	20	21	22	23	24	25	26	27	28	29	30	35	40
HEIGHT (CM)						BODY WEIGHT (KG)								
140	37	39	41	43	45	47	49	51	53	55	57	59	69	78
142	38	40	42	44	46	48	50	52	54	56	58	60	71	81
144	39	41	44	46	48	50	52	54	56	58	60	62	73	83
146	41	43	45	47	49	51	53	55	58	60	62	64	75	85
148	42	44	46	48	50	53	55	57	59	61	64	66	77	88
150	43	45	47	50	52	54	56	59	61	63	65	68	79	90
152	44	46	49	51	53	55	58	60	62	65	67	69	81	92
154	45	47	50	52	55	57	59	62	64	66	69	71	83	95
156	46	49	51	54	56	58	61	63	66	68	71	73	85	97
158	47	50	52	55	57	60	62	65	67	70	72	75	87	100
160	49	51	54	56	59	61	64	67	69	72	74	77	90	102
162	50	52	55	58	60	63	66	68	71	73	76	79	92	105
164	51	54	56	59	62	65	67	70	73	75	78	81	94	108
166	52	55	58	61	63	66	69	72	74	77	80	83	96	110
168	54	56	59	62	65	68	71	73	76	79	82	85	99	113
170	55	58	61	64	66	69	72	75	78	81	84	87	101	116
172	56	59	62	65	68	71	74	77	80	83	86	89	104	118
174	58	61	64	67	70	73	76	79	82	85	88	91	106	121
176	59	62	65	68	71	74	77	81	84	87	90	93	108	124
178	60	63	67	70	73	76	79	82	86	89	92	95	111	127
180	62	65	68	71	75	78	81	84	87	91	94	97	113	130
182	63	66	70	73	76	79	83	86	89	93	96	99	116	132
184	64	68	71	74	78	81	85	88	91	95	98	102	118	135
186	66	69	73	76	80	83	86	90	93	97	100	104	121	138
188	67	71	74	78	81	85	88	92	95	99	102	106	124	141
190	69	72	76	79	83	87	90	94	97	101	105	108	126	144
192	70	74	77	81	85	88	92	96	100	103	107	111	129	147
194	72	75	79	83	87	90	94	98	102	105	109	113	132	151
196	73	77	81	85	88	92	96	100	104	108	111	115	134	154
198	74	78	82	86	90	94	98	102	106	110	114	118	137	157
200	76	80	84	88	92	96	100	104	108	112	116	120	140	160

Table 7. Calculation of Body Mass Index from Height in Centimeters and Weight in Kilograms

WEIGHT (KG)	40	45	50	55	60	65	70	75	80	85	90	95	100	110	120	130	140	150	160	170	180	190	200
HEIGHT (CM)												BODY MASS INDEX (KG/M^2)										
140	20	23	26	28	31	33	36	38	41	43	46	48	51	56	61	66	71	77	82	87	92	97	102
142	20	22	25	27	30	32	35	37	40	42	45	47	50	55	60	64	69	74	79	84	89	94	99
144	19	22	24	27	29	31	34	36	39	41	43	46	48	53	58	63	68	72	77	82	87	92	96
146	19	21	23	26	28	30	33	35	38	40	42	45	47	52	56	61	66	70	75	80	84	89	94
148	18	21	23	25	27	30	32	34	37	39	41	43	46	50	55	59	64	68	73	78	82	87	91
150	18	20	22	24	27	29	31	33	36	38	40	42	44	49	53	58	62	67	71	76	80	84	89
152	17	19	22	24	26	28	30	32	35	37	39	41	43	48	52	56	61	65	69	74	78	82	87
154	17	19	21	23	25	27	30	32	34	36	38	40	42	46	51	55	59	63	67	72	76	80	84
156		18	21	23	25	27	29	31	33	35	37	39	41	45	49	53	58	62	66	70	74	78	82
158		18	20	22	24	26	28	30	32	34	36	38	40	44	48	52	56	60	64	68	72	76	80
160		18	20	21	23	25	27	29	31	33	35	37	39	43	47	51	55	59	63	66	70	74	78
162		17	19	21	23	25	27	29	30	32	34	36	38	42	46	50	53	57	61	65	69	72	76
164		17	19	20	22	24	26	28	30	32	33	35	37	41	45	48	52	56	59	63	67	71	74
166			18	20	22	24	25	27	29	31	33	34	36	40	44	47	51	54	58	62	65	69	73
168			18	19	21	23	25	27	28	30	32	34	35	39	43	46	50	53	57	60	64	67	71
170			17	19	21	22	24	26	28	29	31	33	35	38	42	45	48	52	55	59	62	66	69
172			17	19	20	22	24	25	27	29	30	32	34	37	41	44	47	51	54	57	61	64	68
174			17	18	20	21	23	25	26	28	30	31	33	36	40	43	46	50	53	56	59	63	66
176				18	19	21	23	24	26	27	29	31	32	36	39	42	45	48	52	55	58	61	65
178				17	19	21	22	24	25	27	28	30	32	35	38	41	44	47	50	54	57	60	63
180				17	19	20	22	23	25	26	28	29	31	34	37	40	43	46	49	53	56	59	62
182					18	20	21	23	24	26	27	29	30	33	36	39	42	45	48	51	54	57	60
184					18	19	21	22	24	25	27	28	30	32	35	38	41	44	47	50	53	56	59
186					17	19	20	22	23	25	26	27	29	32	35	38	40	43	46	49	52	55	58
188					17	18	20	21	23	24	25	27	28	31	34	37	40	42	45	48	51	54	57
190					17	18	19	21	22	24	25	27	28	30	33	36	39	42	44	47	50	53	55
192						18	19	20	22	23	24	26	27	30	33	35	38	41	43	46	49	52	54
194						18	19	20	21	23	24	25	27	29	32	34	37	40	43	45	48	50	53
196						17	18	20	21	22	23	25	26	29	31	34	36	39	42	44	47	49	52
198						17	18	19	20	22	23	24	26	28	31	33	36	38	41	43	46	48	51
200							18	19	20	21	23	24	25	28	30	33	35	38	40	43	45	48	50

*Table 8. Normal Range for Body Mass Index by Gender
And Age Group*

AGE GROUP (YR)	AVERAGE RANGE	MEN	WOMEN
19–24	19–24	21–25	18–23
25–34	20–25	21–25	19–23
35–44	21–26	22–26	20–24
45–54	22–27	23–27	21–25
55–64	23–28	24–28	22–26
651	24–29	25–29	23–27

Based on the following sources: 1983 Metropolitan height and weight tables.
Mahan LK, Escott-Stump S (eds): Krause's Food, Nutrition, and Diet Therapy, 9th ed. Philadelphia, WB Saunders, 1996.
Height and weight standards for age used by the United States Army.
The Body Mass Index is primarily useful for population-based studies.
Care should be taken when applying it to individuals.

Table 9. Calculation of Body Surface Area from Height in Inches and Weight in Pounds

WEIGHT (LB) HEIGHT (IN)	90	95	100	105	110	115	120	125	130	135	140	150	160	170	180	190	200	220	240	260	280	300	320	340	360
										BODY SURFACE AREA (M²)														
58	1.30	1.33	1.36	1.39	1.41	1.44	1.47	1.49	1.52	1.54	1.57	1.61	1.66	1.70	1.17	1.78	1.82	1.90	1.97	2.04	2.10	2.17	2.23	2.28	2.34
59	1.31	1.35	1.37	1.40	1.43	1.46	1.49	1.51	1.54	1.56	1.59	1.63	1.68	1.72	1.76	1.81	1.85	1.92	1.99	2.06	2.13	2.19	2.25	2.31	2.37
60	1.33	1.36	1.39	1.42	1.45	1.48	1.50	1.53	1.56	1.58	1.61	1.65	1.70	1.74	1.79	1.83	1.87	1.95	2.02	2.09	2.16	2.22	2.28	2.34	2.40
61	1.35	1.38	1.41	1.44	1.47	1.49	1.52	1.55	1.57	1.60	1.62	1.67	1.72	1.76	1.81	1.85	1.89	1.97	2.04	2.11	2.18	2.25	2.31	2.37	2.43
62	1.36	1.39	1.43	1.45	1.48	1.51	1.54	1.57	1.59	1.62	1.64	1.69	1.74	1.79	1.83	1.87	1.91	1.99	2.07	2.14	2.21	2.27	2.34	2.40	2.46
63	1.38	1.41	1.44	1.47	1.50	1.53	1.56	1.59	1.61	1.64	1.66	1.71	1.76	1.81	1.85	1.89	1.94	2.02	2.09	2.16	2.23	2.30	2.36	2.43	2.48
64	1.39	1.43	1.46	1.49	1.52	1.55	1.58	1.60	1.63	1.66	1.68	1.73	1.78	1.83	1.87	1.92	1.96	2.04	2.12	2.19	2.26	2.33	2.39	2.45	2.51
65		1.44	1.47	1.51	1.54	1.56	1.59	1.62	1.65	1.68	1.70	1.75	1.80	1.85	1.89	1.94	1.98	2.06	2.14	2.21	2.28	2.35	2.42	2.48	2.54
66			1.49	1.52	1.55	1.58	1.61	1.64	1.67	1.69	1.72	1.77	1.82	1.87	1.91	1.96	2.00	2.08	2.16	2.24	2.31	2.38	2.44	2.51	2.57
67			1.51	1.54	1.57	1.60	1.63	1.66	1.69	1.71	1.74	1.79	1.84	1.89	1.94	1.98	2.02	2.11	2.19	2.26	2.34	2.40	2.47	2.54	2.60
68			1.52	1.56	1.59	1.62	1.65	1.68	1.70	1.73	1.76	1.81	1.86	1.91	1.96	2.00	2.05	2.13	2.21	2.29	2.36	2.43	2.50	2.56	2.63
69				1.57	1.60	1.63	1.66	1.69	1.72	1.75	1.78	1.83	1.88	1.93	1.98	2.02	2.07	2.15	2.23	2.31	2.39	2.46	2.52	2.59	2.65
70				1.59	1.62	1.65	1.68	1.71	1.74	1.77	1.80	1.85	1.90	1.95	2.00	2.04	2.09	2.18	2.26	2.34	2.41	2.48	2.55	2.62	2.68
71					1.64	1.67	1.70	1.73	1.76	1.79	1.81	1.87	1.92	1.97	2.02	2.07	2.11	2.20	2.28	2.36	2.44	2.51	2.58	2.64	2.71
72					1.65	1.69	1.72	1.75	1.78	1.80	1.83	1.89	1.94	1.99	2.04	2.09	2.13	2.22	2.30	2.38	2.46	2.53	2.60	2.67	2.74
73						1.70	1.73	1.76	1.79	1.82	1.85	1.91	1.96	2.01	2.06	2.11	2.15	2.24	2.33	2.41	2.48	2.56	2.63	2.70	2.76
74							1.75	1.78	1.81	1.84	1.87	1.92	1.98	2.03	2.08	2.13	2.18	2.26	2.35	2.43	2.51	2.58	2.66	2.73	2.79
75								1.80	1.83	1.86	1.89	1.94	2.00	2.05	2.10	2.15	2.20	2.29	2.37	2.46	2.53	2.61	2.68	2.75	2.82
76									1.85	1.88	1.91	1.96	2.02	2.07	2.12	2.17	2.22	2.31	2.40	2.48	2.56	2.63	2.71	2.78	2.85
77										1.89	1.92	1.98	2.04	2.09	2.14	2.19	2.24	2.33	2.42	2.50	2.58	2.66	2.73	2.80	2.87
78											1.94	2.00	2.06	2.11	2.16	2.21	2.26	2.35	2.44	2.53	2.61	2.68	2.76	2.83	2.90
79												2.02	2.07	2.13	2.18	2.23	2.28	2.37	2.46	2.55	2.63	2.71	2.78	2.86	2.93
80												2.04	2.09	2.15	2.20	2.25	2.30	2.40	2.49	2.57	2.66	2.73	2.81	2.88	2.95

Table 10. Calculation of Body Surface Area from Height in Inches and Weight in Kilograms

HEIGHT (CM) \ WEIGHT (KG)	40	45	50	55	60	65	70	75	80	85	90	95	100	110	120	130	140	150	160	180	200
										BODY SURFACE AREA (M^2)											
58	1.29	1.35	1.41	1.47	1.53	1.58	1.63	1.68	1.73	1.77	1.82	1.86	1.90	1.98	2.05	2.12	2.19	2.26	2.32	2.44	2.55
59	1.30	1.37	1.43	1.49	1.55	1.60	1.65	1.70	1.75	1.79	1.84	1.88	1.92	2.00	2.08	2.15	2.22	2.28	2.35	2.47	2.58
60	1.32	1.39	1.45	1.51	1.57	1.62	1.67	1.72	1.77	1.82	1.86	1.90	1.95	2.03	2.10	2.17	2.24	2.31	2.38	2.50	2.61
61	1.33	1.40	1.47	1.53	1.58	1.64	1.69	1.74	1.79	1.84	1.88	1.93	1.97	2.05	2.13	2.20	2.27	2.34	2.40	2.53	2.64
62	1.35	1.42	1.48	1.55	1.60	1.66	1.71	1.76	1.81	1.86	1.91	1.95	1.99	2.07	2.15	2.23	2.30	2.37	2.43	2.56	2.67
63	1.37	1.44	1.50	1.56	1.62	1.68	1.73	1.78	1.83	1.88	1.93	1.97	2.02	2.10	2.18	2.25	2.33	2.39	2.46	2.59	2.71
64		1.45	1.52	1.58	1.64	1.70	1.75	1.80	1.85	1.90	1.95	1.99	2.04	2.12	2.20	2.28	2.35	2.42	2.49	2.62	2.74
65			1.54	1.60	1.66	1.72	1.77	1.82	1.88	1.92	1.97	2.02	2.06	2.15	2.23	2.30	2.38	2.45	2.52	2.65	2.77
66			1.55	1.62	1.68	1.74	1.79	1.84	1.90	1.95	1.99	2.04	2.08	2.17	2.25	2.33	2.41	2.48	2.55	2.68	2.80
67				1.63	1.70	1.75	1.81	1.86	1.92	1.97	2.02	2.06	2.11	2.19	2.28	2.36	2.43	2.50	2.57	2.71	2.83
68				1.65	1.71	1.77	1.83	1.89	1.94	1.99	2.04	2.08	2.13	2.22	2.30	2.38	2.46	2.53	2.60	2.73	2.86
69					1.73	1.79	1.85	1.91	1.96	2.01	2.06	2.11	2.15	2.24	2.33	2.41	2.48	2.56	2.63	2.76	2.89
70					1.75	1.81	1.87	1.93	1.98	2.03	2.08	2.13	2.18	2.27	2.35	2.43	2.51	2.58	2.66	2.79	2.92
71						1.83	1.89	1.95	2.00	2.05	2.10	2.15	2.20	2.29	2.38	2.46	2.54	2.61	2.68	2.82	2.95
72						1.85	1.91	1.96	2.02	2.07	2.12	2.17	2.22	2.31	2.40	2.48	2.56	2.64	2.71	2.85	2.98
73							1.93	1.98	2.04	2.09	2.14	2.19	2.24	2.34	2.42	2.51	2.59	2.66	2.74	2.88	3.01
74							1.95	2.00	2.06	2.11	2.17	2.22	2.26	2.36	2.45	2.53	2.61	2.69	2.77	2.91	3.04
75								2.02	2.08	2.13	2.19	2.24	2.29	2.38	2.47	2.56	2.64	2.72	2.79	2.94	3.07
76									2.10	2.16	2.21	2.26	2.31	2.40	2.50	2.58	2.66	2.74	2.82	2.96	3.10
77										2.18	2.23	2.28	2.33	2.43	2.52	2.61	2.69	2.77	2.85	2.99	3.13
78											2.25	2.30	2.35	2.45	2.54	2.63	2.71	2.80	2.87	3.02	3.16
79												2.32	2.37	2.47	2.57	2.66	2.74	2.82	2.90	3.05	3.19
80													2.40	2.50	2.59	2.68	2.77	2.85	2.93	3.08	3.22

Table 11. Calculation of Body Surface Area from Height in Centimeters and Weight in Kilograms

HEIGHT (CM)	\ WEIGHT (KG) 40	45	50	55	60	65	70	75	80	85	90	95	100	110	120	130	140	150	160	180	200
									BODY SURFACE AREA (M²)												
140	1.24	1.30	1.36	1.42	1.47	1.52	1.57	1.62	1.66	1.71	1.75	1.79	1.83	1.91	1.98	2.05	2.11	2.17	2.23	2.35	2.46
142	1.25	1.32	1.38	1.43	1.49	1.54	1.59	1.64	1.68	1.72	1.77	1.81	1.85	1.92	2.00	2.07	2.13	2.20	2.26	2.37	2.48
144	1.26	1.33	1.39	1.45	1.50	1.55	1.60	1.65	1.70	1.74	1.79	1.83	1.87	1.94	2.02	2.09	2.15	2.22	2.28	2.40	2.51
146	1.28	1.34	1.40	1.46	1.52	1.57	1.62	1.67	1.72	1.76	1.80	1.85	1.89	1.96	2.04	2.11	2.18	2.24	2.30	2.42	2.53
148	1.29	1.36	1.42	1.48	1.53	1.59	1.64	1.69	1.73	1.78	1.82	1.86	1.90	1.98	2.06	2.13	2.20	2.26	2.33	2.45	2.56
150	1.30	1.37	1.43	1.49	1.55	1.60	1.65	1.70	1.75	1.79	1.84	1.88	1.92	2.00	2.08	2.15	2.22	2.28	2.35	2.47	2.58
152		1.38	1.45	1.51	1.56	1.62	1.67	1.72	1.77	1.81	1.86	1.90	1.94	2.02	2.10	2.17	2.24	2.31	2.37	2.49	2.61
154			1.46	1.52	1.58	1.63	1.68	1.73	1.78	1.83	1.87	1.92	1.96	2.04	2.12	2.19	2.26	2.33	2.39	2.52	2.63
156			1.47	1.53	2.24	1.65	1.70	1.75	1.80	1.85	1.89	1.94	1.98	2.06	2.14	2.21	2.28	2.35	2.42	2.54	2.66
158				1.55	1.61	1.66	1.72	1.77	1.82	1.86	1.91	1.95	2.00	2.08	2.16	2.23	2.30	2.37	2.44	2.56	2.68
160				1.56	1.62	2.36	1.73	1.78	1.83	1.88	1.93	1.97	2.02	2.10	2.18	2.25	2.33	2.39	2.46	2.59	2.71
162					1.64	1.69	1.75	1.80	1.85	1.90	1.94	1.99	2.03	2.12	2.20	2.27	2.35	2.42	2.48	2.61	2.73
164						1.71	1.76	1.82	1.87	1.91	1.96	2.01	2.05	2.14	2.22	2.29	2.37	2.44	2.51	2.63	2.75
166						1.72	1.78	1.83	1.88	1.93	1.98	2.03	2.07	2.16	2.24	2.31	2.39	2.46	2.53	2.66	2.78
168							1.79	1.85	1.90	1.95	2.00	2.04	2.09	2.17	2.26	2.33	2.41	2.48	2.55	2.68	2.80
170							1.81	1.86	1.92	1.97	2.01	2.06	2.11	2.19	2.28	2.35	2.43	2.50	2.57	2.70	2.83
172								1.88	1.93	1.98	2.03	2.08	2.12	2.21	2.29	2.37	2.45	2.52	2.59	2.73	2.85
174									1.95	2.00	2.05	2.10	2.14	2.23	2.31	2.39	2.47	2.54	2.62	2.75	2.88
176									1.96	2.02	2.06	2.11	2.16	2.25	2.33	2.41	2.49	2.57	2.64	2.77	2.90
178										2.03	2.08	2.13	2.18	2.27	2.35	2.43	2.51	2.59	2.66	2.80	2.92
180											2.10	2.15	2.20	2.29	2.37	2.45	2.53	2.61	2.68	2.82	2.95
182												2.16	2.21	2.30	2.39	2.47	2.55	2.63	2.70	2.84	2.97
184												2.18	2.23	2.32	2.41	2.49	2.57	2.65	2.72	2.86	2.99
186													2.25	2.34	2.43	2.51	2.59	2.67	2.74	2.89	3.02
188													2.27	2.36	2.45	2.53	2.61	2.69	2.77	2.91	3.04
190													2.28	2.38	2.47	2.55	2.63	2.71	2.79	2.93	3.06
192														2.40	2.49	2.57	2.65	2.73	2.81	2.95	3.09
194														2.41	2.50	2.59	2.67	2.75	2.83	2.98	3.11
196															2.52	2.61	2.69	2.77	2.85	3.00	3.13
198																2.63	2.71	2.79	2.87	3.02	3.16
200																	2.73	2.81	2.89	3.04	3.18

INDEX

Page numbers in **boldface type** indicate complete chapters.